The New Language
of Psychiatry

Learning and
Using DSM-III

The New Language of Psychiatry

Learning and Using DSM-III

Ronald Levy, M.D.

LITTLE, BROWN AND COMPANY
Boston   Toronto

To Jessie and Joshua,
and to
Maureen and Shannon

Library of Congress Cataloging in Publication Data

Levy, Ronald
  The new language of psychiatry.

  Includes index.
  1. Mental illness—Diagnosis. 2. Psychology,
Pathological—Classification. I. Title. II. DSM-III.
RC469.L46   616.89'075'014   80-25655
ISBN 0-316-522368

Library of Congress Catalog Card No. 80-25655

ISBN 0-316-52236-8

9 8 7 6 5 4 3 2
BP

Published simultaneously in Canada
by Little, Brown & Company (Canada) Limited

Printed in the United States of America

This book is not written or endorsed
by the American Psychiatric Association.

Preface

On June 1, 1980, the entire psychiatric profession began using a new set of names for mental disorders. This official new nomenclature will be used to state the diagnoses of patients and to categorize mental disorders for statistical purposes. Definitions of these new terms and categories are to be found in The American Psychiatric Association's publication: *Diagnostic and Statistical Manual of Mental Disorders, Third Edition,* or, "DSM-III" as it is referred to throughout the psychiatric profession and as we shall refer to it in this book. (The term "DSM-III" is the name of the new nomenclature, as well as the name of the manual that defines it.)

The changeover affects not only the entire field of mental health care with its psychiatrists, psychiatric nurses, psychiatric social workers, psychologists, recreational therapists, occupational therapists, and administrators, but also affects other physicians, nurses, and allied health professionals who need to know what a psychiatrist means when he says that a given patient has a particular psychiatric diagnosis.

In the future, insurance companies may pay benefits only for the care of patients who have a diagnosis found in DSM-III, making this new nomenclature of interest to hospital administrators and persons working in the field of health insurance. Students and teachers of psychiatry, nursing, social work, and other allied health professions will be affected.

The new system is more complicated than the old, substituting not only a new name for an old one, but also establishing new criteria for many diseases and mental disorders, at the same time redefining them substantially.

DSM-III is sufficiently different from the system previously used, that a period of confusion will ensue while those affected make efforts to acquire a working knowledge of the new system. This book is a guide to the new system.

It is intended to be used by psychiatrists, physicians in other specialities, nurses, psychiatric technicians, social workers, psychologists, mental health administrators, insurance workers, and even lawyers, probation officers, and judges, as well as laymen who wish to learn and understand DSM-III.

Students in all of these areas will find this book a guide and study aid to the new language of psychiatry of the '80s.

To get the most from this book, readers are advised to read the self-study sections and to attempt to answer the questions and case examples to be found there (in most cases answers are provided; where they are not, the answer required is information that readers should try to put into their own words). By taking a bit longer to read the book in this way, they can be assured of realizing their goal of acquiring a practical knowledge of the DSM-III system.

The Appendices at the end of the book include a numerical list of DSM-III disorders for use in identifying a diagnosis when only the numerical code is presented; an alphabetical list of disorders, for clerical use in adding the numerical codes to a diagnosis written only verbally; and an extensive set of tables relating DSM-III disorders to the symptoms, or diagnostic criteria, which make up those disorders—for use in identifying expectable symptoms when a diagnosis has been made, or projecting possible diagnoses on the basis of observed symptoms.

The author gratefully acknowledges the assistance of Carolyn Wohlert, whose administrative, editorial, and organizational talents were an invaluable resource.

The typing skills of Patricia Mothersead and the proofreading abilities of Anthony C. Madonia and Camille Stuart are sincerely appreciated.

The author especially thanks Charles Durang and Herbert Nolan of Winthrop Publishers, Inc.; Mr. Durang's literary professionalism and command of his field and Mr. Nolan's precision and industry were of much help in the careful preparation and production of this book. Special thanks go to Paul O'Connell, chairperson of Winthrop, whose determination and enthusiasm for this project encouraged us all.

Contents

part I

The
Multiaxial
System:

How
a Psychiatric Diagnosis
Is Written

MENTAL DISORDER

There is a traditional distinction in medicine between mental disorders and physical disorders. *Mental disorders* are those diseases and conditions that have manifestations that seem mostly to affect a person's behavior, how a person feels, how a person thinks, and how they perceive and view the world around them. Mental disorders are the disorders that are treated by the medical specialists called Psychiatrists and Child Psychiatrists.

DSM-III recognizes that mental disorders as defined above can have causes within the body and also usually have relationships to events in the body. DSM-III needed a term to use to cover all of the diseases of Man that were outside of the terminology of DSM-III; a term that covered all of the conditions that are usually considered as "non-mental medical disorders" was needed. For convenience these are called *physical disorders*. These are the disorders that are usually treated by the specialists called Internists, Pediatricians, Surgeons, Gynecologists, and so on. And these are the diseases that have their major manifestation in damage to the body or in bodily aches and pains.

SYNDROME VERSUS DISORDER

Strictly speaking, what a patient complains about to the physician is called a *symptom;* what the physician finds when he examines the patient is called a *sign.*

If a cluster of patient's complaints, or physicians findings regularly occur together in association with each other, that regular occurrence and association would be called a *syndrome.* Saying that something is a disorder implies something more than just the regular occurrence of a group of symptoms and signs.

Calling something a *disorder* means that physicians have recognized that a group of complaints and/or physician's findings regularly occur in association with each other, have a describable onset and progression, and regularly respond to, or fail to respond most of the time to certain methods of treatment or management.

ONSET AND COURSE

The start of a syndrome or disorder is called its *onset.*

The way a disorder unfolds after the onset is called its *course.*

Some disorders, like heart attacks, have a way of bursting forth upon a patient with serious symptoms and signs. But often, when they are searched for, subtle symptoms and signs were present before the florid period of severe illness.

This period that precedes the dramatic period of apparent onset is a time when the disease smolders and gathers momentum — it is called the *prodromal phase* or *prodromal period* or simply the *prodrome*. The *premorbid period* is the entire period of time before there is any disease (but often what appears to be the premorbid period contains some or all of the prodrome).

A heart attack is then seen as one phase in a larger picture of disease. The heart attack had an onset, but the disease process itself, of which the heart attack was only one part, had an onset that was earlier; the onset of the disease is found at the start of the prodromal period.

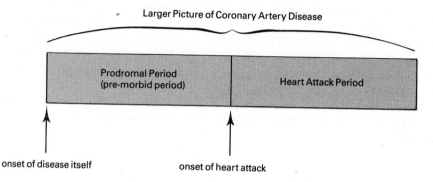

Larger Picture of Coronary Artery Disease

When a heart attack is over, there may be problems that persist afterwards stemming from the heart attack or from other aspects of the larger context of the disease process.

The phase of the disease where some health problems persist, perhaps long afterward, is called the *residual phase* of the illness.

The period just after the onset of the dramatically florid phase of a disorder is often called the "Acute phase," or "Acute period".

When recovery is incomplete, the period after the acute phase cools down to an ongoing disease with persisting health problems and is the part of the disease called the *chronic phase*.

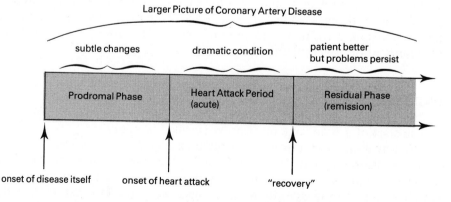

Larger Picture of Coronary Artery Disease

Residual phase and chronic phase are roughly equivalent terms implying a prolonged persisting state of continuing illness, usually less severe than what was seen in the acute phase.

Some disorders, like influenza, can have a dramatic and florid phase (with apparently sudden onset of high fever, chills, generalized weakness, etc.), but recovery can be complete.

Influenza can have a prodromal period, before the dramatic picture of onset of severe flu, where there were various signs that the patient was "coming down with something."

Complete recovery from flu can occur, without any persisting problems, and without persistence of any of the subtle signs of disease of the prodromal period.

Here there is a prodromal phase, an acute phase, but no chronic phase.

Remission is a period of apparent recovery from a disease that can later strike again in acute form.

A disease process with recurring acute episodes is called an *episodic disorder*. When each acute episode subsides into an apparent complete recovery, we say "The disease is in remission."

THE MULTIAXIAL SYSTEM

An important change that came with DSM-III is that a patient's psychiatric diagnosis will *look different*.

In DSM-III every psychiatric diagnosis has five parts. Each part is called an Axis. Each Axis is numbered with a Roman numeral—Axis I, Axis II, Axis III, Axis IV, and Axis V.

The five parts of every psychiatric diagnosis that are to be given for every patient are like a questionnaire that has blank spaces for five answers. Supplying the answer to the correct blank is called "coding" by DSM-III.

Axis I and Axis II cover all of the mental disorders discussed in DSM-III. To give a person a diagnosis of a mental disorder as was done in DSM-III now means supplying an answer for Axis I or Axis II.

Schizophrenia is a name of a mental disorder used in both DSM-II and DSM-III. Although the term schizophrenia has been redefined in DSM-III, there were many persons whose mental disorder was called schizophrenia in DSM-II that will still have their disorder called schizophrenia in DSM-III.

If a person has schizophrenia, DSM-III says that this is to be coded on Axis I and thus is only one part of the whole psychiatric diagnosis required under DSM-III.

In DSM-II there were many circumstances where the term schizophrenia would be considered to be enough of a diagnosis in itself. This is not true in DSM-III.

Supplying a part of the five part diagnosis in DSM-III is called "coding the part".

The mental disorders themselves are divided into two kinds, those coded on Axis I and those coded on Axis II. This separation is made to insure that consideration is given to the possible presence of long-term disturbances that are frequently overlooked when attention is given to a current episode of illness.

The five parts of a DSM-III psychiatric diagnosis are given below.

Axis I - is the part of the diagnosis used to describe the current episode of illness.

Axis II - is used to describe styles of personality traits and kinds of personality disorders in adults (and in some children), and is used to describe specific developmental disorders in children (and in some adults).

Axis III - is used to describe any current physical disorders that are potentially relevant to the understanding or management of the patient.

Axis IV - is used to describe how much environmental stress the patient is under in terms of how much stress an average person would be under in the same situation.

Axis V - is used to describe the highest level of adaptive functioning in the previous year — where *adaptive functioning* is a composite of three areas: social relations, occupational functioning, and use of leisure time.

DSM-III does not make all five Axes mandatory.

Axis IV and Axis V are optional.

The intent of DSM-III is that they should be used, and they probably will be required at University Hospitals, in research studies, and in other settings where psychiatrists and child psychiatrists will make an effort to be careful, thoughtful, and complete.

All health professionals should know what a rating on Axis IV and Axis V means when someone has taken the time to provide Axis IV and/or Axis V.

Under DSM-III, saying that a person has schizophrenia would be filling out the part of the psychiatric diagnosis on that person called Axis I. There are at least two more parts left to be filled out.

A person with acute schizophrenia who always had a compulsive personality disorder, who also had been in a car accident and had multiple fractures, would have schizophrenia coded on Axis I, compulsive personality disorder coded on Axis II, and multiple fractures coded on Axis III.

Axis IV is for describing the stress on the person. If this same person with schizophrenia had just had his or her brother die, we would code death of brother, car accident, and multiple fractures on Axis IV.

When any mental disorder is judged to result as a reaction to a recent stressful event, DSM-III advises (but does not require) that Axis IV be used to list the stressful event.

A disorder in DSM-III that is *always* a reaction to external stress is Adjustment Disorder, because it is *defined* that way.

Adjustment Disorder is the DSM-III disorder that corresponds to what used to be called "Adjustment Reaction".

Because an adjustment disorder is *defined* as being the result of a specific life stress that occurred within the previous three months, is makes sense to put down on Axis IV the stress that was involved, but it isn't "required".

On Axis IV the significant life stresses that are thought to affect a patient's mental health are called *"Psychosocial Stressors"* or just *"stressors"* instead of calling them "stresses" as we have done until now.

Psychosocial stresses are listed on Axis IV together with a rating of the severity of all of them taken together. This is given by rating the total effect of the group of stressors on a seven point scale. A stress rating on Axis IV is a rating number and a descriptive word like "5-Severe."

Case Illustration

A thirty-year-old woman whose dutiful husband left her two weeks ago because she has always been jealous and suspicious and hounded him constantly about his whereabouts, is brought into the emergency room after trying to cut one of her wrists with a dull pen knife. She inflicted a laceration on the left. She is drunk after drinking a half bottle of scotch and the examining psychiatrist believes that her state of mind before and while intoxicated with alcohol is related to the specific life stress of being left by her husband.

Before DSM-III she could have been diagnosed simply as adjustment reaction of adult life and alcohol intoxication.

In DSM-III she would be said to have an adjustment disorder codable on Axis I, paranoid personality traits codable on Axis II, alcohol intoxication coded on Axis I and a lacerated wrist coded on Axis III.

This would be written out on her chart as follows:

> *Axis I:* Adjustment disorder
> Alcohol intoxication
>
> *Axis II:* Paranoid personality traits
>
> *Axis III:* Lacerated left wrist

Because so much of what happened to this woman is related to being left by her husband, specifying that life stress on Axis IV would help the other health professionals who look at this diagnosis to understand what the psychiatrists meant when he listed Adjustment Disorder in her diagnosis.

Notice that two disorders are listed on Axis I.

When more than one mental disorder codable on Axis I is present, the Axis I portion of the diagnosis should list all of them.

Also, *when several diseases are listed on Axis I,* the one that is the major concern at the time should head the list.

A drunken patient with schizophrenia, paranoid sub-type, chronic, who comes to the emergency room would have the Axis I portion of their diagnosis listed as:

> *Axis I:* 303.00 Alcohol intoxication
>
> 295.32 Schizophrenia, paranoid
> sub-type, chronic

Notice that each of the above mental disorders has a decimal number preceding it. In DSM-III, as in the system it replaces called DSM-II, every mental disorder has both a name and a special number called the "code number" or "coding number" of the disease.

This use of the word "coding" when referring to those numbers is not to be confused with the way we have been using the word "coding" to mean "filling out one of the five Axes" as when we spoke of "coding a stress on Axis IV".

The code numbers of mental disorders will be used in this book, but you do not have to learn them. They can be looked up when needed.

More than one disorder can be given on Axis II whenever more than one personality disorder and/or more than one group of personality traits is present in adults (and in some children) and when more than one "specific developmental disorder" is present in children (and some adults).

A *personality trait* is a feature of a person's personality that is enduring and is displayed in a wide variety of social and occupational situations.

A personality trait of a particular person is part of what characterizes that particular person because it endures over the years and it is predictably displayed.

Some people have the personality trait of generally being mistrustful of others, while some people have the personality trait of being perfectionistic. In DSM-III saying that someone has a personality trait of perfectionism means that it is not a new feature of their character, but "they have always been like that." A personality trait endures and it is pervasive in its manifestations.

Because the personalities of children are not rigid, but can change as they develop, children are not usually described as having personality traits *in the DSM-III sense.*

"Children" in DSM-III sometimes means "anyone under eighteen years of age" so that is includes adolescents, and sometimes "Children" in DSM-III means "anyone who is pre-teen or hasn't undergone the changes of puberty", and in those cases, excludes adolescents.

An older adolescent might have a characteristic that for him had been a relatively persistent way of thinking, feeling, or behaving, such as a sixteen-year-old adolescent that was a meticulous perfectionist and had been that way since at least age ten. Such "children" (persons under age eighteen) would have a personality trait in the DSM-III sense.

A *personality disorder* is a cluster of personality traits that are "maladaptive" to the individual's social or occupational functioning or cause him "significant distress" (usually through the way they grate on the people around him).

DSM-III describes eleven personality stereotypes that are each a cluster of personality traits appearing together that are invariably maladaptive.

One of the eleven kinds of personality disorder is paranoid personality disorder. In that personality disorder, one of the personality traits that is part of the cluster is a *pervasive* and unwarranted suspicion and mistrust of other people.

A person who had that particular trait without having the other traits that are part of the stereotype would have a paranoid personality *trait* and would never be said to have a paranoid personality disorder. (Part of the definition of the paranoid personality disorder is that the unwarranted pervasive mistrust and suspicion of others not be due to any other mental disorder like schizophrenia).

The *Specific Developmental Disorders* coded on Axis II for children (all people under age eighteen) are a group of four kinds of difficulties in development that are not the result of any other physical or mental disorder in DSM-III, and are related to specific difficulty in acquiring certain skills such as reading. The category of Developmental Reading disorder contains most children previously described as having "dyslexia".

Such conditions can persist beyond age eighteen and might be prominent enough in an adult with a striking history of similar difficulty throughout childhood and adolescence (again, not due to any other physical or DSM-III mental disorder) that an adult would receive the diagnosis of "315.00 Developmental Reading Disorder".

Why was the separation of mental disorders into those coded on Axis I and those coded on Axis II made?

DSM-III wants you to be sure that consideration is given to the possible presence of long term disturbances that are frequently overlooked when attention is given to a current episode of illness.

DSM-III insists that personality disorders be listed on Axis II, but it doesn't require that personality traits (in the absence of personality disorder) be listed on Axis II.

However, Axis II is intended to be used to list prominent features of an individual personality even when they are not subsumable under a personality disorder diagnosis.

Compulsive traits in a person's personality are not the same as compulsive personality disorder. Most well functioning people have compulsive traits — only a minority of them have compulsive personality disorder.

Knowing about such features as prominent personality traits of the patient should be something that happens often as a result of getting to know the patient. Hence in many cases when there is disorder codable on Axis I, but no evidence for a personality disorder codable on Axis II, the person may yet have prominent personality traits that will emerge through getting to know them.

When There is no Axis I Disorder

A person who has no illness describable as "current episode of something" who comes to the doctor with complaints that are long standing and which fit a personality disorder (or other disorder coded on Axis II) should have Axis I and Axis II filled out as follows:

Axis I: V71.09* No diagnosis or condition on Axis I

Axis II: "name of personality disorder"

If such a person had problems referable to a life long history of borderline personality disorder, the parts of the diagnosis for Axis I and II would be given as:

Axis I: V71.09 No diagnosis or condition on Axis I

Axis II: Borderline personality disorder

Remember the jealous suspicious lady who hounded her husband until he left and then got drunk and cut her wrist? If she had gone to a doctor before her husband left her and was thought to have problems in her life due to her paranoid personality disorder, her doctor would write this as:

Axis I: V71.09 No diagnosis or condition on Axis I

Axis II: Paranoid personality disorder

Axis III: None

When there are prominent personality traits but no personality disorder in an adult or older adolescent, Axis II is to be filled out as follows:

Axis II: Paranoid traits - no disorder

or

Axis II: Paranoid traits - V71.09 No
diagnosis on Axis II.

In addition, the physician can further indicate *that the personality traits are prominent* and say:

Axis II: Prominent paranoid traits - no disorder

or

Axis II: Prominent paranoid traits - V71.09
No diagnosis on Axis II

Notice that since personality traits are not considered mental disorders, we indicate that there is no Axis II disorder.

This is the practice used when there is an Axis I disorder and nothing to be entered on Axis II. Here we could write:

Axis I: "Name of disorder"

Axis II: V71.09 No diagnosis on Axis II

Thus a person with a major depression who had no personality disorder or prominent personality traits would have their diagnosis written:

Axis I: Major depression

Axis II: No diagnosis on Axis II

When both an Axis I and an Axis II diagnosis are given, it is assumed that the Axis I condition is the disorder that describes the current episode of illness.

*For discussion of the V-Codes, see page 13.

To indicate that the current contact with the mental health care system is because of an Axis II condition, when there is both an Axis I and an Axis II diagnosis listed, the doctor writes:

Axis I: "Name of disorder"

Axis II: "Name of disorder," Principal Diagnosis

A patient with a history of recurring major depressions who now was in remission, who had a compulsive personality disorder, and who was now being seen because of that Axis II personality problem would have his or her diagnosis written:

Axis I: Major depression, recurrent, in remission

Axis II: Compulsive personality disorder
(Principal diagnosis)

If the same patient in addition had borderline personality traits, the doctor could additionally indicate this as:

Axis I: Major depression, recurrent, in remission

Axis II: Compulsive personality disorder (Principal diagnosis),
borderline personality traits

RECURRENT, IN REMISSION, AND PRODROMAL

Notice that it is a practice in DSM-III to code Axis I conditions that have been recurrent in a particular patient, even though the patient may now be in remission and appear to be relatively free of problems from the disorder, or has only some residual symptoms.

DSM-III would also like the doctor to code Axis I conditions that are often recurrent but where a particular patient may have had only one episode and then recovered. Examples are:

Axis I: Major depression, in remission

or

Axis I: Schizophrenia, in remission

or

Axis I: Alcohol dependence, in remission

A major mental illness may be so dramatic that the usual features of a person's personality may be overwhelmed and unrecognizable. DSM-III urges doctors to specify the features of the patient's personality before the acute illness occurred by writing down on Axis II those personality traits or personality disorders that existed before the acute illness, followed by the word, "premorbid".

A man who had a paranoid personality disorder and then developed a schizophrenic disorder where he became catatonic and sat mute and motionless for days, would have his diagnosis on Axis I and II written as:

Axis I: Schizophrenic disorder, catatonic

Axis II: Paranoid personality disorder, premorbid

LEVELS OF UNCERTAINTY IN DIAGNOSIS

When there is not enough information to make a diagnosis, DSM-III provides a way to write this. This can be done in several ways.

The writing of a specific diagnosis is avoided altogether by writing, *"Diagnosis deferred"* on the appropriate Axis, indicating that either not enough information is available to decide whether a mental disorder exists or that if one does, the doctor has avoided even a guess at what it might be.

Here, if the Axis I diagnosis is avoided, the doctor would write:

Axis I: 799.90 Diagnosis or condition deferred on Axis I.

and if Axis II was the issue, the doctor writes:

Axis II: 799.90 Diagnosis deferred on Axis II.

Although "Diagnosis Deferred" is not a diagnosis at all, it has a code number, 799.90.

When the doctor thinks that there is a mental disorder and that he has enough information to take a guess at the diagnosis, this can be written several ways.

He can write his guess at a specific disorder, and add the phrase *"Provisional diagnosis"*, after it. Thus,

Axis I: Schizophrenia disorder (provisional)

He can further *indicate the other possibilities he plans to rule out* before his diagnosis could be more solid by additionally writing:

(rule out "name of disease to be considered")

Thus,

Axis I: Schizophrenic disorder (provisional –
　　　　 rule out bipolar disorder, manic,
　　　　 with psychotic features)

or for Axis II,

Axis II: Borderline personality disorder (provisional)
　　　　 or
Axis II: Borderline personality disorder (provisional –
　　　　 rule out histrionic personality disorder)

When the doctor believes that there is an Axis I mental disorder present accounting for the current episode of illness that does not involve a psychosis, (see page 161 for a discussion of psychosis) but cannot pin it down further, at that time he can write:

Axis I: 300.90 Unspecified mental disorder
　　　　 (non-psychotic)

He could of course also use the other ways we have discussed above such as writing "Diagnosis deferred" or taking a guess at the disorder and writing "provisional" after it.

THE WORD ATYPICAL

When the doctor believes that there is an Axis I diagnosis that accounts for the current episode of illness, and that it is a psychotic condition, but the doctor can't at that time specify the disorder any further, he can write:

Axis I: 298.90 Atypical psychosis

Here the word *Atypical* has a special meaning unique to DSM-III. The adjective *Atypical* does not mean "strange" or "unusual". For DSM-III *Atypical* is used to mean "all of those kinds that can't be specified any further."

An atypical anxiety disorder is one that cannot be specified as one of the types that are defined, and does not mean that the "Atypical anxiety disorder" is in any way "weird" or "strange" or even that it is unusual.

The patients that are classified as having atypical anxiety disorder may, in certain settings, even outnumber the patients who have the disorders that are defined.

CONDITIONS NOT ATTRIBUTABLE TO
A MENTAL DISORDER (V-CODES)

When after a full examination, there is no evidence of any disorder codable on either Axis I or Axis II, the diagnosis of:

V71.09 - No mental disorder on Axis I (or Axis II)

or one of the conditions in DSM-III from the section, "Conditions not Attributable to a Mental Disorder" should be given.

The conditions listed under that section are interpersonal problems or life circumstance problems that are not severe enough in themselves to justify a diagnosis of a mental disorder like adjustment disorder but where contact with the health delivery system occurred and the reason had to be noted.

A patient who was found to have no mental or physical disorder would have this conclusion written as:

Axis I: V71.09 No diagnosis on Axis I

Axis II: V71.09 No diagnosis on Axis II

Axis III: None

or

Axis I: V71.09 No diagnosis on Axis I

Axis II: V71.09 No diagnosis on Axis II

Axis III: No physical disorder

Notice that both Axis I and Axis II are written down as specifically having no diagnosis.

Some ways that the "conditions not attributable to a mental disorder" categories of DSM-III might be used are given below.

The code numbers of all such categories begin with a capital letter "V" as in "V71.09 No diagnosis or condition on Axis I," or "V71.09 No diagnosis on Axis II.

Important -

In DSM-III there is now no V-code called "V71.00 No mental disorder". There was such a code when DSM-III was being written. It was then possible, in the case of a patient with no mental disorder on axis I or II and no physical disorder, to write:

> V71.00 no mental disorder
>
> *Axis III:* no physical disorder

This is now changed, and Axis I and Axis II are now to be individually specified as having no mental disorder by always writing out: V71.09 No diagnosis or condition on Axis I or V71.09 no diagnosis on Axis II on the respective axis despite the use of the same coding number of V71.09.

The reason for this is to force consideration of possible Axis II disorder when no Axis I disorder is found, and force a search for Axis I disorder when no Axis II disorder is found.

When there is no disorder on either Axis I or Axis II we write:

> *Axis I:* V71.09 No diagnosis or condition on Axis I
>
> *Axis II:* V71.09 No diagnosis on Axis II
>
> *Axis III:* (whatever is relevant)

When any other V-codes are used, the V-code appears on Axis I and Axis II is also evaluated and written out. We will now give some examples of this.

Case Illustration

A physically healthy woman is told to see a psychiatrist by her clergyman after she phones him about arranging an appointment to discuss an argument she had with her husband. She goes to a psychiatrist and he determines that she has no mental disorder.

The psychiatrist could write:

> *Axis I:* V61.10 Marital problem
>
> *Axis II:* V71.09 No diagnosis on Axis II
>
> *Axis III:* No physical disorder

If instead she had phoned the clergyman about her relationship with her child and was not having any marital problems, the psychiatrist could write:

> *Axis I:* V61.20 Parent-child problem
>
> *Axis II:* V71.09 No diagnosis on Axis II
>
> *Axis III:* No physical disorder

If the problems with her child had settled down by the time she saw the psychiatrist and the real issue was a problem she had getting along with her clergyman, this physically healthy woman with no mental disorder could be given the diagnosis:

Axis I: V62.18 Other interpersonal problems

Axis II: V71.09 No diagnosis on Axis II

Axis III: No physical disorder

This category of "V62.18 other interpersonal problems" is not used for parent-child or marital problems.

If problems with relatives other than spouse or child are the reason the patient sought or was referred to the mental health care system, and the patient does not have a mental disorder, the category of "V61.80 Other specified family circumstances" is used.

Case Illustration

A Protestant man married a Catholic woman whose mother had always disapproved of the marriage and had continually urged the wife to convince her husband to convert to Catholicism.

After an argument with his mother-in-law, she announced that she thought "he was crazy" and persuaded the wife that he needed "to see a psychiatrist". The man's wife pressured him to go to the psychiatrist and even phoned and made an appointment for him, which he kept to please her. The psychiatrist found that the man had no mental disorder (and not even prominent personality traits).

The man had had a complete physical examination one month earlier and the psychiatrist had a copy of the medical report that described the man as being healthy.

The psychiatrist's diagnosis was:

Axis I: V61.80 Other specified family circumstances

Axis II: V71.09 No diagnosis on Axis II

Axis III: No physical disorder

The reaction to the death of a relative can be severe, but eventually subsides within a year of the loss. Usual social and occupational functioning are resumed by that time in most people.

Since all persons are expected to go through a period of grief following the death of a close tie, the bereavement reaction of most people falls outside the subject of mental disorder. The picture of the grief stricken person can resemble the picture of major mental disorder, such as major depression.

A person suffering from severe grief may ask for help from a psychiatrist or may be urged to "go get help for yourself" by relatives and friends who cannot bear to see the person undergo such misery. If the judgement is made that the person suffers from grief and that no other mental disorder is present, this is called "uncomplicated bereavement".

The doctor would write:

Axis I: V62.80 Uncomplicated bereavement

Axis II: V71.09 No diagnosis on Axis II

Axis III: (whatever is relevant)

A man who saw a psychiatrist because he was dissatisfied with his job and was found to have no mental disorder would be diagnosed on Axis I as:

V62.20 Occupational problem

A woman who was given "water pills" (diuretics) by her family doctor and refused to take them because they upset her stomach was sent to a psychiatrist by her medical doctor who said that she was "going to do damage to herself" by not taking the medicine he prescribed for her mild high blood pressure.

If the psychiatrist concluded that she had no mental (or physical) disorder responsible for her behavior, he could write:

Axis I: V71.09 No disorder on Axis I

Axis II: V71.09 No disorder on Axis II

or he could specify further what happened and say:

V15.81 Noncompliance with medical treatment

This category also covers people who refuse to comply with kinds of medical treatment because of their religion (when they are found to have no mental disorder).

AXIS III

When a physical illness is directly related to the DSM-III mental disorder in a current episode of mental illness, the physical illness *must* be listed on Axis III.

A Vietnam war veteran who had erratic and bizzare behavior due to a delirium during an attack of malaria with high fever, could have his diagnosis written as:

Axis I: Delirium

Axis II: Any noteworthy Axis II information

Axis III: Malaria

Delirium is a mental disorder described in DSM-III. We will discuss it later on.

Isolated explosive disorder is another new disorder discussed in DSM-III. It is a condition where a person who previously appeared to have no mental disorder and no previous history of violence commits a catastrophic act of violence and where the person cannot be shown after the violent act to suffer from any other DSM-III mental disorder.

When it is shown that such a patient suffers from a physical disease that can account for the behavior, the physical disease is written on Axis III.

Case Study

A twentytwo-year-old graduate student with no problems in social or academic functioning and who had not suffered any recent life stress, suddenly shot seven people with his roommate's pistol and then shot himself in the head and died.

An autopsy revealed a large brain tumor.

This man's psychiatric diagnosis could be written:

Axis I: Isolated explosive disorder

Axis II: V71.09 No diagnosis on Axis II

Axis III: Brain tumor

When real physical disease is thought to be caused or aggravated by psychological factors, we write *Psychological factors affecting physical condition* on Axis I and write the name of the physical illness on Axis III.

Psychological factors affecting physical illness is a DSM-III mental disorder that inherits what were previously called "psychosomatic disorders" or "psychophysiologic disorders".

A patient with compulsive personality traits and a peptic ulcer, who was judged to have real ulcer symptoms whenever he got into an argument with his wife or boss, would be diagnosed as follows:

Axis I: Psychological factors affecting physical condition

Axis II: Compulsive personality traits -
no diagnosis

Axis III: Peptic ulcer disease

AXIS IV

This part of DSM-III diagnosis is optional.

The current use of Axis IV provides two things, a list of the stressful events that the physcan believes to be important to the exacerbation or development of the current disorder, and also Axis IV gives a rating of the combined stress these events put on the individual. The rating has two parts also. It has a number from 0 to 7 together with a word. A stress does not have to be an event that has actually happened. It can be something that a patient believes will happen. An eleven-year-old girl whose best friend was going to move away is an example. Axis IV for her could look like this:

Axis IV: Psychosocial stressors:
Anticipated loss of closest friend
Severity: 4 Moderate

Notice that the word "Psychosocial stressors" is written out with the stressor (stressful, actual or anticipated events) written below it, and then the word "severity" together with the rating. In the rating, a number is written before the rating word.

Notice that the stressors are not just precipitating factors, but can be the results of a problem that themselves then become a stress.

In the case just cited of a man with peptic ulcer disease see above, the man's ulcer, while the result of psychological factors (including the arguments with wife and boss) now becomes itself a stressor.

His abdominal pain, frequent and distracting belching, and his knowledge that every painful attack may be moving him closer to a severe complication, constitute a stress in addition to any other stresses in his life.

If we consider that he has marital trouble, the combined severity of the two stresses of peptic ulcer disease and marital difficulty deserve a higher severity rating when taken together than either one alone.

Axis IV when written out for these two stresses, where we give them a combined severity rating of "5 Severe" would look like this:

> *Axis IV:* Psychosocial stressors:
> Marital difficulty
> Peptic ulcer disease
> Severity: 5 Severe

A *stressor* is a real or anticipated event that puts stress on the patient.

Knowing the psychosocial stressors on a patient with a mental disorder can help in planning treatment. A treatment plan could focus on ways to remove the stresses or help the patient develop better ways of coping with them.

If having a physical illness is a stressor on a patient with a mental disorder, a treatment plan for that patient could include ways to help the patient get rid of the physical illness or include ways to help the patient cope with the physical illness.

Axis IV information is probably useful in *prognosis* (the predicting of outcome) because a person who develops a mental disorder when there is little or no stress, probably has a poorer chance of complete recovery than a person who develops similar symptoms while under great stress.

KINDS OF STRESSORS AND THE SEVERITY RATING SYSTEM

What is a stress to one person may not be a stress to others. Going on vacation may be somewhat a stress to certain people while it may be no stress at all to others. The ratings give the stress that an average person of the same age would experience from the combined effect of all of the stressors listed for that patient.

When rating single individual stresses the most severe rating is "7 - Catastrophic" while the least severe rating is "1 - None". This rating of "1 - None" means "no apparent psychosocial stressor".

Zero means "no information", or "not applicable" and does not mean that there is no stress. We would here write:

> 0 - Unspecified

If you list even a single stressor, it cannot be rated as 1 - None or as 0 - Unspecified.

A person who had no mental disorder, no physical disorder, and who was under no stress could be given a diagnosis of:

> *Axis I:* V71.09 No diagnosis or condition on Axis I
> *Axis II:* V71.09 No diagnosis on Axis II

Axis III: No physical disorder
Axis IV: Psychosocial stressors
>>no apparent psychosocial stressor
>>Severity: 1-None

The hedger in a diagnosis where there was no psychosis could use:

Axis I: 300.90 Unspecified mental disorder (nonpsychotic)
Axis II: 799.90 Diagnosis deferred on Axis II
Axis III: Not enough information
Axis IV: Psychosocial stressors
>>not enough information
>>Severity: 0-Unspecified

(Please don't do this — DSM-III gives you ways to hedge, but the intent of the system is that you would try to be more explicit and more careful.)

The rating numbers and rating words are:

0-Unspecified
1-None
2-Minimal
3-Mild
4-Moderate
5-Severe
6-Extreme
7-Catastrophic

For children, (persons under eighteen) the death of a parent or sibling within the previous year when listed as the only stress would be expected to be given the value of 6-Extreme.

In the case of adults, death of a parent, death of a spouse, death of a child, death of a brother or sister, is rated as 6-Extreme if it has occurred in the previous year.

The rating of 7-Catastrophic for adults and for children is used when there have been multiple family deaths, concentration camp experiences, or devastating disasters like the Managua Earthquake or the Guyana Mass Suicide.

Case Illustration

A seven-year-old Vietnamese boy who is brought to you because of difficulty in school is found to have witnessed the death of his entire family in an air raid shortly before coming to this country. Without going into the complete list of the psychosocial stressors that describe his tragic circumstances, you would know that the severity rating for the list would be 7-Catastrophic.

Case Illustration

A father brings his ten-year-old son to see you because the son refuses to speak to him at all. You learn that the boy's mother (father's wife) died three weeks ago. Each of these people would receive an Axis IV severity rating of 6-Extreme. (The boy's parent died — one family death, the father's spouse died — one family death.)

For children, death of a friend (peer) is rated as 5-Severe but is rated as 4-Moderate in the case of adults.

Death of a parent for both adults and children is rated as 6-Extreme.

The point is that death of a close relative or friend is not considered to be less severe than 4-Moderate.

An arrest is usually rated alone as 4 or 5 in an adult and as 5 in a child. A jail term alone would be rated as 6 in both children and adults.

A man arrested for drunk driving could be given a 4-Moderate or 5-Severe. (Perhaps it would be 4-Moderate while he was intoxicated changing to 5-Severe when he sobered up.) If he was immediately jailed away from home, and three days elapsed before he was bailed out, we could rate the stressor as 6-Severe.

For an adult, Divorce is rated as 6-Extreme while Marital Separation is rated as 5-Severe. Obviously this is a matter of judgment. The point is that divorce is usually as significant a life stress on the average adult as is the death of a relative.

For children, divorce of parents is equivalent to death of a peer and rated as 5-Severe.

Parental fighting, or change to a new school, or illness of a close relative, or birth of a sibling is rated as 4-Moderate.

For a child, change in a teacher or the start of a new school year is rated as 3-Mild.

A vacation with the family for a child may be a stressor and would be rated as 2-Minimal.

Stressors become significant in the causation of a psychiatric disorder when the Axis IV total severity level is at least 4-Moderate.

Below this, the contribution to the current episode of disease would be ignored.

Test Your Knowledge

A ten-year-old girl saw her dog killed by a car last spring. Her mother and father helped the griefstricken child bury the dog in the nearby field. One week later she developed what her pediatrician diagnosed as her first attack of hay fever. Now, whenever she is saddened by real or imagined losses, she regularly develops hay fever. When you see her, she is having an attack brought on by the knowledge that her bestfriend is moving out of town. When she is having an attack, between sneezes, she looks with her watery eyes and runny nose strikingly like someone who is crying at a funeral. She doesn't feel sad, and claims she is not crying. She is sensitive on allergy panels to springtime pollens like those found in the field where her dog is buried. This girl could be diagnosed as:

_____

_____

(optional) _____

Answer: *Axis I:* Psychological factors affecting physical condition
 Axis II: (not enough information in above example)
 Axis III: Allergic rhinitis (hay fever)
 Axis IV: Psychosocial stressor: Anticipated
   loss of best friend
   Severity: 5-Severe (or 4-Moderate)

In the case of children, the large number of psychosocial stressors is frequently not appreciated.

For children, the stressors would be as follows:

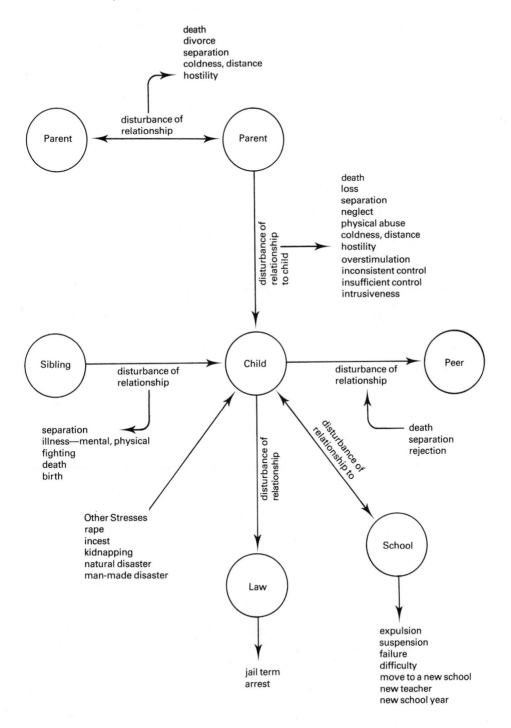

AXIS V

Axis V is optional.

Axis V considers the highest level of adaptive functioning in the previous year. Like Axis IV, Axis V gives a rating number and a rating word. They are:

1-Superior
2-Very Good
3-Good
4-Fair
5-Poor
6-Very Poor
7-Grossly Impaired
0-(Same)

0 means that there is no information.

To write out an Axis V rating, you write:

"Axis V: Highest level of adaptive functioning: 4-Fair"

The rating 0-Unspecified means that you don't know enough about the person to give them a rating.

Average functioning or functioning with *slight* impairment is rated a 3-Good, while average to better than average functioning is rated as 2-Very Good. 1-Superior is reserved for truly exceptional functioning.

Most impairments in functioning that tend to be significant to the psychiatrist begin with 4-Fair.

Highest level of adaptive functioning in adults and in children are to be rated on the three categories of:

1. Social relations – relations with all other people with emphasis on family and friends.

2. Occupational functioning – functioning as worker, student, housewife, complexity of task is to be considered.

3. Use of leisure time – range and depth of involvement in recreation or hobbies.

Since average functioning or functioning with slight impairment is pegged at 3-Good, an adult who did well at a difficult job but who had only one or two friends could be rated as 3-Good.

A child who does well at school but gets sent home occasionally because he picks on younger children could also be rated as 3-Good. Both of these cases have slight or possibly slight impairment of social relations but no problems in occupational functioning (school is children's work).

For the adult, the slight impairment here is having only one or two friends. For the child, the slight impairment is picking on younger children.

A child who was at the top of her class, was popular and well liked by teachers and peers, and had good relations with everyone in her family, and really excelled in sports would be given a rating of 1-Superior.

A man who was chosen as top salesman, who was an excellent husband and father, and was a civic leader would be given a rating of 1-Superior.

The child doing well at school with only a few friends who hits younger children could be given a rating of 3-Good.

If this child does well in school but has no friends, or does poorly in school with adequate family and peer relations, they are rated as 4-Fair.

If a child fails at school and has trouble getting along with peers, he could be rated as 5-Poor. If a child has no peer relations and cannot function at all in school without special help, the rating is 6-Very Poor. The category "7-Grossly Impaired" is used for a person who is impaired enough to receive a rating of 6-Very Poor and additionally requires continual supervision, so as to prevent self-injury or to provide for personal hygiene.

Social Relations

And	no impairment	slight impairment	moderate impairment	marked impairment
no impairment	2 very good	3 good	4 fair	5 poor
slight impairment	3 good	4 fair	4 fair or 5 poor	5 poor
moderate impairment	4 fair	5 poor	5 poor	5 poor
marked impairment	5 poor	5 poor	5 poor	6 very poor

(left axis label: Occupational Functioning)

The table above illustrates the use of the rating terms. Marked impairment in both Social Relations and Occupational Functioning, such as an adult that hadn't worked most of the year, had no friends, and had been thrown out of the house by the family because they couldn't stand him any longer, would be rated as 6-Very Poor.

Trouble doing tasks at a job rates 4-Fair. Trouble keeping the job itself rates a 5-Poor. For a child, trouble getting average grades and trouble doing assignments rates a 4. Getting asked to leave the school rates 5, at least, depending on the circumstances.

No social relationships rates at least 5, trouble with social relationships such as arguments or fights, rates a 4.

Judgment has to be used about how serious the troubles are. We will give some examples for you to rate.

SELF-STUDY QUESTIONS, PART I

1. A ten year old girl is doing poorly in school but has good family and peer relations. How would you rate her on Axis V?
Answer: 4-Fair

2. She hasn't been suspended or expelled from school. If you know that she had been expelled, how would you rate her?
Answer: 5-Poor She still has good peer and family relations and wouldn't rate a 6 because that would require a serious impairment in both occupational and social functioning. If she were in need of supervision to provide basic care of herself, she would be rated 7-Grossly Impaired.

3. A housewife who has no friends cannot seem to keep up with her family and is letting everything go around the house. She argues with her husband and children. How do you rate her?
Answer: Could be a 4, 5, or a 6 depending upon what we mean by "letting things go" and by "argues". If the degree of impairment is very serious in both social and occupational areas (her occupation is housewife and mother — that's a very complex job) it would rate a 6-Very Poor. If both housework and family relations were not suffering that much, she would be rated as 4-Fair. Between these two, use your judgment — housewife and mother is so complex that when a woman does well at it, she rates a 1-Superior if she is able to have any leisure time for herself which she uses to devote to an activity not directly related to housework or to child care.

CASE STUDY WITH QUESTION

A successful businessman is picked up for driving while intoxicated. He goes to see you because he hopes his seeing a psychiatrist might work in his favor since the authorities want to suspend his driver's license. You conclude only that he has compulsive personality traits. He fits the criteria, however, for the DSM-III diagnosis of 303.9x Alcohol dependence (alcoholism).

He has some degree of cirrhosis of the liver. He functioned very well at work all year but had a lot of arguments with his entire family over his drinking. He copes with increased stress by drinking more.

How would you diagnose him on the five Axes?
Answer:

Axis I: 303.9x Alcohol dependence
Axis II: V71.09 No disorder on Axis II, Compulsive Personality Traits
Axis III: Hepatic cirrhosis (mild to moderate)
Axis IV: Psychosocial stressors:
　　　Arrest for driving while intoxicated
　　　Anticipated loss of driver's license
　　　Knowledge of hepatic cirrhosis
　　　Arguments with family
　　　Severity: 5-Severe
Axis V: Highest level of adaptive functioning: 4-Fair

part II

The Cardinal
Manifestations
of Mental Disorders

INTRODUCTION

By defining the mental disorders, the whole of DSM-III now defines what is and what is not a mental disorder.

By defining each mental disorder by a characteristic group of signs and symptoms, DSM-III now defines what signs and symptoms are possible signs and symptoms of mental disorders.

Each mental disorder in DSM-III is a cluster of signs and symptoms. No one symptom carries such weight that by itself it can do more than raise questions about whether something is the matter with a person who shows such a symptom or sign.

Furthermore, no single symptom or sign in DSM-III is so characteristic of a particular mental disorder that when taken all by itself it allows an immediate diagnosis to be made.

This point is so important that it will be further explained.

"Low-grade fever" is not a sign of any mental disorder in DSM-III. Low-grade fever can be a sign of any one of a large number of physical illnesses. Fever of 100 F taken by itself does not carry enough significance to mean that physical illness is present. Ovulating women and teething babies often have low-grade fevers and are only two of many examples that could be given of how fever alone does not mean that physical illness is present. Furthermore, low-grade fever is not enough, even when a part of physical illness, to point directly, by itself, to the presence of a specific illness.

Low self-esteem appears in each of the cluster of symptoms of several mental disorders in DSM-III. Each of these disorders that includes low self-esteem as part of the cluster also includes other symptoms. It is the cluster that defines a DSM-III disorder, not any one particular symptom.

Low self-esteem, taken by itself, does not allow the diagnosis of any DSM-III mental disorder.

Furthermore, low self-esteem can appear in individuals with no mental disorder as part of their way of coping with disappointment.

A patient's complaint about low self-esteem, or an examiner's conclusion that some of the observations point toward low self-esteem, does not, in itself, either indicate mental disorder, or indicate that a specific mental disorder is present.

However, by defining each mental disorder as a characteristic group of signs and symptoms, DSM-III has now spread out before us those signs and symptoms that can be part of a mental disorder.

Whenever information is gathered about patients, whether by direct interview of a patient, or by a report by someone who knew the patient, or by a report by someone who knew the patient, DSM-III now defines what signs and symptoms are important.

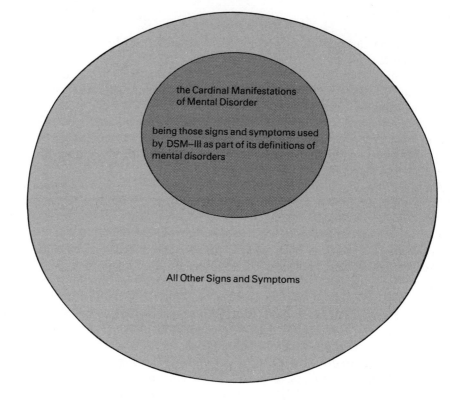

As depicted in the above diagram, the special signs, symptoms, findings, complaints, and reports of specific disturbance that are used by DSM-III to create its definitions of disorder will be set off and given a special name in this book.

The special term we shall use is *"cardinal manifestation."*

When we discuss a "cardinal manifestation of mental disorder," we shall mean a sign or symptom of mental illness that appears somewhere in DSM-III as part of the definition of a mental disorder. Any other signs and symptoms that are not "cardinal manifestations of mental disorder" are not covered by DSM-III.

As these cardinal manifestations of mental disorder are covered, there will appear questions and answers that the reader is urged to use to test his knowledge.

This Chapter discusses impairments in social relating, academic areas, and occupational roles, alertness, attention, memory, thought, emotion, speech, and sensory perception, problems of self-esteem, overall level of activity, impulsiveness, confusion about ones identity, and kinds of odd or peculiar behavior. And, we will examine specific physical complaints such as fatigue, pain, insomnia, premature ejaculation, and paralysis, looking at complaints about physical illness that have a physical condition underlying them, as well as those where after thorough search, medical doctors can find no physical disease.

The reader is again warned that no single manifestation can be taken out of context of the cluster of manifestations that defines a DSM-III mental disorder, and that no single manifestation should be looked at out of the context of the life of the particular patient where some individual symptom might be found.

As we proceed, we will whenever possible begin creating various groupings that will help the reader to understand the DSM-III classifications. Such groupings are at a higher level of clustering than is a single symptom, but they will usually fall short of the full cluster required in any specific DSM-III diagnosis. These partial clusterings may receive names.

In some cases we will have, in these early clusters, all that is required for some DSM-III diagnosis.

In order to cover these manifestations of mental illness in a logical way, we will present them under several headings. At times, the same manifestation of a mental disorder may be covered under more than one heading where the author feels that it makes sense to do so. Thus, outbursts of rage may be covered under "Difficulties in Social Relating" and it may also be discussed under the heading of "Emotion".

chapter 1

Disturbance of Adaptive Functioning

Adaptive functioning or simply "functioning" cover all of a person's social relationships, occupational or school functioning, and use of leisure time, and includes their level of self-care including their personal hygeine, grooming, and capacity to feed and take care of themselves when they are required to be independent.

In children it includes, at certain ages, their ability to feed themselves, dress themselves, take themselves to the toilet, and to be able to function and perform comfortably in certain situations where they are away from their families.

The term "adaptive functioning" covers almost every conceivable situation in which a person can find him or herself. In covering this huge area we will break it down into:

1. social functioning or social relationships
2. functioning and performance in an occupational role or in an academic setting
3. use of leisure time
4. self-care

These are not clearly delimited areas and a person's difficulty in one of them may cross over into their difficulty in another. A person whose self-care is poor, giving them a dirty disheveled appearance and a strong body odor, may have difficulties in social relationships.

The importance of adaptive functioning in DSM-III is firstly that many of the symptoms of mental disorder that we will discuss can be viewed as particular ways that adaptive functioning can be impaired, and secondly, when DSM-III presents a cluster of symptoms that characterize a particular mental disorder, the decision as to whether the appearance of this cluster is a given patient is sufficiently severe to warrant the diagnosis of mental disorder, often depends on whether it is judged to interfere with adaptive functioning: socially or occupationally.

SOCIAL RELATIONS

Social relations, social functioning, and interpersonal relations comprise the most important of the areas of adaptive functioning. Each mental disorder in DSM-III can be viewed as a different kind of impairment in social relationships. Social relationships concern whether individuals have friends. If they do not, we wonder why. Do they seek friends or do they isolate themselves, avoiding opportunities to meet people? A person who isolates him or herself and avoids opportunities to meet people or who avoids meeting them when provided with opportunities, and shrinks from social interaction, manifests *social isolation* or *social withdrawal.*

Does a patient behave in ways that repel people, being overly demanding, mistrustful, wanting things done only their way, or lacking warmth? Do they talk in a strange way or talk about odd things? Do they have emotions that others have difficulty coping with such as outbursts of anger, irritable moods, complaints about fears, or about guilt, complaints about sadness or about physical illness that other people don't want to hear?

We can discuss social relations in terms of quantity and in terms of quality.

Quantity

When we look at a person's amount of social relating, there are several levels, and each is a symptom that can be found somewhere in DSM-III.

There is, firstly, the level of no relations with people in spite of opportunities to have them. Secondly, there is social relating confined to what DSM-III calls *"peripheral social contacts"*. At this level there is an amount of social relating where social contacts are confined to ones that are either essential to performing one's job or to one's self-care (such as dealing with the neighborhood grocer in order to buy food). Then there is a level where close relations with people are confined to only one person outside of one's own family, and where in spite of an opportunity to meet other persons, the formation of close relations with others has stopped at one or two people.

Then there is a level where there may be more interpersonal relations, more contacts between people, which begins to approach a quantity of social relatedness that DSM-III feels does not constitute impairment. Here, when impairment is present, it lies in the quality of the relationships.

Lastly there is a level where there is a lot of social relating, to the extent that there is an over-involvement and over-pursuit of social contacts, and this excessiveness is another manifestation of some mental disorders.

Quality

The quality of social relationships is another focus. Does a person use other people and manipulate them for his or her own selfish purposes?

Is there a lack of empathy? Is there a lack of concern about the feelings of others so that the patient does things or demands things without realizing the effect that this could have on how other people view him or her? (How many times people have to break their "word of honor" until other people become indifferent to their promises?)

Is there undue suspiciousness and mistrust of others? Are there feelings and attitudes about other people such as over-valuing them, under-valuing them, devaluing them, showing excessive clinging to others, or trying to steer other people into a relationship where they will take care of the patient who can then become dependent upon them?

Does the patient try to dominate others? Is he or she viewed by other people as shallow and insincere? Is he or she hostile towards other people, so that others are wary of the patient, fearing that the patient will do something to take advantage of them, or physically hurt them?

There are manifestations of mental disorder in this book that are not discussed. Under the category of impairments in social relationships, but which should nevertheless be considered whenever an impairment in social relations occurs. For example, a person whose social relating suffers because he cannot pay attention to what others are saying to him, does have an impairment in social relations. Insomnia causing a habitual lack of sufficient sleep might result in a diminished capacity to concentrate on what other people are saying because the patient is so sleepy. A patient who suffers from intense auditory hallucinations (hearing a voice that carries on a running commentary about his or her behavior) might also be unable to pay attention to what a real person is saying to him or her and so suffer from a problem that would interfere with social relatedness.

Varieties of Social Withdrawal

Looking once again at the quantity of social relatedness: *social isolation* or *social withdrawal* is a cardinal manifestation of mental illness.

The avoiding of people because of persistent irrational fear of, and compelling desire to avoid a situation in which the individual is exposed to possible scrutiny by others, and fears that he or she may act in a way that will be humiliating or embarrassing, is another cardinal manifestation of mental illness.

Individuals who avoid public places because they fear that they will become incapacitated and will be unable to escape, such as in a crowd, in a tunnel, on a bridge, or in a vehicle of public transportation, who constrict their social relations because of these fears, perhaps even to the point of their staying home and having only the peripheral of social relations, is another cardinal manifestation of mental illness.

Withdrawal from social relations because of complaints of physical illness, whether founded or unfounded, is another cardinal manifestation of mental illness.

Being withdrawn from others because of a preoccupation with a feeling, idea, or hallucination, is a symptom.

Learning that a patient has few of no friends requires some exploration. Does it result from markedly odd or peculiar behavior, such as talking to himself, wearing peculiar clothing, expounding on strange ideas, or from some of the things that will be discussed below under the heading of delusions (such as telling people that he thinks he is Jesus Christ)? Do people avoid *him?*

Does the examiner experience anything in the interview, or hear of anything in the history about the patient, that would make it understandable why the patient is socially isolated? Thus social isolation and social withdrawal can occur either because the patient avoids people, or avoids certain social situations, because the patient is *indifferent* to whether he sees people or not, or can result because other people understandably avoid *him*.

Some kinds of social isolation can occur because of difficulty in a particular area, such as sexual relationships. An individual's preferred mode of sexual activity can cause him to have few or no social contacts. In the case of voyuerism, the principal mode of sexual activity is by watching other people undress or have sexual relations, and the patient may have no need for an intimate social relationship with another person where sexual behavior would be part of the relationship.

Social Bonding

Returning now to the subject of social relating, of special concern is a lack of capacity to form intimate and enduring relationships with other people that are mutually enjoyable and satisfying. Many of the problems of adult patients that involve lifelong difficulties in social relations of various kinds come under this heading. These difficulties are also seen in children and adolescents.

In children we speak of *failure to establish a normal degree of affection, empathy, or bond with others* as shown by no more than one of the following indications of social attachment:

1. has one or more peer group friendships that have lasted over six months

2. extends himself or herself for others even when no immediate advantage is likely
3. apparently feels guilt or remorse when such a reaction is inappropriate (not just when caught or in difficulty)
4. avoids blaming or informing on companions
5. shows concern for the welfare of friends or companions

This is an important manifestation of mental disorder. We will call it the *"attachment criterion of conduct disorder"*.

In adults, inability to maintain an enduring attachment to a sexual partner as shown by two or more divorces and/or separations (whether legally married or not), desertion of spouse, promiscuity (ten or more sexual partners within one year), is what we will call the *"sexual attachment criterion of adulthood"*. It is a cardinal manifestation of mental disorder.

OCCUPATIONAL OR ACADEMIC FUNCTIONING

Depending on the occupation, or on the type of academic setting, problems in social relating can translate into reduced occupational performance. If the person can't deal with people, or doesn't want to, or is afraid to, or repels them, he won't do well in a job that depends on how he meets the public.

Under occupational or academic functioning, we look at whether the abilities required are absent, or are present but not utilized, or were present at one time but are declining.

Are there emotions, thoughts, or behavior that impair performance?

Are the individuals having trouble making decisions? Is there inability to pay attention or to concentrate? Do they show illogical thought or illogical speech? Do they have speech that is overly vague, confusing, metaphorical, or digressive so that their capacity to respond to questions or to organize their work is impaired?

Do they jump from one task to another? Is ther over-attention to little details, without being able to see the "big picture"? Is there an irritable "making mountains out of molehills"?

Is there a problem with rules, obligations, promises, or dealing with authority - either open rebellion against authority, provacative defiance, or resisting authority by procrastinating, dawdling, or by exhibiting "intentional inefficiency"?

Is there impairment of occupational functioning because of complaints of physical illness where medical examinations can find no disease, or where medical examinations reveal that patients should be able to function at their occupation despite diagnosed disease?

Is there a decline in occupational performance because of fatigue, "lack of energy", diminished enthusiasm, or diminished ability to think clearly?

Is work interrupted by episodes of tearfulness, or by persistent irrational fears? Is there a desire to avoid situations that are part of the job where there may be unreasonable fears of social embarrassment or of physical harm?

Reduced occupational and/or academic performance for whatever reason means that the individual is not doing well at his or her job or not doing well in school.

Antisocial Work Manifestation

This is an important cardinal manifestation of mental disorder and means that the patient has one of the following:

1. too frequent job changes (meaning three or more jobs in five years not accounted for by nature of job or economic or seasonal fluctuation
2. significant unemployment meaning six months or more in five years when expected to work
3. serious absenteeism from work meaning an average of three days or more of lateness or absence per month
4. walking off several jobs without other jobs in sight

Similar behavior in an academic setting during the last few years of school can substitute for the above manifestations in the antisocial work problem.

USE OF LEISURE TIME

The most important areas of adaptive functioning are social and occupational (or academic) functioning and the issues of self-care, personal hygiene, grooming, and personal cleanliness.

Use of leisure time may be of concern when it involves alcohol or drug use, engaging in excessive or unusual varieties of sexual activities, and when it involves impulsive pursuits or reckless behavior that have a potential for harm or self-injury (reckless driving, playing russian roulette, or attempting feats that are dangerous and for which the individual is not qualified by training or experience).

Of concern also is loss of pleasure, interest, or enthusiasm in what once were recreational pursuits or leisure time activities that the patient used to enjoy. This includes loss of, or decline of interest in the patient's usual sexual activity.

As a cardinal manifestation of mental illness, lack of pleasure involving activities includes loss of interest or failure to derive pleasure from the level of social relatedness (friendships) that had been previously satisfying.

Under this heading should also be included any activities that the individual engages in while not on the job that are themselves manifestations of mental illness, such as setting fires and watching them burn, stealing from stores, or excessive gambling that disrupts social relations or causes financial trouble.

In the case of children and adolescents, vandalism, theft, juvenile delinquency, running away from home, unusually early or exceptionally frequent casual sexual relationships and recurrent physical fighting are cardinal manifestations of mental disorder.

For children, inability to enjoy recreation or to perform in school when they are away from their parents, apparently suffering from the effects of being separated from them, is of concern.

Any situation in which a person seems to have no recreational pursuits and no leisure time activity, has a cardinal manifestation of mental disorder.

Any person who has markedly excessive involvement in recreational or leisure time activities to the extent that is impairs functioning on the job, or impairs important social relationships with spouse, children, or friends, has a cardinal manifestation of mental illness.

SELF CARE

Self-care consists of personal hygiene and grooming, but includes, in addition, a person's effectiveness and efficiency, in taking care of himself in situations where others expect him to be independent: feeding themselves, and obtaining help for, and giving themselves special care when they have a physical illness or injury. A cardinal manifestation of mental disorder is a level of personal hygiene that is below the accepted norms for the individual's social group. Patients who do not wash, never change their clothes, or who walk around seemingly indifferent to an infestation by lice, are examples.

Standards of grooming vary among various social groups and sub-cultures. Adolescents in almost every decade of this century and in almost every era that has given us some piece of writing that describes the adolescents of that period have shown a tendency of adolescents to deviate significantly from adult norms of acceptable dress and even grooming. The beatniks and bohemians of earlier decades sometimes even deviated from norms that, at the time, were considered standards of personal hygiene.

DSM-III applies to individual persons, not to groups in our society. Only by assessing an individual patient in the context of their particular environment can these kinds of deviation be properly considered.

Some sub-cultural groups do not dress in accordance with what a larger number of people consider either fashionable or appropriate. This kind of deviation must also be seen for what it really is. And again, the individual patient must be assessed in the context of their own environment in order to determine whether a breakdown has occurred in the level of care that people are expected to give to themselves.

The level of care that people give themselves for illnesses and injuries needs to be considered also in the context of religious beliefs and social behavior that they share with the group of which they may be a part before it is held that they are victims of their own self-neglect.

When these considerations have been met, and the individual's departure from standards of personal hygiene, grooming, dress, or self-care for injury and illness goes beyond what can be explained by religious beliefs or local social norms, it is a cardinal manifestation of mental disorder.

Individuals who live alone and who do not buy food for themselves, do not feed themselves, or who eat a markedly bizarre or inadequate diet, or who fail to maintain an adequate level of hygiene in their living quarters show a cardinal manifestation of mental disorder.

We need to call attention as well to the individual whose standards of personal hygiene, grooming, or dress, level of self-care in regard to illness and injury, and behavior within their own personal living environment reaches a level of excessive fastidiousness. Here there can be excessive neatness and over-concern about disarray, messmaking, dirt, germs, or an excessive striving for a level of perfection that is appreciated only by the patient. Excesses in each of these areas are cardinal manifestations of mental disorder.

MONEY MANAGEMENT

It is often supposed that when patients begin to talk about sex, they are discussing a topic of great importance.

The author believes that if an examiner can get a patient to start talking about money, then the patient is talking about an area that is more important than sex.

How persons handle their finances, their financial obligations, how well they budget their money, and what they choose to spend it on, and what prompts them to make a purchase, is of tremendous importance in assessing an individual patient for cardinal manifestations of mental disorder.

Why is this so?

Because these issues about how people handle their own money can reveal much about how they think of themselves and how well they are able to care for themselves and for their dependents. Hidden in these ideas and feelings about money can lurk many issues related to social and occupational functioning, use of leisure time, and issues related to self-care.

Persons who go on foolish spending sprees, or make foolish business and financial commitments may be in serious financial trouble. Financial difficulties of patients should be sifted for this kind of foolishness to determine whether it results from recklessness that is motivated by an overoptimism, or whether it is a recklessness that results because the person "just doesn't care any more about what happens to them" and is related to a pessimism or bleak view of the future.

Financial trouble needs to be examined for indications that the patient is defaulting on obligations as part of a pattern of defrauding others, defaulting on other obligations, rule breaking, and disregard for the law.

Financial trouble needs to be sifted for signs that the individuals are spending their money on expensive drugs, or are gambling their money away because they are gripped by a larger need.

On the other hand, patients whose financial situation is relatively good, or even superior, can hide cardinal manifestations of mental disorder such as over involvement with work and productivity to the exclusion of recreational and social relationships ("workaholics"). Some patients who are doing extremely well financially may be doing something illegal, or may have achieved success by being ruthless or inconsiderate of other people and by taking advantage of them.

The Care of Dependents

Adaptive functioning in social and occupational roles also includes a person's capacity to provide care for dependent persons such as children, unemployed spouses, and aged persons living in the home.

The capacity to provide care for children is of particular concern. Care of children means providing them with adequate food, shelter, and appropriate level of hygiene, sufficient stimulation to promote their psychological and social development, and providing them with special care for illness, injury, or special handicap. It includes making sure that children attend school, and includes showing appropriate concern about children who, by their behavior at home, with peers, or in school, are themselves showing cardinal manifestations of mental disorder.

It includes providing an appropriate level of discipline, through the setting of limits, and the use of punishments that are consistent without being cruel and likely to cause injury.

Lack of ability to function as a responsible parent would be evidenced by one or more of the following:

1. child's malnutrition
2. child's illness resulting from lack of minimal hygiene standards
3. failure to obtain medical care for a seriously ill child
4. child's dependence on neighbors or non-resident relatives for food or shelter
5. failure to arrange for a caretaker for a child under six when the parent is away from home
6. repeated squandering of money on personal items while neglecting purchases of household necessities

THE WAY THE PATIENT BEHAVES TOWARDS OTHERS

A cardinal manifestation of mental disorder in relations with other people is a repetitive and persistent pattern of conduct in which the basic rights of others are violated. This is an important manifestation of mental disorder. Here we look at two kinds, an aggressive kind and a non-aggressive kind.

Aggressive Violation of the Rights of Others

This is a repetitive and persistent pattern of aggressive conduct in which the basic rights of others are violated as shown by either one of the following:

1. physical violence against persons or property (not to defend someone else or one's self) for example, vandalism, rape, or breaking and entering, fire setting, mugging, assault
2. thefts outside the home involving confrontation with the victim (for example, extortion, purse snatching, gas station robbery)

Non-aggressive Violation of the Basic Rights of Others

This is a repetitive and persistent pattern of non-aggressive conduct in which either the basic rights of others or major age appropriate societal norms or rules are violated as manifested in children by any of the following:

1. chronic violation of a variety of important rules (that are reasonable and age appropriate for the child) at home or at school (persistent truancy, substance abuse)
2. repeated running away from home overnight
3. persistent serious lying in and out of the home
4. stealing not involving confrontation with the victim

The cardinal signs of *"aggressive violation of the rights of others"* and of *"non-aggressive violation of the rights of others"* are of particular importance in discussing children and adolescents.

But in order to discuss some adults (persons eighteen or older) an assessment of their past performance in relation to people and in relation to school performance, conformity to rules, honesty and respect for the law, is important.

An important group of cardinal manifestations are: truancy, expulsion, or suspension from school, juvenile delinquency, running away from home overnight, lying, repeated casual sex, repeated drunkeness, substance abuse, thefts, vandalism, and school grades that are way below expectations, chronic violations of rules at home and/or at school (other than truancy), and starting fights.

Having a history of three or more of the above before the age of fifteen is the cardinal manifestation of mental illness that we will call *Early Antisocial History*. (Truancy means missing at least 5 days of school per year for at least two years, not including the last year of school; expulsion of suspension from school must be for misbehavior; delinquency means "arrested or referred to juvenile court because of behavior"; running away from home overnight must occur at least twice while living in the parental home of the parental surrogate; lying must be persistent; school grades are markedly below expectations in relation to the estimated or known IQ and low grades may have resulted in repeating a year of school; the violation of rules at home or at school, other than truancy, must be chronic and repeated.)

Relations with Authority

Social relatedness does not include only relationships that occur horizontally with persons on one's level such as peers and friends. Social relatedness also involves the ways a person behaves toward real of imagined authorities that could compel the individual to observe rules or laws.

For children and adolescents this includes parents and school personnel, and may include neighbors and persons who supervise recreational activities such as scout leaders, etc.

Adults too, may have impairment of social relatedness and of occupational/academic performance because of problems with authority, such as with bosses, foremen, teachers, or with rules and regulations.

A person may break rules and have problems with authority because of his intent to defy, or attempt to provoke the authority, and in situations where "the person knows what is expected of him" but defies the authority or breaks the rule because he doesn't care whether he hurts other people or feels that the rule should not have to apply to him. Such persons must be distinguished from patients who appear to be behaving in the same way but suffer from mental disorders that produce distinctive symptoms such as hallucinations that tell them to break rules.

Oppositional Behavior

Oppositional behavior is a pattern of disobedience, negativism, and provocative opposition to authority figures as shown by at least two of the following cardinal manifestations:

1. violation of minor rules
2. temper trantrums
3. agumentativeness
4. provocative behavior
5. stubborness

Passive-Aggressive Cardinal Manifestations

This is a different problem in relation to authority. This is an indirect resistence to demands for adequate performance in both social and occupational functioning, as contrasted with direct confrontation.

Resistence to authority is said to be "passive-aggressive" when it is expressed indirectly through at least two of the following:

1. procrastination
2. dawdling
3. stubborness
4. international inefficiency
5. "forgetfulness"

Patients who display these manifestations can include persons who always come late, always make promises that they fail to keep, and always seem to forget things that other people want them to remember. These passive-aggressive manifestations of resistence to authority need to be distinguished from other kinds that are more open and direct.

A mother who doesn't buy food that she needs to stock the house because she dawdles and puts things off as a persistent pattern of behavior, manifests a cardinal sign of mental disorder. But is is a different manifestation than a mother who cannot *in any way* assume the role of a responsible parent as we have described above under caring for dependents (see page 39).

These ways that an individual resists authority without directly challenging the authority through arguments or open defiance, if pervasive and long standing, could lead to a ineffectiveness in both social and occupational functioning. An example would be an individual who was not promoted to a higher paying job because he had been intentionally inefficient as part of a pattern of defying authority or not conforming to rules of the job.

Unwarranted Suspiciousness and Mistrust of People

As a way of relating to others, being suspicious and mistrustful of them without any reason may impair interpersonal relating and could effect performance in certain occupations. This kind of behavior toward others can involve a belief that a lover or spouse is unfaithful, and can lead in such cases to an inability to maintain a lasting relationship with particular sexual partners.

Behaving cautiously and guardedly when there is no reason, as though others meant to harm or in some way trick the patient, can impair social and occupational functioning. Questioning the loyalty of others when there is no reason can lead to similar difficulties.

Being over-concerned with other people's ulterior motives, finding reasons to be suspicious and mistrustful by taking things they say out of context or failing to give proper weight to medications that they do not intend to be disloyal and mean no harm to the patient are manifestation of mental disorder and can cause social and occupational difficulties.

A particular manifestation called *hypervigilance* which is a continual scanning of the environment for signs of threat is a symptom. Taking unnecessary precautions to safeguard one's self against harm, trickery, disloyalty, or infidelity in relations with others is a sign of mental disorder.

Some patients may tend to be easily slighted and quick to take offense, and their reactions may be way out of proportion to what is said or done. This too is a cardinal sign of mental illness.

The exaggeration of one's difficulties, for example "making mountains out of molehills" or "being defensive" are also a problem. "Defensive" people are ready to counterattack when any threat or slight is perceived by them. This is an important manifestation: The overreaction to minor events.

OTHER PROBLEMS IN RELATING TO PEOPLE

Coldness

Coldness, or aloofness, or lack of warmth, or inability to express warm and tender emotions is a cardinal manifestation of mental disorder. Here a person is perceived by others as cold, or distant, or aloof, and with an absence of warm and tender feelings. Other people may find it difficult to be close to such a person who seems to have difficulty being colse to them.

This manifestation of mental disorder sounds like another which is discussed below under intensity of emotional expression and may need to be distinguished from it (see page 101).

Another problem in social relating is seen in individuals who are truly indifferent to other people. Such a manifestation means that not only do they perhaps have few or no friends, or have no social involvements, but they basically don't care about having any, and they often ignore both criticism and praise and flattery, not responding to the solicitations and invitations of others who may attempt to have a social relationship with them.

Appearing cold and unemotional is a cardinal manifestation of mental illness.

A lack of a true sense of humor is another manifestation.

Persons who take pride in being objective, rational, and unemotional are displaying a symptom. Any person who has an absence of passive, soft, tender, and sentimental feelings has a cardinal manifestation of mental illness. A person with a restricted ability to express warm and tender emotions may appear unusually conventional, serious, formal and stingy.

A serious form of difficulty in social relating occurs in individuals who fail to make eye contact, while being aloof and cold. They do not establish an adequate rapport in face-to-face social interaction. An important cardinal manifestation of mental illness is failure to make adequate eye contact or failure to have adequate face-to-face rapport.

Manipulation of Others

This is a problem in social relatedness, involving a variety of manifestations, where other people seem to be manipulated for the patient's own purposes. The motive may lie in getting other people to feel admiration and appreciation for the patient or may lie in an attempt to obtain goods or money, whether by an openly hostile and aggressive act or by a subtle and clever fraud.

Some persons feel entitled to special favors by others without assuming reciprocal responsibilities, and may become surprised and angry that other people will not do as wanted. This is a manifestation of mental illness called *"Entitlement"*.

When others are manipulated, there is often a lack of empathy (a lack of ability to recognize how other people feel). An example of a lack of empathy is that of a husband, whose wife had just returned home from the hospital to convalesce after having a major operation, who became upset that she would not come and pick him up at a lodge meeting when he was having car trouble, having asked him to take a bus.

Demands Made on Others

Some individuals have an expectation that others will appreciate them as being special, unique, and very important, and become upset when they do not receive such special treatment. A manifestation of mental disorder is an incessant drawing of attention to one's self which can be through actions, through exaggerated expressions of friendliness and involvement (which might be perceived by others as shallow and empty), perhaps dressing in a dramatic and flamboyant way, while scanning the environment to determine whether the appropriate degree of attention and interest is being given.

Slights By Others

Having an overreaction to feeling that one is being slighted by others or to real slights and criticism is a cardinal manifestation of mental disorder. The individual's reaction may be intense embarrassment and humiliation, it may be rage, with irrational angry outbursts or tantrums, or it may be to react with a sense of inferiority or emptiness.

Some individuals suffer from what lay people always called shyness where they have a desire for affection and acceptance by others that causes them to be unwilling to enter into relationships with other people unless they are given unusually strong guarantees of uncritical acceptance.

There are circumstances in which people *are* rejected by others! For example, some women do not accept every proposal for marriage, and some employers do not accept every job applicant. Being hypersensitive to rejection is a manifestation of mental disorder, especially when individuals search the environment for signs that they are being put down by others, and interpret innocent remarks and actions as a sign that they are being ridiculed.

Apprehensive alertness to signs of rejection by others is another aspect of hypersensitivity to rejection.

Constant seeking of reassurance from others is another source of difficulty in social relationships and another sign of mental disorder.

Hypersensitivity to real or imagined criticism can result in nervousness, worrying, uneasiness, and inability to relax in social situations, sometimes to such a degree that this tension in itself interferes with interpersonal relations; the over-concern with being slighted or with being liked uncritically creates circumstances that make it difficult for the patient to relate to others, or make it awkward for other people to relate to the patient comfortably.

Clinging, Overvaluing and Devaluing - Instability

The intensive clinging and intense overvaluing and devaluing of people and their significance for the patient in their social relations, sometimes swinging back and forth between intense overvaluation and devaluation of the same person, is a cardinal manifestation of mental disorder.

Inability to tolerate being alone, with constant craving for relations with people, and frantic efforts to avoid being alone are other cardinal manifestations.

A feeling of emptiness and depression when alone is another symptom.

The kind of manifestations we are describing here focus on an instability in a patient's feelings towards others, so that relations with others may be unstable, being at times intense, and may also consistently involve using others for one's own ends, such as to avoid being alone and having to feel unpleasant feelings.

In such cases the patient may call upon a particular person, but it is not that particular person who is wanted. Any person would do, who would help the patient alleviate their unpleasant and unsettled feelings while they are alone. This is, therefore, using another person for one's own purposes, where real intimacy with them, and real caring for another person, as a unique individual, with their own feelings and their own life to live, is not possible for the patient.

Instability in interpersonal relations can involve sudden displays of emotion such as irritability and anger, so that relations with others are difficult because of the patient's unpredictable mood.

Specific problems in relating to others that have not yet been mentioned include cardinal manifestations of mental illness that are equally important. A patient who refuses to talk to anyone in his or her environment will have impaired adaptive functioning.

So also will individuals who suffer from some sensory impairment, such as deafness, or some physical handicap, such as paraplegia, where social relating and attempts to relate to others may not only be impaired by the handicap but may be complicated by the patient's reactions to it. Difficulties in social and occupational functioning in such individuals need to be carefully examined to determine what role is played by the physical problem and what role is played by a manifestation of the mental disorder.

UNCOMPLICATED BEREAVEMENT

Individuals who are undergoing uncomplicated bereavement, the normal reaction to the loss of a loved one, may for a time lose interest in their usual activities, lose interest in associations with friends, and be unable to perform effectively at their job or at school. Such problems are not, when they are due to uncomplicated bereavement, the manifestation of a mental disorder.

Catastrophic Stress

Some individuals have been exposed to stresses so far beyond what is in the experience of most normal people that they suffer reactions that can involve a disengagement from the environment, including social relations and activities that used to give them pleasure. This is a major manifestation of a mental disorder in DSM-III.

Individuals who suffer from real damage to the brain, from whatever cause, may have a declining ability or deficiency in comprehending what is said, or observing social norms, and who show poor judgment in social situations (urinating in public). Elderly people who suffer from what laymen call "senility" may have impaired social relations, and be impaired in other areas of adaptive functioning.

CHILDREN

Children are impaired in adaptive functioning when at any period of their development they cannot behave in an age-appropriate fashion for any sustained period of time. For example, a seven-year-old child who needed to be taken to the toilet and wiped whenever he or she had a bowel movement would be said to have an impairment in adaptive functioning. *Any child who is not at all bowel trained after the age of four or any child who has frequent episodes of wetting his or her pants or wetting the bed after the age of five has a cardinal manifestation of mental disorder.*

In summary, we wish to concentrate on the quantity of social relationships: whether there are no companions, or only one or two, and why;
and to look at the quality of social relations including: difficulty in getting
along with others owing to suspiciousness and mistrust, indifference to
others, fear of rejection with humiliation and embarrassment, the selfish
using of other people, the disregard for the rights of others, the problems
in relation to authority, acts of violence committed against others, and
situations where the individual wishes to assume an unreasonable and
self-indulgent relationship such as wanting to be dependent on another
person and have that person take all responsibility for the patients' life and
make all decisions for the patient.

We have looked at occupational and academic functioning and have
discussed various problems in the use of leisure time and self-care.

SUBSTANCE USE AND ABUSE IN PERSONS WITH
IMPAIRMENT IN ADAPTIVE FUNCTIONING

Difficulty in social relationships also includes individuals who have social
impairment because they are frequently intoxicated with a drug that
prevents them, because of its effect, from being accepted in the
opportunities that are present for social contacts.

On the other hand, individuals with problems in relation to people are
among those individuals who may turn to the use of drugs and alcohol,
and may exhibit maladaptive behavior in association with the use of these
substances. Such individuals may have further problems in social relating
because of the maladaptive behavior (needing to mug other people in order
to obtain money, or disrupting the relations within the family because of
dependent and maladaptive behavior associated with a drug like alcohol).

Substance use and abuse in patients with problems in adaptive functioning
should be looked for, and DSM-III makes no assumption as to what is the
cause and what is the effect in patients where both problems are found.
The careful examiner who discovers that a patient is a substance abuser
looks further for the manifestations of mental disorder that could have
created problems in adaptive functioning. When individuals are present
with problems of adaptive functioning let us not forget that such patients
may, in their distress, turn to the use of a drug for relief.

SELF-STUDY QUESTIONS, CHAPTER I

1. Define adaptive functioning.

2. What are four areas of adaptive functioning?

3. Which area of adaptive functioning do you think is the most important?

Answer: Social relatedness. When rating individuals on Axis V for highest level of adaptive functioning in the previous year, the highest level of social relatedness in the previous year has the greatest significance in predicting outcome for a person who suffers from a mental disorder.

4. What are the two kinds of violation of the rights of others?

Answer: Aggressive and non-aggressive.

5. What is the difference between the aggressive and the non-aggressive types?

Answer: The aggressive type involves activities where acts of aggression are committed directly against people such as committing robberies where people are directly confronted during the act of the crime.

6. What is important about the way an individual handles money?

Answer: It contains many issues related to how individuals feel about themselves and the world, and may yield additional information about certain kinds of reckless involvement or certain kinds of not caring about their future, and can show some of the ways that the patients might hurt other people or fail to take care of people who depend on them.

7. What would a person be like who appeared to others as "cold?"

8. What are some of the manifestations of mental disorder involving social relating where a person would use others for their own purposes?

9. Cite two important manifestations of mental disorder where persons are used for the patient's own ends.

Answer: Others may be defrauded for the purpose of obtaining goods or money, or may be needed to allay chronic concerns about loneliness, or they may be needed to provide the patient with feelings that he is admired and is special, etc.

10. What is responsible child-care? What are some of the signs in the care of a particular child, that show that their parent is not performing as caretaker of a dependent person?

11. What are the things involved in the early manifestations of antisocial behavior (incidents and acts committed before age fifteen)?

12. What is the antisocial work manifestation?

13. What is entitlement?

14. How could poor social relating affect occupational performance? Give an example.

15. What are oppositional manifestations of mental disorder?

16. What are passive-aggressive manifestations? Give an example.

Answer: Always coming late, procrastinating, etc.

17. A cardinal manifestation of mental disorder is swinging back and forth between overvaluation of people, and _____ .

    Answer: devaluation.

18. This is an example of what?

    Answer: Instability or unpredictability in social relationships.

19. A patient who threatens a friend or close family member saying "if you don't do what I want, I'm going to kill myself" is attempting to do what?

    Answer: Manipulate the other person.

    Note: Note that the manipulation of others can include suicidal threats, and even what are called *suicidal gestures:* where the person does not really intend to kill himself, but really wants to manipulate or change the way another person feels.

chapter 2

History
of Life Stress

In the history of a patient (the history is the general term used in psychiatry and medicine for what is true about the patient or what we know about the patient in the past), the occurrence of the kinds of psychosocial stressors that were mentioned in our previous discussion on how to use Axis IV of the multiaxial system (see page 17) are cardinal manifestations of mental disorder. That is, the occurrence of a significant life stress, especially a stress that has a relationship to the patient's current problem, is a piece of data that, while not in itself indicating the presence of a mental disorder, may nevertheless be a piece of data that is required in one of the DSM-III clusters that define a particular mental disorder. Such a history of recent stress would need to be present in the patient's history in order to correctly use some of the diagnoses in DSM-III.

When there are life stresses that are related to the onset or worsening of a physical illness, when there are extraordinary psychosocial stressors that lie far beyond what would occur in the life experience of most normal people, and when there are stresses such as death, divorce, loss of a job, expulsion from school, or arrest, that occurred *within three months* of the onset of the patient's current episode of illness, our knowledge of that stress is a cardinal manifestation of mental disorder and it may be necessary to making the diagnosis of certain DSM-III disorders.

The absence of any history of significant stress is likewise an important piece of information and is also a piece of data that taken together with the other cardinal manifestations of mental disorder in a particular patient, may help to exclude specific DSM-III diagnoses from being applied to the particular patient.

chapter 3

Alertness, Attention, Orientation, and Memory

These four terms: alertness, attention, orientation, and memory, will be covered together because cardinal manifestations of mental disorder involving one, can usually be assessed correctly, only by knowing about the other three.

There are clusters of symptoms under this grouping that are particularly important, and which we will name as we describe them.

ALERTNESS AND ATTENTION

A cardinal manifestation of mental disorder is a disturbance in a patient's alertness and level of consciousness. Here we are concerned with the patient's level of awareness of what is going on around him. The patient's awareness of what is going on around him can be related to his capacity to focus his attention, hold his attention on stimuli in the environment, and to shift his attention and then focus it and sustain it again.

DISTURBANCES OF ATTENTION

Inattention in Children

Some children have persistent problems in paying attention. Such children often fail to finish what they start, they often don't seem to listen, they may be easily distracted and have difficulty concentrating on school work or other tasks requiring sustained attention, and they may have difficulty sticking to a play activity. When at least three of the above are present, we say that a person has a cardinal manifestation of *inattention*.

Distractability means that patients cannot hold his or her attention on one thing in a sustained way, being unable to exclude other stimuli in the environment from the task at hand.

Attention is therefore closely related to *concentration,* which is sustained attention on a particular task or problem.

Decreased attention and decreased concentration is a cardinal manifestation of mental disorder.

Likewise, unusually sharpened and heightened concentration is another sign of mental disorder. At times *hyperattentiveness* (increased attentiveness) can result in distractability. Here patients are so attentive to every detail in the environment that they move rapidly from one thing to another, and have difficulty in concentrating.

Individuals who show *hypervigilance and scanning of the environment* for such things as signs that they are being rejected by others, or for signs that other people mean them harm or are going to trick them, may also have difficulty paying attention to a particular task.

Attention that focuses excessively on minute details and trivia to the exclusion of the larger context is also a defect in attention, and is a cardinal manifestation of mental disorder.

Alertness can be described on a spectrum going from a state of being alert and fully conscious, down through levels of diminished alertness and clouded consciousness that are described by terms such as stupor, obtundation, semi-comatose, and coma.

A patient suffers from "clouding of consciousness" when he is not fully alert while not yet being semi-comatose.

Clouding of consciousness is a cardinal manifestation of mental disorder.

ORIENTATION

Orientation is the patient's capacity to know where he is in time and place and to know who the people are that he is dealing with.

Disorientation refers to an impairment in orientation.

Disorientation to person means that the person does not know who he is dealing with, thus he might not be aware or understand that a doctor asking him questions was really a doctor.

Disorientation to place means that the patient does not know where he is. Thus a patient in a hospital who exhibited disorientation to place would not know that he was in a hospital and might either seem confused when asked where he was or might say that he was at home.

Disorientation to time means that the patient doesn't know what day it is, and that he might not even know what month or year it was. Some patients severely disoriented for time do not even know what season of the year it is.

Patients who are severely *disoriented for place* might not know what town they are in.

Disorientation is a cardinal manifestation of mental illness.

Each of the three kinds of disorientation is a cardinal manifestation of mental illness.

MEMORY DISTURBANCE

There are three kinds of memory: *immediate recall, short-term* or *recent memory,* and *long-term* or *remote memory.*

The three kinds of memory are partially defined by ways that they are tested.

Immediate recall

Immediate recall is an ultra-short term memory that can sometimes persist even when short-term memory is impaired. It is tested by giving the patient a small amount of data to be repeated back immediately.

Immediate recall could be tested by saying to a patient, "Here are three objects I want you to remember: a red ball, a chocolate cookie, and a white cloud. Say those back to me now." When the patient says them back to the examiner without making a mistake, the patient is displaying immediate recall.

A more precise way of testing immediate recall is to say: "I'm going to say some numbers to you, and I want you to say them back to me. So if I say 1, 2, 3, then you say 1, 2, 3. Let's try it now." Then the examiner would say a string of digits to the patient, and ask the patient to repeat the string back to him.

Most adults tested in this way should be able to repeat back to an examiner a string of numbers containing seven digits. A seven digit number is a phone number. Normal functioning in today's world requires that a person be able to repeat back immediately a phone number that is told to them.

Immediate recall can be further tested by giving a patient a string of digits and asking him to repeat the string backwards.

Most six-year-old children can repeat back to an examiner a six digit number going forward and can repeat a three digit number backwards. It could therefore be said that any adult patient who cannot perform that well has immediate recall that functions below that of a six-year-old child.

Recent Memory

Recent memory is a memory faculty that can hold information considerably longer than the faculty of immediate recall. Recent memory, when intact, allows a patient to remember small pieces of information that were given to him a few minutes ago. Some examiners adopt the convention that if small bits of information cannot be recalled after five minutes, then short-term memory is impaired.

Short-term memory can be tested by saying to the patient (as above) "Let me give you some things I want you to remember, a red ball, a chocolate cookie, and a white cloud. I'm going to ask you about them in a little while." Five minutes later the examiner would ask the patient to repeat these items back to him. If a patient failed this test, and gave an answer like, "A red something, I don't know what it is, and a chocolate chip cookie," short-term memory would be said to be impaired.

Long-term Memory

Long-term memory is the capacity to recall information that was known in the past, and which might be tested by asking the patient about events of the previous day. A patient in the hospital could be asked: "What did you have for supper last night?" Long-term memory also refers to the ability to recall events from childhood or adolescence.

Impairment of any one of the three kinds of memory is a cardinal manifestation of mental disorder. Furthermore some mental disorders of DSM-III involve memory impairment of a characteristic kind. For example, memory impairment resulting from prolonged and excessive use of certain drugs can impair short-term memory and leave immediate recall intact. This is characteristic of the DSM-III disorder called *alcohol amnestic disorder.*

Patients who intoxicate themselves with certain substances can experience "blackouts" with inability to recall events that occurred during the period of intoxication. This is an impairment in long-term memory.

Registration versus Recollection

The reader should note that memory, as we have been discussing it, is a combination of two mental capacities: the capacity to register or record events in the memory, and the capacity to recall events or data that was previously recorded. The tests for immediate recall and for short-term memory, and even the questions put to a patient about what the person had for dinner the previous night, assume that this information was recorded in the person's memory. Obviously if there is something that interferes with the recording of information while the examiner asks his questions, such as an inability of the patient to focus his attention on what the examiner is saying, then the patient will not be able, five minutes later, to tell the examiner what the information was that the patient is expected to remember.

In the same way, if the patient last night did not record in his memory what he had for dinner, he will be unable to tell the examiner today what was on the menu.

Similarly, a disoriented patient who has hospital personnel that come in and out of his room and inform him where he is and what day it is, may seem disoriented to an examiner if the patient has not recorded the information so generously supplied by the hospital personnel.

Although we can theoretically distinguish between the four different faculties of: level of alertness, attention, orientation, and memory, the situation with a real patient who suffers from clouding of consciousness may be one where it is difficult to determine whether one of the facilities has survived intact and is simply untestable because the other three are not working properly.

Some patients have a clear consciousness and are fully alert and can be shown by appropriate testing to suffer from one or another impairment of memory or even of orientation.

Some patients seem fully alert but their capacity to sustain their attention fluctuates. This too can be tested by a careful examination.

Amnesia

Amnesia is a partial or complete inability to recall events in the past. It relates specifically in DSM-III to effect on long-term or remote memory. Amnesia is of four kinds.

Localized or circumscribed amnesia is an inability to recall all of the events occurring during a circumscribed period of time. The period of time is usually the first hours following an experience that is deeply disturbing. The author once experienced this kind of amnesia himself, having rescued a patient from a hospital fire and being unable to recall the events of the rescue until several days later.

The second kind, called *selective amnesia,* is an ability to recall only some of the events that occurred during a circumscribed period of time. If the author had suffered from selective amnesia, he would have been immediatly able to recall some of the events of the rescue, but not others.

The third kind of amnesia is called *generalized amnesia,* in which the patient is unable to recall any of the events of his entire life.

The fourth kind of amensia, *continuous amnesia,* is one where the patient has lost his entire memory from some particular point in the past up to the present moment.

This last kind of amnesia where the individual "loses" his or her memory from some point in the past up to and including the present moment is called *anterograde amnesia.*

Memory loss of the kind that covers the period of time for some period prior to an event is called *retrograde amnesia.* When a person is hit on the head and suffers post-concussion amnesia, the disturbance in memory, although circumscribed, usually encompasses a period of time before the blow to the head and not afterward.

Psychogenic amnesia is almost always anterograde, and covers a period of time following an upsetting event or serious incident.

chapter 4

Organic Versus
Functional Disease

We now make an important distinction between organic versus functional disease. This distinction can be confusing and DSM-III does not really devote much space to explaining it. To understand the important of the cardinal manifestations of mental disorder that we have discussed in clouding of consciousness, disturbance of attention, disorientation, and disturbance of memory, the reader must understand the distinction between organic and functional disease.

All mental disorders are divided into two classes: organic mental disorders and functional mental disorders.

Organic mental disorders are those with a known cause, related either to structural damage or operational malfunction of the brain. The kind of disease process that falls under this heading is a condition like that seen in some elderly patients whose mental disturbances are related to structural changes in the brain.

Organic mental disorders also include all of the mental disorders that have a demonstrable metabolic disturbance in the body as their cause. Examples are the emotional and behavioral changes associated with chronic renal disease, hyperthyroidism, and so on. Disorders of emotion, thought, and behavior that result from intoxication with a drug or from withdrawal from a drug, or that result from the effect of continual excessive use of a substance are also considered to fall into the category of organic mental disorders.

The functional mental disorders contain, as a category, all of the mental disorders for which there is not yet a well established cause.

The functional category contains all of the mental disorders where we cannot at this time reliably point to either structural damage in the brain, or to metabolic or biochemical disturbance of the brain, as the cause of the condition.

The distinction between organic versus functional disorders in DSM-III should not be interpreted as implying that any of the group of functional disorders is believed to arise without some basis in the brain or in brain functioning.

What causes the functional mental disorders? Some of the mental disorders that are considered to be functional, when we wonder what basis in brain functioning they might have, are probably better conceptualized as having their roots on another level of brain function than the level that is responsible for organic mental disorders.

A crude way to explain this idea is to think of a computer that is made out of a lot of complex electronic parts, and which also does what it does because it has a particular program that has been given to it.

If the computer doesn't do what it is supposed to do, the reason is because either something is the matter with the electronics or because something isn't right with the program or both.

The kind of malfunction that is caused by improper programming is the kind that might be thought of as analogous to what is thought to be the matter in some theories about the origin of disorders of the personality (coded on Axis II).

Programming problems might also be thought of as analogous to the kind of malformation that underlies the factitious disorders, where persons throughout most of their life will fake the signs of either mental or physical illness for no other purpose than to assume the role of being a patient in a hospital, having no more motive than that, and having little insight or understanding of their behavior.

This kind of malfunction, namely, something the matter with the program, is to be constrasted with the kind of malfunction due to real physical damage to the electronic structure of a computer machine. Real physical damage to the electronic structure of a computer is the kind of damage that in this crude and oversimplified analogy corrosponds to the group of disorders that we called the "organic type".

The distinction between organic and functional disorders often runs into trouble in cases such as mild mental retardation, where the cause of the problem in a particular child may be a neglectful mother who did not provide the child with sufficient environmental stimulation and sufficient affection. Are these problems more on the side of bad programming? How are they to be completely separated from the effects on a child's growth of the poor diet given to the child by such a neglectful mother? Poor diet during the early phases of a child's growth can be responsible for certain kinds of subtle structural or biochemical damage from malnourishment of the nervous system during this crucial period.

The important point is that we understand what is meant by the distinction between organic versus functional disorder, because *in the use of DSM-III the question about whether a patient has an organic mental disorder is the most important!*

It is a question that should always be asked, and should always be carefully answered by giving consideration to what is actually known about the patient, and the state of the patient's physical health.

Theraputic techniques such as psychotherapy, crisis intervention, family therapy, and behavior modification, that can be well suited to the management of some of the functional mental disorders, are of little or no value in dealing effectively with organic mental disorders that have a specific cause such as hyperthyroidism or normal pressure hydrocephalus.

The presence of an organic mental disorder (a mental disorder arising from structural damage in the brain) does not exclude the possibility that there are in addition other mental disorders present in the same patient that would be listed in the functional category. A patient can have both an organic mental disorder and a functional mental disorder at the same time. A patient with a mild organic mental disorder who reacts to a major stressful life event by becoming mildly to moderately depressed in the face of the stress (e.g. being placed in a nursing home and separated from the family with whom he lived for many years) is an example.

The four cardinal manifestations of mental disorder that we have discussed in this section, (disturbance of attention, alertness, orientation, and memory), when all of them occur together, point in the direction of an organic rather than a functional disorder.

Even when only one of them is present to a significant degree, the presumption that an organic mental disorder is present is often made until it can be shown otherwise.

chapter 5

Intellectual
Abilities

Intelligence has always been a very difficult thing to define.

One way to define intelligence is the score one receives on an IQ test.

Another way to define intelligence would be: the capacity to handle a new situation by finding a new response that represents an adaptation. This is an ability that might be tested by giving a person problems to solve.

ABSTRACT THINKING

In DSM-III the emphasis is on *"abstract thinking"* which is a capacity to understand and handle abstract ideas and words.

It could be tested by giving a patient a proverb to explain, such as "don't cry over spilled milk". An example of how this proverb might be poorly explained by a patient who would be judged to have an impairment of intellectual ability would be an answer like, "When the milk is on the floor, that's the end of it. There is no reason to cry over it." Such an answer does not go beyond the concrete aspects of the situation presented. Which is: "don't cry over milk on the floor", to the abstraction which would be the application of a principle as shown by a patient without such an impairment who said: "When something bad happens, don't be upset about it; forget about it." A further example of abstraction from the same proverb might be: "Don't dwell on past misfortunes."

Impairment of abstract thinking as tested by interpretation of proverbs is a cardinal manifestation of mental illness.

Abstract thinking can also be tested by asking a patient the meaning of words, or asking a patient about the similarity or difference between the meanings of two words.

To test abstract thinking in relation to similarities, the examiner might ask, "How are an apple and an orange the same?" An answer that was concrete, but nevertheless true, would be, "You can eat them both," or "They both have seeds." Both of these answers miss the main point, which would be apparent in the abstraction, namely: apples and oranges are both fruit. Another kind of answer that would reflect difficulty with abstract thinking would be seen in the case of a patient who stubbornly maintained that an apple and an orange were different, and that there was nothing the same about them. Here the impairment in abstract thinking would be inferred from the patient's apparent inability to go beyond the concrete differences in the appearances of the two fruits to the abstraction that they both belonged to the same class of thing.

Significant impairment on this kind of testing involving the meanings of words is also a cardinal manifestation of mental disorder.

Obviously a patient's background, and social and economic level in society, needs to be appreciated as part of the context in which this kind of testing and its interpretation are to be done.

LOW IQ

A low score on an IQ test, which means a score of 70 or below on an individually administered IQ test, is also a major manifestation of mental disorder.

chapter 6

Judgment

This is a difficult concept to define. It is used in DSM-III. Judgment can be related to the capacity to act reasonably and wisely in social relations and occupational and self-care functions.

A history of poor judgment in social relations might include inappropriate sexual advances, starting an argument with a policeman and threatening him with a knife when the individual had no intention of using it and was "just trying to scare him", or allowing a small child to play with a power tool.

Poor judgement is relation to one's own safety and welfare, such as smoking a cigarette near an open container of gasoline (assuming the individual was aware that such behavior constituted a clear and present danger) or piling a lot of items on a stove and turning a burner on with the intention of boiling water and then going out to shop for groceries, is a serious sign.

Judgment, the capacity to act wisely and circumspectly in life situations, when impaired, is a cardinal manifestation of mental disorder.

SELF-STUDY QUESTIONS, CHAPTERS 2–6

1. What is meant by "clouding of consciousness"?

2. What is meant by disorientation of time? to place? to person? Give examples of each.

3. How would you test for immediate recall? for short-term memory? for long-term or remote memory? To your questions, what would be a good answer? what would be a poor answer?

4. Explain how a patient whose attention was disturbed might appear to have a problem with memory?

5. Explain the difference between organic mental disorder and functional mental disorder.

   Answer: Organic mental disorders have a known physical cause. Functional illness does not as yet have a known physical cause.

6. When DSM-III calls a disease a functional mental disorder, does that imply that there is no basis for the disease in what goes on in the brain?

   Answer: Absolutely not.

CASE STUDY WITH QUESTIONS

A sixty seven-year-old alcoholic who was being treated at a municipal hospital in New York City called to his doctor from his bed, shouting, "Waiter, waiter, would you please bring me an order of herring?" The doctor asked the patient where he was and the patient replied, "I'm in a hotel on the Volga River and I'd like to try some of your herring." The patient did not know what day, what month, or what year it was.

1. What cardinal sign of mental disorder is being demonstrated by this patient?

   Answer: Disorientation.

2. We know that the patient did not know what day, month or year it was. This means he was disoriented for _____.

   Answer: Time.

3. Does he show evidence for any other kinds of disorientation? If so what are they? How do you know?

   Answer: The patient was *disoriented for place* because he did not realize that he was in a hospital, he thought that he was in a hotel. Furthermore, he thought he was on the Volga River, and did not seem to be aware that he was in New York City.

   The patient was also *disoriented for person* believing that the doctor taking care of him was actually a waiter running a room service.

4. If the doctor told the patient where he was and what day it was, and the patient could not remember it five minutes later, that would be a disturbance of what?

   Answer: Short-term memory (assuming that the patient was able to pay attention to what the doctor said to him).

5. Would the patient still be disoriented?

   Answer: Yes, since he would not be able to recall what the doctor said to him, he would still not know where he was and what day it was.

6. If a patient was asked: "How are a pair of scissors and a saw the same?", and he said: "they are both tools," what could you make out of that answer?

   Answer: That he was able to abstract or think abstractly. (Performance on only one proverb may not indicate a lot. It suggests that further testing may be necessary.)

7. A patient who was told a phone number, and could not immediately recite it back to the examiner, would show evidence of what?

   Answer: Impairment in immediate recall, one of the disturbances of memory.

8. What IQ score is a major manifestation of mental disorder?

   Answer: 70 or below on an individually administered IQ test.

chapter 7

Disturbances
of Sensory Perception

Here we discuss the cardinal manifestations of mental disorder that include hallucinations, illusions, distortions of sensory experience, and certain misinterpretations of sensory perceptions.

HALLUCINATION

An *hallucination* is a false sensory perception that has no basis in any real, external stimulation of a sense organ.

However, the hallucination is experienced as though what the person perceived had really taken place. Hallucinations are categorized by the sense organ through which they are allegedly perceived: Visual hallucinations consist of sights, while auditory hallucinations consist of things that are heard, and so on.

ILLUSION

Illusions are false sensory perceptions that do have some real stimulation of a sense organ from the external environment as their basis. The difference between a hallucination and an illusion lies in whether the sense organ involved received any stimulation from the environment related to what was allegedly perceived.

For example, a person who stood talking to someone when there was no one there, might be having an hallucination, or might be having an illusion. If there was really nothing there in the place where the individual appeared to be addressing a person, and he explained to you that someone was standing there, talking to him, this would be an example of an hallucination. Furthermore, it would be an example of a visual hallucination (because he believed that he saw someone), and also an example of an auditory hallucination since he heard and talked to the imaginary person.

A patient who is heavily intoxicated with alcohol who said "hello" to a lamppost, who when asked about it, said that he greeted someone, would be said to have had an illusion. He had a false sensory experience (seeing a person) but it had a basis in the stimulation of the sensory organ involved (his eye was stimulated by the presence of the lamppost).

We need to distinguish between illusions—misinterpretations of real sensory experiences—and hallucinations—apparent perception when there is nothing corresponding to it in external reality, not even a neutral stimulus.

Both hallucinations and illusions are cardinal manifestations of mental disorder.

Some patients can experience hallucinations extremely vividly. Some patients who experience hallucinations may take action because of them. Hallucinations are a particularly serious manifestation of mental disorder.

"UNUSUAL SENSORY EXPERIENCES"

There are some unusual kinds of feelings that do not fit into the catagories of illusions or hallucinations, such as sensing the presence of a force or a person not actually present. An example would be a person who described feeling the presence of a dead relative in the room.

Such an experience is not a hallucination because no one was *actually* seen, heard, or felt, and so no false sensory experience was involved. Yet the story given by such a patient may sound suspiciously as though a hallucination may have taken place. It is important to distinguish hallucinations and illusions from such unusual sensations.

VISUAL HALLUCINATIONS

Visual hallucinations are sights or visions. The person may see formed images as in the case of a patient who saw a deceased relative who appeared in front of him.

Visual hallucinations may be unformed images that consist of balls of fire, lights, or flashes of color.

AUDITORY HALLUCINATIONS

Auditory hallucinations are those involving sounds. What is heard can be noises, music, or can be voices speaking words.

When the patient hears voices, they may be perceived as coming from the external environment, or they may be perceived as coming from inside of his own head. (Some investigators have tried to limit the concept of auditory hallucinations only to voices perceived as coming from an externally located source; however, DSM-III expresses the opinion that this distinction is not usuful in general because its clinical significance has not yet been completely established.)

A patient who hears voices may hear the voice of a man, women, or child. The voice may be familiar or unfamiliar.

The patient may hear several voices talking at the same time, either to him directly, or carrying on a conversation that he can overhear, or the patient may hear a single voice that calls him names or insults him.

When a patient has an auditory hallucination of a voice that gives him instructions or commands, that kind of hallucination is called a *command hallucination*. Command hallucinations can concern a variety of topics, including instructions to the patient that he should perform acts of violence, command him to perform sexual acts, or even commit suicide.

Patients who hear voices that carry out a running stream of talk may become terrified or they may become very angry. Some patients are not troubled at all about hearing voices when the voices are the result of long standing mental disorder, and they may treat them as old friends.

OLFACTORY HALLUCINATION

This is an hallucination involving the sense of smell. A patient may smell something unpleasant, such as garlic, or may smell something burning.

GUSTATORY HALLUCINATION

These are hallucinations of taste. The tastes that are falsely perceived are usually unpleasant.

TACTILE HALLUCINATION

Tactile hallucinations involve the sense of touch or the sensation of feeling something under the skin or on the skin.

SOMATIC HALLUCINATION

Somatic hallucinations involve a sensory perception localized within the body such as the feeling of electric shocks running up and down one's body.

Phantom Limbs

The phantom limb is the most common somatic hallucination that results from a physical disorder. It needs to be distinguished from the other kinds of somatic hallucinations we have discussed.

In this case the patient has had a limb amputated from which he cannot now receive any sensations. The phantom limb is the sensation that he still has a limb, and he may report painful and unpleasant sensations in the space where a limb used to be.

Phantom limbs occur in about ninety five percent of all amputations that are done after the patient is six years old.

The phantom limb may not correspond to the previous perception of the limb. It may be shorter or it may consist only of the furthest portion so that a patient who has lost an entire arm might have a phantom sensation of only a hand, and the hand may seem to arise directly from the shoulder.

Some patients have very painful sensations that seem to them to arise from the phantom limb. These may be very difficult to manage. This is not a cardinal symptom of mental disorder.

STRANGE INTERPRETATIONS OF HALLUCINATIONS

We need to distinguish between the hallucination, which is the false sensory experience, and the fantastic and strange interpretation of these experiences.

For example, to have the hallucination of an unpleasant smell, like the smell of garlic, and report it, needs to be distinguished from cases that would involve the bizarre interpretation of an unpleasant smell. One patient complained before entering the doctors office, that he smelled a dead body rotting under the floor of the waiting room.

Another patient claimed that he felt as though someone were running their hands up and down his guts. Such a report is more than just a somatic hallucination, it is a bizarre and fantastic interpretation of a sensation occurring within the body.

Some patients experience tactile hallucinations that consist of sensations as though pins and needles were being stuck into their bodies. To report such tactile hallucinations is one thing, it is another for a person to report that he could feel an invisible vampire sticking pins into him in order to withdraw blood.

All hallucinations of whatever kind are cardinal manifestations of mental disorder.

CHARACTERISTIC HALLUCINATIONS OF SCHIZOPHRENIA

Certain auditory hallucinations are characteristic of schizophrenia.

Auditory hallucinations where a voice carries on a running commentary about the individual, his behavior, and thoughts, or where two or more voices talk to one another, is particularly characteristic.

Auditory hallucinations on more than one occasion consisting of more than one or two words at a time, where the content of the hallucination has no apparent relation to feelings of depression or of elation (elevated mood which will be discussed below under emotion), are also characteristic.

Auditory hallucinations are the modality of hallucination that is characteristic of schizophrenia, particularly voices that speak directly to the patient, carry on a continual commentary on the patient's thoughts or behavior, or that issue commands to the patient that he obeys.

Other kinds of hallucination can occur in schizophrenia, such as olfactory, gustatory, and visual hallucinations, but usually auditory hallucinations occur as well.

CHARACTERISTIC HALLUCINATIONS OF ORGANIC MENTAL DISORDER

When a patient experiences olfactory, gustatory, visual or tactile hallucinations without any experience of auditory hallucinations, this should always raise the possibility of organic mental disorder (a disorder due to a physical illness). This possibility should be carefully considered and all evidence related to the patient carefully sifted.

A hallucination is a cardinal manifestation of mental disorder; however, hallucinations by themselves do not point to any particular mental disorder. Even the hallucinations that are extremely characteristic of schizophrenia do not point to that particular disorder taken by themselves, but require that other manifestations of mental disorder be present.

Illusions are of particular concern when they are recurrent. Isolated illusions can occur as transitory experiences in patients with no mental disorder when they are extremely tired, and when they are under the influence of certain drugs.

SELF-STUDY QUESTIONS, CHAPTER 7

1. What is a hallucination?

2. How is it different from an illusion?

3. What is a command hallucination?

4. What are the various kinds of hallucinations? (Hint: you name them by the organ that has the false sensory experience.)

5. Which modality of hallucination is most characteristic of schizophrenia?

6. An auditory hallucination that is most characteristic of schizophrenia would consist of which one of the following:
   (a) noises
   (b) the sound of rushing water
   (c) human voices

7. An elderly man leaving his apartment building to go out on a walk, who was observed by the doorman to say "hello" to a potted plam in the lobby, is an example of what? Why?

   Answer: An illusion, because there was a real stimulus in the environment to his false sensory perception of a person, namely the potted palm.

8. A very tired automobile driver slowed his car down on the freeway at night to avoid hitting a person walking along the road. As he approached he saw that what he had thought was a person was actually a highway sign.
   This person had (a) an hallucination
                    (b) an illusion
   Pick the right answer. Explain your answer.

   Answer: An illusion.

9. A man who had several teeth extracted in a dentist's office while under the influence of a general anesthetic and who was given medication for pain before leaving the dentist's office, drove home in the rain. He suddenly became alarmed when it seemed to him that he vividly heard the sound of many geese quacking and honking. He realized that the sound he heard was actually the sound his tires made on the wet road surface.
   This patient had (a) an hallucination or
                    (b) an illusion?
   Explain why.

10. A patient complained that he could feel the hands of the Angel of Death around his neck. If we grant that this patient had an hallucination, what kind of hallucination is it? What do you think about the patient's interpretation of the hallucination of a bodily sensation?

    Answer: The patient had a somatic hallucination if he experienced the sensation inside his neck.
        If he experienced something touching his skin or moving on his skin, it was a tactile hallucination. His interpretation of the hallucination is bizarre.

11. What kinds of hallucinations are characteristic of the class of organic mental disorders?

    Answer: Any kind other than auditory.

12. If a patient tells you that he or she has experienced the smell of burning rope when there was no basis for this sensory experience in an environmental stimulation, is this an hallucination or an illusion? What kind of hallucination or illusion is it? What is the first thing you should think of?

Answer: It is an hallucination because there was no external stimulation to the nose. It is an olfactory hallucination because it was an hallucination of smell, and the first thing that you should think of is that the patient may have an organic mental disorder.

chapter 8

Speech

Problems with speech are major manifestations of mental illness, and certain problems with speech may be signs of physical disease.

The cardinal manifestations of mental disorder are concerned with the quantity of speech, whether there is too much *(loquacity)* or too little *(impoverishment)*. We are concerned with the *rate of speech,* whether it is spoken expremely slowly. We are concerned with the lengths of the pauses between words and sentences. We are concerned with the pronunciation of words, whether the words are distinctly pronounced or whether they are slurred and hard to understand. We are concerned with the tones of voice that predominate in the speech that signal distinctive emotions, and with the effectiveness of speech as a method of communicating (which concerns the form of the speech and the way ideas are expressed).

DEVELOPMENT OF SPEECH PROBLEMS IN CHILDREN

The development of speech in children can be abnormal. By about the age of two, most children can speak in two word utterances. By the age of three, most children can speak well enough to tell a simple story. Children who have not acquired that degree of facility in spoken language by the age of three may have an impairment.

Delayed language development needs to be distinguished from the cardinal sign of mental illness where a child who had previously learned to speak now refuses, and may now communicate only by gestures, by nodding or shaking his head, or in some cases by one word or one syllable utterances. Such children refuse to talk in almost all social situations, including at school, but have the ability to comprehend spoken language *and to speak.*

This is a cardinal sign of mental disorder and can occur in adults; it is called the manifestation of *elective mutism.*

LANGUAGE DISORDER IN CHILDREN

Children have other types of language disorder. There can be a failure to acquire any language at all. There can be acquired language that is difficult to understand, or difficult for the child to use, and there can be delayed acquiring of language (where language ability does develop, but it develops relatively late).

Children who acquire no language at all are unusual and in such cases it is almost always the result of severe neurological problems associated with profound mental retardation.

Language disabilities that are *acquired* after the child learns to speak and has some language ability are nearly always the result or neurological disease or injury to the brain.

Delayed language acquisition is the most common type of language disorder in children. It involves either the difficulty in expressing verbal language *(expressive type developmental language disorder),* or in comprehending spoken language without having any impairment of hearing *(receptive type developmental language disorder).*

Children who can understand spoken language, but cannot seem to speak and who have difficulty with articulation (producing the particular sounds of a language) can have a severely limited vocabulary. When such difficulty in acquisition of language is not due to profound mental retardation, to a hearing impairment, or to physical damage to the nervous system, it is a cardinal manifestation of mental disorder.

Some children acquire language but have peculiar speech patterns. *Echolalia* is a peculiar speech pattern where the child repeats back exactly what is said to him. He sounds like an echo. Some children have strange ways of saying things, called *pronominal reversal,* where the child uses the pronoun "you" when the pronoun "I" is what he intends. Some children may have a peculiar grammatical structure to their speech that is not what is expected for their level of development. Some children may have what is called *"metaphorical language"*, which means that they make statements where the usage of words is unique to them and whose meaning is not understood. Some children have abnormal speech melody and they may raise their voice in a question-like way at the end of a statement.

All of these disturbances in speech are cardinal manifestations of mental disorder.

Aphasia is a whole area of disturbance and disorder affecting the comprehension and production of language. Acquired expressive aphasia concerns the production of language, and can be a cause for a diminished quantity of speech. The patient may say little or nothing, or may be able to respond not with words, but only with unintelligible noises and grunts. Aphasia of other kinds (invariably the result of neurological damage or disease) can cause peculiar sounding speech. The patient may produce plenty of speech, but it may make no sense.

The production of a lot of speech that makes no sense is one of the cardinal signs of mental disorder. Therefore it needs to be distinguished from neurological problems that can produce a similar picture. This book will not explain how to make that distinction. But the question of whether the speech problem represents a physical disorder is a question that should always be asked.

Anomic aphasia can be a disturbance that relates specifically to the naming of things, leaving other aspects of speech undisturbed. This too is a neurological disorder. Certain kinds of aphasia and anomia (inability to name objects) can occur in organic mental disorder.

Being less talkative than usual, including a slowing down of speech, increased pauses between words and statements, and a lowering of the volume or loudness of speech, are cardinal manifestations of mental disorder.

Being more talkative than usual, including a speeding up of speech with decreases pauses between words and statements, and a raising of the volume of the voice, is also a cardinal manifestation of mental disorder.

Pressured speech describes the speech of patients who show a pressure to keep talking. They are usually more talkative than usual, and show the kind of speeding up of speech we have discussed above.

The tones of voice that are expressed in speech are of major importance. Cardinal manifestations of mental disorder can involve predominant tones of sadness and unhappiness expressed in speech (as a predominant finding), or involve predominant tones of elation and continuous good mood.

The combination of slowed speech, increased pauses between words and/or sentences, lowered volume of speech together with a sad tone to the voice is a clustering of speech problems that is a major manifestation of mental disorder.

Similarly a patient who shows pressured speech that flows rapidly from one subject to another, where the voice is either loud or dominated by a marked over-enthusiasm that is incessant, or by tones of irritation is a symptom-cluster of considerable significance.

STUTTERING

Stuttering is a symptom where there are frequent repetitions or prolongations of sounds, syllables, or words, or frequent unusual hesitations and pauses that disrupt the rhythmic flow of speech. It is considered a cardinal sign of mental disorder in DSM-III. In DSM-III stammering and stuttering are synonyms.

THE CONTENT OF SPEECH

The content of speech refers to what it expresses and what it contains. In this area the discussion of speech blends in with the discussion of thought, for it is by talking with a patient that we find out how he thinks and what he thinks. We will discuss this area further under the subject of thought.

The *tones of voice used in speech* are closely related to the expression of emotion. Speech that is unusually empty of emotional expression, or speech that is spoken in a monotone conveying little feeling, is a cardinal manifestation of mental disorder and is discussed under the subject of emotion.

chapter 9

Disorders of Thought, Part 1

As with speech, thought is considered from the standpoint of quantity, the flow and the rhythm of thought (stream of thought), and the content of thoughts and ideas is also examined.

THOUGHT AND SPEECH

The discussion of thought is in some ways also a discussion of speech since the examiner discovers the patient's thought through the window of speech. When we look at the rate of thought, we are actually talking about the rate of speech, and about inferences made concerning the rate of thought by listening to the patient. When the patient is described as having thought that is markedly speeded up in its flow, with one idea following the other so rapidly that the thought is said to be "racing," he has a cardinal manifestation of mental disorder.

The examiner can learn about the patient's markedly increased rate of thought either by a direct report from the patient, who informs the examiner that he feels as though his thoughts are "racing", or the examiner can conclude from a patient's pressured speech and rapid movement from topic to topic that the patient's thought is indeed speeded up.

There are two cardinal manifestations of mental disorder connected with problems in rate of speech. There is the cardinal manifestation that comes from the patient's self report, and there is the cardinal manifestation that comes from direct observations and interviews with the patient; these need to be distinguished.

RATE OF THOUGHT

Similarly when patients are said to have thought that is markedly slowed down, so that ideas come very slowly, the examiner can learn of this either through the patient's own report that his thoughts are, or feel slowed down, and that it is hard for him to think, or the examiner can listen to a patient and conclude from the markedly slowed speech and prolonged pauses between words and sentences, perhaps with lowered volume to the voice, that the patient indeed has thought that is slowed down and that it is hard for the patient to think.

Perseveration is a disorder in thinking where a mental operation or thought tends to persist past the point where it is relevant, and further movement in thought is prevented.

Thus a patient was asked who the president was, and he said, "Carter". Then when asked "who was the president before him?", the patient replied, "Carter, no I mean Carter." This is an example of perseveration where the word "Carter" is being inappropriately repeated - where the thought of Carter as president has persisted past the point where it is relevant. This is perseveration in speech and in thought.

Perseveration can also be reflected in behavior where a persistence of a thought or idea blocks further progress, so that a patient asked to copy a row of five circles continues to make circles long after he has made five of them, and makes them until he writes off the edge of the paper. That is an example of perseveration that affects behavior, where a mental operation lasts beyond the point where it is relevant and halts further progress in thinking.

Blocking is observed when the train of thought comes to a sudden stop, perhaps in the middle of a sentence, a kind of blank or empty space occurs and an entirely new thought may then start.

It is to be distinguished from the rather common experience of ordinary people where they suddenly lose their train of thought, especially when they are tired and very upset. One of the ways blocking may be distinguished is that some patients become very terrified when it occurs, indicating that it is an experience rather different from the ordinary.

DISORDER IN ASSOCIATION

When a person speaks and thinks, one topic usually bears some relationship to the next that is understandable and makes sense. The connection between one thought and another is what we call association.

Loosening of associations means that the connection between one thought and another has become harder to follow. The thought is described as loose, meaning that one thought is less tightly connected to another.

The examiner learns of a loosening of associations not through a patient's report, but by speaking with the patient and listening to how the patient expresses himself. When thoughts are loosely related, the patient is not usually aware of this lack of logical connection between thoughts, but speaks as though he were making good sense.

Incoherence is a cardinal manifestation of mental disorder where the loosening of associations becomes so marked that speech is unintelligible; the patient's speech then shows a complete lack of any meaningful relationship between words, phrases, or sentences.

An example of loosening of associations that is not severe can be seen in the case of a thirty-two-year-old inpatient of a state hospital in New York City, who told his psychiatrist, "Say listen, I know where the plot to kill Kennedy was hatched. Look what you've got-Lee Harvey Oswald, . . . Lee Harvey Oswald, . . . What have you got? L. . .D. . .L. . .D. . .D,L. . . the first letter is L, the last letter is D. . .D-L. Dill! You've got downtown and Long Island. It happened right here, and that's the whole thing. And that's the whole story right there."

The logical association between the first letter of Lee Harvey Oswald's name and the last to the thought of downtown Manhattan or the thought of Long Island and the assertion that the sharing of letters by words is the basis for concluding that President Kennedy's assassination was plotted in New York City definitely lacks logic. The association between ideas is not logical; the way one thought is based on another does not follow logical principles.

A more severe loosening of associations which could be described as approaching incoherence is the remark of a patient who, when asked how he was feeling, who replied: "My poor hole is in America. And this Tuesday I've got five believers. That's my head that is being squeezed. If I have any money at all it's in the radio."

Because loosening of associations and incoherence appear as a disorder in the *form* of thoughts, that is, in the way one thought follows another, it has been referred to as a *"formal thought disorder"*. Formal thought disorder is a cardinal manifestation of mental disorder.

A speeding up in the tempo of thought where the patient moves rapidly from one idea to another, together with some loosening of association and pressured speech has often been described as *"flight of ideas."*

The distinction between flight of ideas and the loosening of associations in formal thought disorder is not a distinction that is of relevance to DSM-III. While much has been made of the distinction between flight of ideas and formal thought disorder, this distinction in practice is often difficult to make and is usually not useful in everyday situations with patients.

DISORDER IN THE POSSESSION OF THOUGHT

The *possession of thought* refers to a person's sense that his thoughts are his own, and belong to him; it includes the feeling that thoughts belong in his mind as opposed to the feeling that thoughts are unwanted and appear in his mind against his conscious wishes.

Thoughts and ideas that are unwanted and repeatedly intrude into the mind are called *obsessions*. They are a cardinal manifestation of mental disorder. Obsessions are recurrent, unwanted thoughts, images or urges that are commonly experienced as forcing their way into the mind and that may be completely uncharacteristic of the individual's moral value system or how the individual views himself.

An example of a patient with an obsession is a twenty three-year-old mother who loved her baby and had always behaved as a responsible parent, and who sought help from a psychiatrist because of complaints that, "The idea kept coming into my head that I could kill my baby by throwing him out the window." She displayed alarm and concern saying, "How could I ever *think* such a thing?"

This patient felt the unwanted thought about throwing the baby out the window as an intrusion on her usual stream of thought, and had no difficulty continuing to behave as a responsible parent. She recognized the senselessness of the thought and saw it as highly uncharacteristic of her.

The patient with an obsession, while feeling that the thought appears against his will, feels that it can be resisted—and recognizes that although it does intrude on his mind, and he does not want to think it, it is nevertheless his own thought.

A different problem, that should not be confused with obsessional thoughts, are experiences of thoughts of being under the control of an outside agency, or feeling that other people are participating in one's own thinking.

Thought insertion is an experience where the patient believes that thoughts are being inserted into his mind, and sees them as being foreign and coming from outside of him.

In *thought withdrawal,* the patient has the experience while he is thinking of his thoughts suddenly disappearing, and feels them as being withdrawn from his mind by a foreign outside influence.

Thought broadcasting is when the patient is sure that as he is thinking, everyone else is thinking together with him or knows his thoughts; he is able to broadcast his thoughts to others.

The experience of having one's thoughts under control of an outside alien force, which is part of what is meant by *delusions of being controlled* (see the section on delusions below), are all cardinal manifestations of mental illness that are thought to be extremely characteristic manifestations of the mental disorder called schizophrenia.

Compulsions are repetitive, unwanted acts which the individual recognizes as silly, unnecessary, or foolish, but nevertheless feels obligated to perform.

Compulsions are often associated with obsessions. The urges to do the compulsive act intrude upon the mind, and can be regarded by themselves as obsessions (obsessional urges).

An example of a compulsion is that of a patient who had to count the number of panes of glass in any window that he happened to be looking at, and who recognized the silliness of such behavior, but who spent a good part of the day counting panes of glass in windows.

Patients who experience obsessions and/or compulsions feel considerable anxiety (see anxiety below under section on emotions, page 107) and may have severe distress when they try to resist performing the compulsive acts, or are prevented from performing them by other people.

Just as compulsions (acts) can be associated with obsessions (thoughts), in the same way, loosening of associations and illogical flow of one idea to another can be reflected in illogical, meaningless, and senseless behavior.

DISORGANIZED BEHAVIOR

Disturbances in behavior are discussed in a separate section, but it is important to mention that in many patients who exhibit this kind of disorganization of behavior, a corresponding disturbance in the association of thoughts is present.

Looseness of associations as reflected in the patient's speech should be distinguished from problems with attention where individuals are easily distracted by external stimuli, forming their current thought around whatever strikes them at the moment. An example of such thought is found in the following remark made by a patient, "I like your tie, it's red, not quite the color of that wall over there. How come that door is open? Maybe the other patients are going to eat dinner. It's beautiful weather we're having now outside. The trees out in front don't look so good this year. You don't look so good either."

SELF-STUDY QUESTIONS, CHAPTER 9

1. By what age have most children acquired enough spoken language to be able to tell a simple story?

   Answer: Three years old.

2. A child who once was able to talk, understand spoken language, and has stopped speaking might be suffering from a physical problem. If you know that he is not, what cardinal manifestation of mental illness does he display?

   Answer: The manifestation of elective mutism.

3. If the child does have a physical problem which has caused him to suddenly stop speaking, name two conditions that it could be the result of.

   Answer: Neurologic disease, or injury to the nervous system.

4. Describe stuttering.

5. Describe echolalia.

6. Describe pronominal reversal. Give an Example.

7. Of all the mental disorders of children that affect language, how common is delayed language development?

   Answer: It is the most common.

8. What are the two kinds of delayed language development?

   Answer: The expressive type and the receptive type.

9. What is the difference between these two types?

10. Describe acquired aphasia.

11. What are the cardinal manifestations of mental illness that concern the quantity of speech?

12. Describe pressured speech.

13. What is meant by articulation in speech?

14. Of what significance is the patient's tone of voice?

   Answer: It expresses the person's feelings while he or she talks.

15. A person who talks in a monotone expresses what about their feelings?

   Answer: Very little.

16. Describe loose associations. How is incoherence related to loose associations?

17. What is meant by formal thought disorder? What is an obsession? What is a compulsion?

18. Explain the difference between an obsession and thought insertion.

   Answer: An obsession is a repetitive and unwanted thought that the patient cannot resist, that he usually recognizes as different from his usual thought, but which he nevertheless feels is his own, despite feeling that it is forced upon him. In thought insertion the patient has the experience of having thoughts inserted into his mind, but does not experience them as his own and feels that they are coming from an outside alien power. Furthermore, he may be unable to resist them.

19. What is thought broadcasting?

20. What is thought withdrawal?

21. In the examination of patients, how is the patient's speech related to his thought?

CASE STUDY

A disheveled twenty eight-year-old man was taken to a local hospital after a policeman observed him for about a half hour. The policeman said the man stood near an alley and seemed to walk aimlessly back and forth between some garbage cans, sometimes walking over to a brick wall and tracing his finger along the spaces between the bricks. Returning once again to the garbage cans, he would open one, stare at it, and proceed to rearrange the trash in the can. When approached by the policeman and questioned, the man made no sense and instead of understandable speech produced what the policeman described as, "a lot of words thrown together without any regard for which word went where."

1. What can be said about the patient's speech?

   Answer: It was incoherent.

2. What can we say about the patient's behavior?

   Answer: It makes no sense, and appears disorganized.

3. What inference can you make about the patient's thought from his behavior and from his speech?

   Answer: The patient suffers from a disorder in the association of ideas. His thought is illogical as reflected in his speech and grossly disorganized behavior.

22. Thought insertion, thought broadcasting, thought withdrawal, and the experience of having one's thoughts controlled by an outside alien force are each said to be characteristic of what group of disorders in DSM-III?

    Answer: The schizophrenic disorders.

chapter 10

Disorders of Thought, Part 2

DELUSIONS AND PECULIAR IDEAS

A *delusion* is a false, unshakable belief that is out of keeping with the patient's social and cultural background.

A delusion is a false idea.

A delusion is unshakable and is maintained by the patient despite any evidence and proof to the contrary.

A delusion is out of keeping with the patient's social and cultural background, and is therefore to be distinguished from beliefs that are ordinarily accepted by other members of the patient's culture or sub-culture, such as religious beliefs (which to some people might be considered false and firmly maintained despite incontrovertible evidence).

Delusions are to be distinguished from *overvalued ideas* and *delusion-like ideas* in which an unreasonable belief or idea resembling one of the kinds of delusions to be described below is held by the patient, but not as firmly as is the case with a delusion.

Delusions are cardinal manifestations of mental disorder, as are overvalued ideas and delusion-like ideas that are not as firmly held as delusions.

An example of a patient suffering from a delusion is seen in the case of a twenty seven-year-old woman who told the examining psychiatrist that she was the Virgin Mary. Before seeing the psychiatrist, she had gone to her parish priest and told him that she was the Virgin Mary. He attempted to talk her out of her belief, attempting to explain Catholic theology, showing her portions of the Bible, and suggesting that she might be committing a sin by saying such things. She became violent, attacked the priest, who managed to escape from the Church after a struggle, and phoned police.

We will now discuss some of the common kinds of delusions, realizing that each type of delusion is a cardinal manifestation of mental disorder.

Delusions of Being Controlled

These are delusions where the person has the experience that his thoughts or his feelings, his urges or his actions, are not felt as being his own, but are experiences being pushed upon him by some outside influence.

(The patients who experience thoughts being forced upon them by an outside influence and not felt as being their own were discussed above on page 78.)

An example is a man who insisted that homosexual urges that he was currently feeling were coming to him from outer space.

This kind of delusion must be distinguished from beliefs that some people have that God is helping them to live their lives in certain ways, or the belief that some people have that they are God's representative in a socially accepted situation such as in the role of minister or missionary.

Delusions of being controlled should be distinguished from some people's belief that their lives are affected by a "fate," or where people have the belief that a curse or hex has been placed upon them and such beliefs are socially acceptable in their sub-culture.

Delusions of being controlled are said to be present only when the patient has the experience that his or her thoughts and feelings are being operated by an external force.

Two varieties of delusions of being controlled are *thought insertion* and *thought withdrawal.* These have been discussed above (page 78).

An example of thought insertion is a man who said that the F.B.I. was putting thoughts into his mind and making him into a secret agent.

In a case where a person has the experience that God is placing thoughts into his mind, an examiner needs to use his judgment before deciding that the patient is having a delusion of being controlled, because the patient's beliefs might be part of a socially accepted religious teaching.

Thought withdrawal is another experience that one's thoughts are under outside alien control. Such a person may say that they have a reduced number of thoughts in their head because thoughts have been taken out of their mind, and they may indicate that some particular outside force is responsible for this.

Bizarre Delusions

These are delusions that are so bizarre and fantastic that they could have no basis in reality.

An example is a man who believed that during an operation for a hernia repair, the doctors had made some adjustments to his penis so that he could only have an erection with a sexual partner who was a lesbian.

Grandiose Delusions

Grandiosity is an exaggerated and inflated feeling of one's self importance and self worth, where a person may exaggerate their accomplishments, and minimize their failures and faults. A grandiose person has an inflated self-esteem.

A *grandiose delusion* is one that involves inflated notions of one's importance, knowledge, power, or identity.

These would include delusions where someone believes that he is the savior of the human race, or that he has the power to influence the weather, or control future events, or something of this kind.

Religious Delusions

This is a delusion with a predominantly religious theme but where the religious concept is extraordinarily personal, idiosyncratic, and not related to beliefs generally held by any recognized religious organization or by society. An example of a religious delusion was the woman mentioned above who stated that she was the Virgin Mary.

Persecutory Delusions, or Delusions of Persecution

These are delusions where the content is that the patient is a victim and is being attacked, persecuted, harassed, gypped, or ripped-off by somebody or some group of people.

This delusion includes ideas of being plotted against by people who intend to do harm to the patient or cause the patient to come out on the short end in some way, and it involves the belief that one is being picked on and singled out for this kind of treatment.

Sometimes delusions of persecution have a grandiose quality.

When delusions of persecution have a grandiose quality, the delusion makes the patient sound or feel as though he is someone special, even though he believes he is going to be treated badly at the hands of others. The patient feels he is specially singled out from others for this kind of treatment.

Delusions of Jealousy

This is the delusion that someone's sexual partner is unfaithful. A delusion of jealousy is unshakable in the face of evidence to the contrary. It is to be distinguished from *ideas* that the partner is unfaithful that may be based on fact, or that may be worries that the patient can be talked out of when confronted with reasonable evidence.

Patients who suffer from delusions of jealousy often tie together a lot of pieces of circumstantial evidence that are not logically related in order to make a case that the partner is unfaithful.

Delusions of Reference

These are delusions where the theme is that objects, people, and events in the patient's immediate surrounding have a special and unusual significance meant just for him.

Delusions of reference need to be distinguished from *ideas of reference,* where the patient also thinks that objects, people and events in his immediate environment have a special and unusual significance that is meant just for him, but where an idea of reference is held less firmly than a delusion.

The point of view that events in a patient's surroundings may have a special significance for him is called *"self-reference".*

The self-referential viewpoint can be illustrated by the following example: A person who saw an unusual light in the night sky, and thought that it was a flying saucer would be distinguished from a person who saw an unusual light in the sky and also concluded that it was a flying saucer but believed that people from outer space were coming specifically to talk with him or harm him.

The latter idea involves self-reference. The event revolves around the patient and has special meaning and significance for him.

An example of delusion of reference is seen in a patient who believed that a particular newscaster, who made a habit of ending his broadcast by smiling and winking at the audience, was actually directing his winking and smiling at the patient personally, and that this was a personal message intended for him, and having some special significance.

When delusions of reference contain themes of persecution as well, a delusion of persecution is said to be present in addition to the delusion of reference.

A patient received a phone call late at night from a person who had accidentally dialed the wrong number, apologized, and hung up. The patient made frantic attempts to contact his psychiatrist claiming that someone was checking on him to see if he was home in order to kill him.

Notice how the delusion of reference and the delusion of persecution occur together. The delusion of reference involves the patient's belief that the phone call has special significance for him, although it is only a person who accidentally dialed the wrong number. The delusion of persecution is seen in the patient's belief that someone now intends to kill him.

Somatic Delusions and Hypochondriacal Delusions

These are delusions that relate to the patient's body. Somatic delusions involve the belief that *specific changes in the functioning or structure of the body* have taken place, and are to be distinguished from *hypochondriacal delusions* that involve the *fear* of having an incurable disease such as cancer or syphilis.

A patient who believed that his penis was shrinking and moving up into his stomach is an example of a somatic delusion.

A post-menopausal woman's belief that she was pregnant is another example. A patient who believed that his intestines were rotting away is yet another.

Delusions about ill health can involve not just the patient but could concern the patient's spouse or children.

A mother who suffered from the delusion that she had infected her children with an incurable disease might even attempt to murder them in the mistaken belief that she was putting them out of their misery.

Included under *hypochondriacal delusions* would be cases where patients believed that they were becoming incurably insane and who had refused to be admitted to psychiatric hospitals in the belief that once they were admitted they would be incarcerated for life.

The term "somatic delusion" can be applied also to individuals who make extreme judgments about their own body that have no basis in fact. An example is a girl who dieted and fasted to the point where she was as emaciated as a concentration camp victim and insisted that she was "horribly and terribly fat."

Nihilistic Delusions

These are delusions whose theme is nonexistence of the self or part of the self, others, or the world, such as, "I don't have a brain," or "There is no world."

Nihilistic delusions of the body are to be distinguished from somatic delusions.

A person who believed that his brain was rotting away would be having a somatic delusion, but a person who believed that he no longer had a brain inside of their head would be said to have nihilistic delusions.

Delusion of Poverty

This is the delusion that a person is or will become completely without any money or material possessions.

Sexual Delusion

This is a delusion that centers around themes of sexual identity, sexual practices, sexual ideas, and sexual impulses, and doesn't include delusions about pregnancy or jealousy.

An example of this kind of delusion is a delusion involving gender identity, where a woman believed that she was gradually changing into a man.

Systematized versus Fragmented Delusions

The distinction between systematized versus fragmented delusions is a method of comparing delusions along a spectrum of how well the ideas are organized to one another.

Systematized delusions are delusions where several delusional ideas together with facts and pieces of "evidence" are tied together in an apparently logical and coherent way, provided that you grant, in a few places, the truth of some of the things that the person believes.

Systematized delusions are contrasted with *fragmented delusions* where the relationship between one delusion and another is much harder to follow, or where the relationship between a delusion and some of the other incidents it is related to is not very well organized or is much more illogical.

An example of a systematized delusion is that of a man who believed that there was a plot at his place of employment to get him fired in order that the patient's boss could have an affair with the patient's wife. The patient believed that particularly difficult work was being given to him that could only be completed if he worked late at his office, and he believed that during the time that he was working late, certain signs were present indicating that the boss was making time with his wife. On one of the nights that he had to work late, his wife had told him that she was going out with some of her friends. He called the home of the boss whose wife said that the boss was out playing tennis.

Despite much evidence to the contrary that the wife and boss were doing exactly what they said they had been doing, this patient continued to believe that all of these and similar signs pointed to an elaborate conspiracy.

This kind of complicated delusional system should be contrasted with one where the patient would have, perhaps, several delusions that his wife was unfaithful, that the F.B.I. was putting wires into his head to use him as an instrument to gather information, and where he was getting signs from God which were coming to him over his car radio, that were not tied together or organized in any logical fashion.

Mood Congruent and Mood Incongruent Delusions

These are two categories of delusions created in DSM-III. We have not yet discussed mood (see emotion below on page 100). These new categories of delusions were created to clarify some of the differences in the kinds of delusions that occur in extreme forms of mental disorder that affect mood, and to contrast these with delusions that occur more characteristically with the group of disorders termed schizophrenic disorders.

The basic idea is that a mood congruent delusion has themes that seem to be related to the patient's predominant mood, which may be either a depressed mood or a manic mood (markedly euphoric and pleasantly expansive).

Nihilistic delusions and delusions of poverty would be mood-congruent with depression. Grandiose delusions would be mood-congruent with the euphoric and expansive mood of mania.

A mood-incongruent delusion is just what it sounds like: the delusion content and themes do not seem to be consistent with, or have an understandable relationship to, the prevailing mood that the patient has, be it depressed or euphoric or irritable.

Encapsulated Delusion

An encapsulated delusion is a delusion involving any theme that is relatively isolated from the rest of the person's thought and functioning, which behaves as though it were enclosed within a capsule and separated from the rest of the person's mind.

An example of an encapsulated delusion would be a patient who had an unshakable belief, (not a hallucination), that he had a body odor that was unpleasant to other people, and who took special precautions in the form of taking and using deodorant soap, and where he experienced no other difficulty in social or occupational functioning, and had no other delusions or disorders of thought.

Characteristic Delusions of Schizophrenia

There are certain delusions that are now held to be so characteristic of schizophrenia that when they occur, their presence alone strongly points to the possibility that the patient suffers from schizophrenia, (even when there is presence of other cardinal manifestations of mental disorders that point to major disorders of mood).

These are delusions of being controlled, thought withdrawal, thought insertion, thought broadcasting, and bizarre delusions. However, having one of these delusions does not make the diagnosis; it is a cardinal manifestation of mental illness that points strongly towards the possibility that a schizophrenic disorder is present.

Peculiar Ideas and Overvalued Ideas

These are ideas that are false, and are out of keeping with the individual's social or cultural background, but which are not as unshakable as delusions.

They are classified and named in a way that parallels the naming of delusions. False beliefs that involve self-reference would be called *ideas of reference* when they were not as firmly held as delusions of reference.

Ideas of persecution are false beliefs, out of keeping with a person's social and cultural background, where the individual believes that other people are out to get him, but where the idea is not as firmly held as a delusion of persecution.

An *overvalued idea* is an unreasonable belief, more shakable than a delusion, that the individual is so preoccupied with that it takes precedence over all other ideas and maintains this importance to him for a long period of time.

It may be difficult in some cases to distinguish between a delusion and an overvalued idea.

Magical Thinking

Magical thinking is a kind of thinking characteristic of prepubertal children who believe that their thoughts and wishes can have a direct effect on events in the world around them without the necessity of any actions having to be performed by them.

> An example is a child who wished to receive a bicycle for Christmas and never told anyone of his desire (believing that if he told someone that the wish would not come true), and firmly expected to receive a bicycle despite his not having told his parents that he wanted one.

Often children in anger think or express the wish that their parents would die or go away. After making such a wish they frequently experience great distress owing to their belief that wishes can come true.

These are both examples of magical thinking.

Magical thinking in adults occurs, and is commonly found in the belief of some people that if they allow themselves to experience too much joy and happiness on a particular occasion that this indulgence will immediately cause some misfortune to befall them. Such patients make efforts to deliberately restrict the degree of joy and pleasure that they permit themselves in life, fearing that to do otherwise would lead to a catastrophe with great personal suffering.

Such magical thinking is not delusional because most such people will readily admit that such behavior and thinking is foolish or silly.

Peculiar Ideas

Under this heading we include ideas related to magical thinking, including superstitiousness, clairvoyance, telepathy, belief in a "sixth sense", belief that others can feel one's feelings, and in children and adolescents we include bizarre fantasies and preoccupations.

> A six-year-old child who spent several hours a day imagining ways that her mother could be killed (by being hit by a car, being roasted in an oven, etc.) and who while absorbed in such fantasies often was observed to smile and laugh, would be said to have a bizarre fantasy or preoccupation.

Under hallucinations we discussed briefly the case of a person who senses the presence of a force or a being not actually present, such as someone who feels that his or her dead mother is in the same room. Such feelings are also a cardinal manifestation of mental illness. They seem to fit more closely into the thinking disorder section since they are beliefs that a force or a person is present without any sensory experiences in the form of hallucinations or illusions that accompany it.

Bizarre Behavior Resulting from Delusions

In the same way that illogical behavior might accompany markedly illogical thinking, so bizarre behavior may accompany delusions.

A thirty-year-old man who was arrested for standing in a busy intersection and throwing popcorn on the passing automobiles took off his shoes and became violent when the policemen would not accept them as gifts. The patient believed that he was, "An anointed messenger of the seventh archangel of the Pentecost and was therefore the true Pope." He said that the Pope in Rome was an imposter and that he was out in the street blessing the automobiles to insure that the drivers would eventually enter heaven. By refusing to accept his shoes as gifts, the patient said: "The policemen had thrown away their one and only chance for salvation."

SELF-STUDY QUESTIONS, CHAPTER 10

1. Define a Delusion.

   Answer: A delusion is an unshakable false belief that is out of keeping with the patient's social and cultural background.

2. Describe a delusion of reference.

   Answer: A delusion of reference is a delusion whose theme is that events, objects, or people have special and unusual significance to the patient—they refer to, and revolve around, him.

3. Explain the difference between a delusion of reference and an idea of reference.

   Answer: They have the same theme, namely that events, objects, and people have special and unusual significance for the patient and revolve around him, but an idea is more shakable than a delusion. It is less firmly held.

4. Describe delusions of being controlled. What is thought withdrawal? What is thought insertion? What is thought broadcasting? What are bizarre delusions?

5. What do all five of these delusions have in common that is of special importance to DSM-III?

   Answer: DSM-III holds that these delusions and disorders of thinking are particularly characteristic of schizophrenia and point toward the possibility that schizophrenia is present.

6. Explain a somatic delusion.

   Answer: It is a delusion whose theme is that changes in the body have taken place.

7. Distinguish a somatic delusion from a nihilistic delusion.

   Answer: Where a somatic delusion is a belief that changes in the body have occurred, a nihilistic delusion is the belief that some part of the body is totally absent.

8. A man complained that he had "no insides." What kind of delusion is this?

   Answer: A nihilistic delusion.

9. Match up the names of delusions in the left hand column with the statements in the right hand column:

Delusion of persecution	"My wife when she is out walking the dog, is getting into taxi cabs, driving off, and having sex with all the cab drivers."
Delusion of jealousy	"You, and all of the doctors are trying to poison me."
Somatic delusion	"I alone can save the countries of the world from self-destruction."
Grandiose delusion	"My heart has stopped beating."
Religious delusion	"I am Jesus Christ."

10. Describe magical thinking. In what group of people does it constitute an expected and normal mode of thought?

11. What is a delusion of jealousy? Explain how a delusion of jealousy differs from an idea of jealousy.

    Answer: A delusion of jealousy is a false unshakable idea out of keeping with one's social and cultural background whose theme is that one's sexual partner is unfaithful. It differs from an idea of jealousy in being unshakable. Ideas of jealousy may be open to persuasion by presentation of sufficient evidence to the contrary.

12. Explain an encapsulated delusion.

chapter 11

Disorders of the Experience of Self and of Identity

DEPERSONALIZATION

Depersonalization is a feeling of being estranged from one's self or the feeling that one's self is not real, seems unfamiliar, or seems strangely different. The feelings of unreality in relation to one's self may be terrifying, and may cause the patient to instantly conclude that he is going insane, a conclusion that may terrify him further.

Depersonalization is a cardinal manifestation of mental disorder.

Depersonalization may involve a variety of other peculiar sensations and experiences, such as feeling as though one is in a dream, or the feeling of not being in control of one's own behavior.

Depersonalization is often accompanied by feelings of *derealization,* which is a feeling that the world is not real, or that the world has become strange and unfamiliar and may possibly include feelings that other people have become strangely unreal.

While depersonalization is a cardinal manifestation of mental disorder, studies have shown that depersonalization commonly occurs in as many as two-thirds of young adults in mild form at some time.

The essential feature of depersonalization is that the usual feeling of the reality of one's own self is lost and replaced by a feeling of unreality.

FUGUE AND MULTIPLE PERSONALITY

Two other cardinal manifestations of mental disorder are *multiple personalities* and *fugue*. In both of these disorders the individual changes his identity and appears for a time to become another self.

Fugue

Fugue is a sudden unexpected travel away from home together with the assuming of a new identity and an inability to remember one's previous identity. A fugue is a discrete episode that has a beginning and an end, and after a fugue the patient may have no memory of what happened during the fugue.

More frequently fugue is not so complex, and the new identity is only partially assumed during the period of travelling away from home, which may then appear purposeless, and where social relationships involve only peripheral contacts or do not occur.

Multiple Personality

Here there exists within the individual two or more distinct personalities each of which can be dominant at a particular time.

The personality that is dominant at any particular time determines the individual's behavior and each individual personality is complex and integrated, having its own unique behavior patterns, social relations and unique memories. Multiple personalities is a cardinal manifestation of mental disorder.

PROBLEMS WITH GENDER IDENTITY

Problems involving gender identity are a cardinal manifestation of mental disorder. Here we distinguish between anatomical sex, biological sex, and gender identity.

Anatomic sex is the sex that a person is said to have by virtue of possessing either male or female genitalia. It really could be subdivided into *"apparent anatomic sex"* which is the sex the person appears to have upon inspection of external genitalia, as opposed to *real anatomic sex,* which would involve the issue of whether the patient has either ovaries or testes or possibly both (that is, whether the individual has *internal* reproductive apparatus characteristic of a particular sex).

Biological sex is the sex the patient is said to have on the basis of chromosomal studies that attempt to identify whether the person has sex chromosomes indicating that the cells of their body are male or female.

Gender identity is a person's basic feeling of belonging to a particular sex: of knowing "I am a Man," or "I am a Woman."

Gender role is distinguished from gender identity. Gender role involves everything that is displayed to others—all of what is said and what is done in sexual encounters and social relationships that are the ways that a person expresses the belief that he or she belongs to a particular sex.

Gender identity is an inner experience of belonging, while *gender role* could be said to be the way that the inner sense of belonging to a particular sex is shown to others. It includes what causes the patient to become sexually excited.

Gender identity disturbance is a cardinal manifestation of mental disorder. It involves feelings that one belongs to the sex that is the opposite of one's anatomic sex, as in the case of a man who said, "I've always been a girl, even from the time I was litte. I never wanted to be a boy. I am not a boy. I am a woman in a man's body. Operate on me so I can become what I really am."

Gender identity disturbance must be distinguished from the rather frequent occurrence of failing to fulfill one's expectations in regard to gender role. Here the patient, say a man, feels inadequate in relations with women, believing that a "real man" would be more popular with women than he was, but knows he is a man, and has no confusion about that.

Transsexualism

Transsexualism is a cardinal manifestation of mental disorder. It is not to be confused with *transvestism* which we will explain in a moment.

Transsexualism involves *two* cardinal manifestations of mental disorder. The first is a sense of discomfort and inappropriateness about one's own anatomic sex, and the second is a wish to be rid of one's own genitals and to live as a member of the other sex. Transsexualism is the occurrence of both of those individual symptoms together.

Transsexualism is to be distinguished from homosexuality. In homosexuality the patient has no desire to be a member of the opposite sex, but the patient's preferred or exclusive mode of sexual behavior (becoming sexually excited and achieving orgasm) is with a person of the patient's own sex.

Cross-dressing

Cross-dressing is wearing clothes of the opposite sex. It is a cardinal manifestation of mental disorder.

Transvestism

Transvestism is recurrent and persistent cross-dressing by a heterosexual male who uses the cross-dressing for the purpose of becoming sexually excited, at least in the early manifestations; there is intense frustration when cross-dressing is interfered with—the person, always a male, is completely certain that he belongs to the female sex.

Transsexualism as defined here is a major manifestation of mental disorder.

Gender Identity Disorders in Childhood

These problems affecting children are a strong and persistently stated desire to be a member of the opposite sex, or an insistence that they are a member of the opposite sex, which in girls goes beyond merely a desire for obtaining cultural advantages that are perceived as going along with being a boy.

Thus one major manifestation of mental disorder in children is the desire to be a member of the opposite sex or the statement that they are a member of the opposite sex.

Another major cardinal manifestation of mental disorder is a persistent repudiation of their own anatomic structure, which in girls means at least one of the following signs: she says that she will grow up to become a man *(physically,* and not merely to have a male role in society); she says that she is biologically unable to become pregnant, or that she will not develop breasts, or that she has no vagina, or that she has, or will grow a penis.

In boys the persistent repudiation of male anatomic structures is manifested by one of the following signs: that he says he will grow up to become a woman, *(physically* and not merely to assume a female role in society), that his penis or testes are disgusting or will disappear, or that it would be better not to have a penis or testes.

Another cardinal manifestation in the case of boys is a preoccupation with female sterotypical activities as manifested by a preference for either cross-dressing or simulating the attire of women, or by a compelling desire to participate in the games and pastimes of girls.

Concerns about Homosexuality

Issues about gender identity are to be distinguished from issues involving a preference for sexual partners of one's own sex. As discussed above, gender identity disturbance involves a sense that one belongs to the opposite sex, in spite of one's anatomic sexual attributes.

Homosexuality, on the other hand, involves sexual excitement leading to orgasm with members of the same sex, and homosexual feelings can include feelings of becoming sexually aroused towards members of one's own sex. These are issues about sexual preference, but they can be a source of considerable distress to some patients, and DSM-III relates them to other kinds of confusion about one's identity, viewing identity as a complex concept, that is comprised, at least in part, of how one sees oneself in relation to others.

IDENTITY DISTURBANCE

Identity disturbance is a severe subjective distress regarding uncertainty about a variety of issues relating to identity including three or more of the following: long-term goals, career choice, friendship patterns, sexual orientation and behavior, religious identification, moral value systems, and group loyalties. This is the major cardinal symptom of identity disturbance.

A more serious kind of identity disturbance would include in addition, confusion about gender identity.

Persons with identity disturbance ask questions such as, "Who am I?" or "Who am I really?." Some patients may say that they actually feel like someone else.

SELF-ESTEEM AND SELF-CONCEPT

A cardinal manifestation of mental disorder is either an exaggerated sense of self-esteem or a low self-esteem.

In low self-esteem patients may devalue his achievements, and may be overly dismayed by personal shortcomings. He may emphasize his faults, may feel inadequate, and even express feelings of being worthless.

Exaggerated self-esteem, sometimes called inflated self-esteem, is the opposite. Here there may be a grandiose sense of self-importance, with exaggeration of one's past achievements, and a minimizing of one's failures and difficulties. This too is a major sign and a cardinal manifestation of mental disorder.

SELF-CONFIDENCE

Self confidence is often discussed in relation to self-esteem.

A lack of self-confidence is shown in individuals' apprehension and anticipation of failure, and in emphasizing their lack of ability and their faults. They may lack poise and self-assurance, especially in everyday situations where they have little to fear. Some patients are overconcerned with embarrassment and ridicule by others. Overconcern with the opinion and possible criticism of others is a cardinal manifestation of mental disorder.

Exaggerated self-confidence, where the individual engages in activities in a reckless and foolhardy manner, seemingly exhibiting the attitude that "he can do anything", is also a cardinal manifestation of mental disorder. Such individuals may take on too much and get themselves into serious financial and social trouble.

OPTIMISM VERSUS PESSIMISM

The next jump from self-confidence is to a global attitude affecting all of an individual's behavior in a wide variety of situations that are subsumed under the heading of optimism versus pessimism.

In *pessimism* there is a global feeling that things will never work out, and that one can never be happy in the world.

Optimism can be a source of strength, allowing the individual to face difficulties and persevere. It is a trust and belief that by relying on oneself and hanging on in the face of hardship that difficulties can be surmounted.

Overoptimism, however, is a cardinal manifestation of mental disorder, where individuals do not view situations realistically, and do not give proper weight to the risks and possibilities for harm.

Overoptimistic individuals do not display reasonable caution. Overoptimism, as a manifestation of mental disorder, is a kind of global overconfidence that can lead the patient into serious difficulties.

DISTURBANCES IN BODY IMAGE

These are ideas, sometimes reaching delusional proportions, that some part of the body is ugly or disfigured, or that one is fat when one is in fact thin.

While amendable to persuasion in the face of appropriate evidence and facts, such ideas are nevertheless cardinal manifestations of mental disorder, although they are not as serious as delusions that involve the body image.

DEPENDENCE AND THE BELIEF THAT
ONE CANNOT FUNCTION AUTONOMOUSLY

A cardinal manifestation of mental disorder is a person's idea or belief or feeling that he cannot function independently in the world, and involves a wish to assume a role where he depends upon another person who takes care of him. The manifestation of mental disorder is in the seeing of oneself in relation to others as a perpetual dependent and is a form of "never growing up" and being able to stand on one's own feet.

SELF-STUDY QUESTIONS, CHAPTER 11

1. Explain depersonalization.

2. Explain derealization.

3. What percentage of normal young adults have had mild depersonalization at some time?

Answer: At least two-thirds.

4. Explain a fugue. What is multiple personality?

5. How are fugues and multiple personality instances of disturbance of identity?

6. Explain transsexualism.

7. Distinguish transsexualism from homosexuality.

8. What is cross-dressing?

Answer: Dressing in clothes of the opposite sex.

9. What is the difference between gender identity and gender role?

10. What common occurrence needs to be distinguished from problems with gender identity?

Answer: The common experience of inadequacy in meeting one's sexual role expectations while having an unshakable sense of belonging to the sex that is consistent with one's anatomic endowment, which is a problem in inadequacy of fulfilling gender role expectations.

11. What cardinal manifestations of mental disorder involve self-esteem, self-confidence, optimism, and pessimism?

Answer: Low self-esteem and exaggerated self-esteem, lack of self-confidence and exaggerated self-confidence, and excessive pessimism and excessive optimism (overoptimism).

12. Explain the cardinal manifestation of mental disorder called disturbance in identity.

Answer: It is a persistent feeling of severe subjective distress related to a variety of issues involving identity and including at least three of the following: long-term goals, career choice, friendship patterns, sexual orientation and behavior, religious identification, moral value systems, group loyalities.

13. What further problem in identity would indicate a more serious condition if it occurred in relation to two of the other symptoms that are part of the manifestation of identity disturbance?

Answer: Confusion of gender identity.

14. Describe two features that are common to gender identity disturbances in boys and girls (children)?

Answer: A strong and persistently stated desire to be a member of the opposite sex or the insistence that they are a member of the opposite sex, and secondly a repudiation of the anatomic structures of their own sex (involving the belief that they will grow up to be physically an adult of the opposite sex - not merely have an opposite sex role, that their own anatomic structures will either fail to develop or will change into those of the opposite sex or will disappear.)

15. Which sex does transvestism occur in?

16. Describe transvestism.

17. How is transvestism different than transsexualism.

> *Answer:* In transvestism there is cross-dressing with sexual excitement at least in the early phases, together with marked frustrations when cross-dressing is interferred with. It occurs only in males, and the man believes that he is a member of the male sex. In transsexualism there is a belief that one really belongs to the opposite sex; transsexualism can occur in either sex.

chapter 12

Emotion, Part 1

Emotion is a composite concept comprised of three ways of describing what we call emotional experience.

There is first of all an inner subjective feeling which we term *affect*.

There is a *physiological component* which includes all of the bodily changes usually associated with a particular emotion (for example, the characteristic physiological responses to fear, to anger, to sexual excitement, etc.).

And there is a *behavioral component* which includes facial expression, characteristics of speech, (including the rate at which speech is spoken, the length of time taken in pauses between one word and another, the loudness of speech, the quantity of speech, and the predominent tones of voice expressed).

The *behavioral component* of emotion includes the total level of physical and motor activity exhibited by the patient, including whether he could be described as *hyperactive* (overactive) or *hypoactive* (underactive); it includes bodily posture, and everything that we would subsume under the concept of "body language".

MOOD

Weather stands in relation to climate as emotion stands in relation to mood.

Mood is a prolonged or sustained emotion or a predominant emotion. In the same way that we would talk about a part of the world having a warm climate, we would talk about an individual having an irritable mood, a depressed mood, an anxious mood, an expansive mood, or euphoric mood.

The various moods that are cardinal manifestations of mental disorder are discussed below.

EMOTION VERSUS AFFECT

Frequently the subjective inner experience of a person (called affect) is associated with a particular emotion that is inferred from an observation of his behavior and physiologic responses. Thus from fear-behavior and from physiologic responses characteristic of fear (rapid heart rate, rapid respiration, trembling and shaking, and an urge to empty the bladder) it would ordinarily be concluded that the person was afraid and was also experiencing the affect that is characteristic of fear.

It is unfortunate that many psychiatrists use the terms "emotion" and "affect" interchangeably, and some even use "mood" and "affect" interchangeably. In talking about affective disorder, what DSM-III is really talking about is emotional disorder, because affective disorder in DSM-III is really a clustering of symptoms and signs that come from *all three* of the components of emotion: affect, physiologic changes, and behavior characteristic of the emotion.

The behavior and physiologic changes characteristic of a particular emotion can be said to be the expression of the inner affect associated with that emotion.

Intensity of Affective Expression

Because of the interchangeability of the terms "emotion" and "affect", this is sometimes called *emotional expressivity*. It refers to the intensity with which the patient displays all emotions. A cardinal manifestation of mental disorder is a reduced expression of all emotions, so that the individual appears to have diminished feelings of all sorts. When this appears, we speak of *blunted* or *constricted affect*. When there is absolutely no expression of emotion and the patient has an expressionless face and speaks in monotone, seeming to show no emotions (no anger, no fear, no joy, no sorrow) we speak of *flat* affect.

A diminished expressivity of emotion is a cardinal manifestation of mental disorder.

INTEREST

Interest involves the individual's subjective experience and outward behavior that are part of his wish to become involved in some situation or in some activity.

There are patients who do carry out occupational activities, and possibly only peripheral social contacts, and who, because they perform at their occupation with reasonable efficiency, are said to show an interest in their occupation, but who nevertheless have blunted or flat affect.

Interest also involves the concept of an anticipation of pleasure through the involvement in the activity in which the patient wants to become engaged, whether social, occupational, or recreational.

Therefore, lack of interest bears a relation to an inability to derive pleasure from activities.

A state of profound lack of interest is called *apathy,* and may involve some reduced emotional expressivity.

INAPPROPRIATE AFFECT

Inappropriate affect refers to a display of emotion that is either not appropriate to the content of the person's thoughts and speech, or not what would be considered socially and culturally appropriate for this person in a particular situation.

For example, a patient who laughs loudly upon being told that his mother has died, is showing inappropriate affect. (Some psychiatrists would wish to call this "inappropriate behavior" and restrict the use of the term "inappropriate affect" to emotions that are not consistent with the content of the person's *own speech or ideas,* and not to affects that are inappropriate to *a situation.)* Inappropriate affect would be expressed by a patient who wept as he related an obvious stroke of good fortune. Inappropriate affect is a cardinal manifestation of mental disorder.

LABILE AFFECT

Another cardinal manifestation of mental disorder is labile affect, or "affective ability", where affect changes frequently and unexpectedly, and where the patient seems to have reduced control over emotional expression, such as crying and laughing. Such patients seem to switch from laughing to crying with litte or no provocation and may often, while sobbing, deny that they feel sad.

COLDNESS

In our discussion of adaptive functioning, we discussed problems in social relatedness caused by inability to display warm, tender, affectionate feelings, where the individual appeared to others as aloof, cold, and indifferent. We mention this cardinal manifestation again to emphasize its importance and to point out that a patient with *blunted affect* or *flat affect* would seem cold, indifferent, and lacking warmth.

The kind of coldness of the patient with blunted or flattened affect pervades *every* aspect of the individual's emotional expressivity, whereas some individuals who lack an ability to express warm and tender feelings and appear cold and aloof in social situations, are nevertheless capable of intense emotional expression related to occupational pursuits and recreational activities. They do not show blunted or flat affect in those situations, and should not be described as having "blunted" or "flat" affect at all.

DEPRESSED MOOD

Depressed mood, which DSM-III refers to as *dysphoric mood,* is a prominent and relatively persistent group of unpleasant feelings described as: depressed, sad, blue, hopeless, low, down in the dumps, or irritable. The use of the term "dysphoric" emphasizes the inherent unpleasantness to the patient of his or her mood.

Anxiety is another mood that is also dysphoric. Fear is an inherently unpleasant emotion. Frightened people take immediate steps in an effort to create a situation where their fear can subside. Ther more prominent and the more persistent is a mood, the more serious a cardinal manifestation it is.

When a mood is predominantly sad, hopeless, down in the dumps, or blue, it can be accompanied by characteristic physiologic and behavioral changes that are part of the emotion. The physiologic changes that accompany a depression are each cardinal manifestations of mental disorder, as is also the characteristic behavior.

Physiological changes characteristic of depressed mood include increased or decreased appetite for food, perhaps with change in weight, changes in sleeping patterns, and influence the overall capacity for sustained activity of the body, with a seeming loss of energy or easy fatigability.

The behavior associated with depression involves an underactivity, or at times a restlessness referred to as *"agitation",* and can involve complaints about diminished ability to think or concentrate, slowed thinking or indecisiveness.

Depressed mood can involve feelings of worthlessness, self-reproach or excessive or inappropriate guilt as other cardinal manifestations.

PREDOMINANTLY ELEVATED, EXPANSIVE, OR IRRITABLE MOOD

This elevated or expansive mood is the opposite of the dysphoric mood of depression. Here there is a predominantly elevated and expansive mood where the patient appears to "feel good", and where the heights of pleasure can approach euphoria and ecstasy in severe cases. The mood can also be irritable, particularly when a patient in an expansive mood is thwarted by others.

Such patients are frequently over-confident with inflated self-esteem, feeling that they can do anything. They can become involved in activities where they may encounter resistence by others leading to irritability, rage, or possibly even violence.

This kind of expanded, inflated mood with sustained and predominant euphoric affect, which can at times be irritable, we shall refer to as *manic mood,* or mania (which by the way has nothing to do with the suffix -mania, as in kleptomania), in its most severe form. When it is less severe we refer to *hypomanic mood.* Here the mood is elevated and expansive but does not reach the heights seen in manic moods, and the physiologic changes and characteristic behavior of the emotion are also not as severe.

The characteristic physiologic changes involve diminished need for sleep, and an overall increase in activity, reflected in behavior, speech, and thought.

These people appear to have more energy than usual, and their behavior is hyperactive. They are more talkative than usual and show marked and sometimes extreme gregariousness. They may have heightened interest and involvement in sexual activities and excessive involvement in pleasurable activities, with lack of concern for the potential for painful consequences. Their behavior is characterized by over-activity; their thought is speeded up, and associations are looser. Their speech is pressured and they have a high potential for being impulsive and reckless.

Each of these findings involving activities, speech, thought, behavior, and need for sleep, together with the patients' own reports of their experiences and the observation and self-report of the expanded and euphoric mood are cardinal manifestations of mental disorder.

THE CONTRAST OF DEPRESSIVE MOOD
WITH MANIC AND HYPOMANIC MOODS

It is important to appreciate the contrast between cardinal manifestations that we group together with depressed mood, and cardinal manifestations that are grouped together with manic moods. They lie at opposite ends of a spectrum. They are like the two points at the ends of a line, or like the two poles of a magnet. They are opposites. We can contrast them in terms of:

	depressed mood	manic mood
1 mood	↓	↑
2 sleep habits—need for sleep, quantity of sleep	less sleep or more	wide awake less sleep
3 energy level	↓	↑
4 self-esteem	↓	↑
5 productivity	↓	↑
6 attention, concentration, and thinking	↓	↑
7 social relations	↓	↑
8 sexual interests	↓	↑
9 recreation and involvement in pleasurable activities	↓	↑
10 feelings about tempo of activity	↓	↑
11 talkativeness	↓	↑
12 pessimism versus overoptimism	↓	↑
13 tearfulness or crying, verus inappropriate humor	tears	laughter

Most of the items above are at opposite poles between depression and mania, where lowness, diminishing, and lack characterize the depressed aspect, and increase, heightening, and excess characterize the manic. Sleep habits may be an exception, as inability to sleep in specific ways is typical of depression; but in some cases an increased need for sleep may be present, where the manic patient *invariably* has a decreased need for sleep.

Depressed patients may typically have the cardinal manifestation of either decreased appetite or increased appetite and may additionally have a loss of weight or a weight gain.

PSYCHOMOTOR BEHAVIOR

Psychomotor behavior is a term that covers speech together with observable motor behavior. It does not concern thinking or the rate of thought.

Psychomotor agitation can involve pacing the floor, wringing the hands, restlessness and inability to sit still, and may involve uttering complaints and yelling.

Psychomotor retardation involves a slowing down of physical activity where the patient behaves as though tasks are difficult and tire him out easily. Some patients may seem always tired and "worn out", even without performing any physical activity.

Speech is slowed down, and pauses are increased between remarks. Patients do not speak as loud; there may be a reduced quantity of speech *(impoverished speech* or *poverty of speech)* or there may be no speech at all *(mute).*

GRIEF AND UNCOMPLICATED BEREAVEMENT VERSUS DEPRESSION

Depressed mood and the physiologic changes and behavior associated with it bear a strong resemblence to the emotion of grief that is experienced when a relative dies.

Grief is an emotion that is expressed in response to a real loss, and is part of the normal coping with that particular psychosocial stressor.

Uncomplicated bereavement is not a mental disorder in DSM-III, although it is a category that is available, just as the category of "no diagnosis or condition on Axis I" is available.

The cardinal manifestation of *feelings of worthlessness* is not ordinarily associated with uncomplicated bereavement.

Neither is severe psychomotor retardation or a severe and sustained impairment in adaptive functioning.

In some cases of uncomplicated bereavement, extremely severe symptoms and signs ordinarily associated with depression occur, but there is usually less psychomotor retardation, there is a gradual return to previous levels of adaptive functioning, and usually feelings of worthlessness are in relationship to the deceased person and can involve ideas about what one might have done for the person when they were alive (or feeling that one could have done more to keep them alive).

When this is not the case, severe symptoms can mean that bereavement may be complicated by the presence of a mental disorder.

Similarly, some individuals in some situations may experience exceptional joy with intense emotional expressivity, and their level of enthusiasm and excitement can be marked. Such affect needs to be distinguished from the sustained expansive mood and physiologic and behavioral changes that are cardinal manifestations of manic mood.

MOOD-CONGRUENT VERSUS MOOD-INCONGRUENT DELUSIONS AND HALLUCINATIONS

Delusions and hallucinations whose content is consistent with the predominant mood of the patient are said to be mood-congruent. Delusions or hallucinations whose content is inconsistent with the predominant mood of the patient, are called mood-incongruent delusions or mood-incongruent hallucinations, respectively.

What does this mean?

It means that a patient who is severely depressed who has a delusion or hallucination can have the content of the hallucination viewed in terms of whether the content is consistent or inconsistent with the patient's severely depressed mood.

Therefore, a mood-congruent delusion or hallucination might involve themes of personal inadequacy, guilt, disease, death, deserved punishment, and so on in a severely depressed person. A severely depressed person, for example, might hear a voice accusing him of committing "unspeakable sins", or telling him that he deserves punishment for past actions over which he feels much guilt.

A *mood-incongruent* delusion or hallucination in a severely depressed person might involve issues not particularly related to the severe depression.

In the same way, a patient who suffers from a severe manic mood could be said to have delusions or hallucinations that were either mood-congruent or mood-incongruent, where a mood-congruent hallucination or delusion would involve themes of inflated worth, power, knowledge, identity, or having a special relationship to God or to a famous person, while mood-incongruent delusions or hallucinations would not involve these themes, and might involve themes of being persecuted, or involve sexual issues, where the content appeared to have no apparent relationship to themes of inflated worth, power, knowledge, identity, or having a special relationship to either God or to a celebrity.

> Bizarre behavior resulting from delusions that are mood-incongruent are seen in the following twenty nine-year-old man who seemed depressed and sad-voiced and said that he was "better off dead". He refused to use the toilet, urinating in jars that he stacked neatly in his landlady's trashcan. He said that the communist party was putting wires in his head and was going to use him "as a propaganda tool" and intended to force him to "betray his country" and "poison the water supply" by urinating in the toilet.

Notice this depressed affect. Notice the bizarre quality of the handling of his urine in jars and his refusal to use the toilet.

ANXIETY AND FEAR

Anxiety is an emotion, and is a composite consisting of subjective inner feelings of anxiety, physiologic changes that are characteristic of the emotion, and behavior that is characteristic.

The subjective inner sensation of anxiety is likened to that of fear. The difference between anxiety and fear does not lie in a difference between the subjective inner feelings of the two emotions.

Fear is an emotion that is defined as occurring in relation to a real perceived danger that confronts the individual in his environment that would be considered to be a danger by other people in the same situation (that are part of his social and cultural group).

A person who saw and heard a tornado a few miles away, that was bearing down on his neighborhood and ripping up houses as it moved, would be expected to feel afraid.

The source of the emotion of fear lies in a real danger in the external environment.

The emotion of fear felt by the person who saw the tornado would consist of a subjective inner feeling of being afraid, characteristic physiologic changes, and characteristic behavior.

Physiologic Changes' in Fear

The physiologic changes characteristic of fear consist of a rapid heart rate (tachycardia), rapid breathing (tachypna), dry mouth, sweating, a "sinking feeling" or a "sick feeling" in their stomach, trembling and shaking of the limbs, and an urge to empty the bladder. Some patients may lose control of bladder and bowel function in the fearful situation.

Some individuals may feel dizzy and may feel faint.

Fear Behavior

There are characteristic behaviors that would be exhibited by a person who felt fear while looking at an oncoming tornado. The person would exhibit a frightened facial expression, have a fearful tone in his voice, (the voice may quaver with fear, or the fear-stricken person may scream, yell, or moan), and the fearful person would display characteristic behavior, taking steps to avoid the real external danger—most people would run away from the tornado in attempt to take shelter.

Avoidance behavior: the effort to flee from real danger that is part of the behavioral component of the emotion of fear is called "avoidance behavior".

Anxiety is an emotion identical to fear that occurs in the absence of a real threat or danger from the environment.

The absence of a real environmental danger gives anxiety an irrational quality.

Anxiety is an irrational fear.

Anxiety may be felt in relation to an external object or situation, such as seeing a bug, or eating in public, and in such cases we say that the patient suffers from anxiety in relation to these situations, or that he or she is "afraid of them".

A patient who suffers from anxiety while being in a crowd could be said to be "afraid of crowds".

Anxiety can also be felt when there is no object or situation that seems to be related to it, or to trigger it. In such cases anxiety can be said to *"free-floating".*

Anxiety has the same subjective inner sensation as fear, and anxiety has physiological sensations identical to fear. Anxious people exhibit behavior like that seen in the emotion of fear.

Anxious people have facial expressions that are fearful. Anxious people sound fearful when they talk and anxious people display avoidance behavior when their anxiety is felt in relation to a particular object or situation. A person who had an irrational fear of crowds would avoid crowds.

Panic

Panic is fear that is exceptionally intense.

Whenever anxiety is severe with intense affect and intense physiologic manifestations, DSM-III calls it panic. Such intense episodes of anxiety are called *panic attacks*.

The emotion of anxiety and its characteristic affect, physiologic changes, and behavior, particularly avoidance behavior, are cardinal manifestations of mental disorder.

SELF-STUDY QUESTIONS, CHAPTER 12

1. What are the three components of emotion?

   Answer: The subjective inner experience called affect, the physiologic changes that are characteristic, and the behavior that is characteristic.

2. What is the difference between "Dysphoric Mood" and depressed mood?

   Answer: Any mood that feels unpleasant is a dysphoric mood—fearfulness is a dysphoric mood. Depressed mood is one of the dysphoric moods. However, when DSM-III uses the term "dysphoric mood", it is depressed mood that is usually intended.

3. Describe a dysphoric mood (that is, "depressed") by giving some common words that describe some of the affects associated with it.

   Answer: Sad, worthless, guilty, "down in the dumps", blue, low, "down".

4. What are some of the physiologic changes associated with a depressed mood?

   Answer: Loss of appetite, insomnia, weight loss, compaints of fatigue.

5. Can appetite be increased in depression? Can patients sleep more than usual when they are depressed?

   Answer: Yes, to both questions.

6. Describe manic mood.

   Answer: A mood that is the opposite of depression. It is euphoric, grandiose, expansive, pleasant, sometimes may be irritable.

7. What can often produce an irritable or angry mood in a patient who would be describable as having a manic mood?

Answer: Thwarting the patient from doing things his way, or thwarting him in getting what he wants.

8. How would you compare manic mood with depressed mood in relation to each of the following items?

a. energy
b. self-esteem
c. productivity
d. attention
e. social relations
f. sexual interest and involvement
g. recreational involvements and pursuit of pleasurable activities
h. the patients' report of whether their own activity was speeded up or slowed down
i. quantity of talk (loquacity)
j. attitude toward the future

Answer: Depressed patients show a decrease or diminishing of all of the above, while it is characteristic of manic mood to have an increase or an excess. Attitude toward the future is pessimistic and bleak in the case of depressed mood, and is over-optimistic in manic mood.

9. What is the difference between a manic mood and hypomanic mood?

Answer: Hypomanic mood is a less intense, less severe manifestation of essentially the same kinds of findings seen in manic mood, involving mood itself, level of activity, rate and quantity of talk, interest and involvement in activities, etc.

10. What kinds of trouble could a person with marked features of manic mood get themselves into?

Answer: Some possibilities are: financial trouble, social problems, occupational difficulties, etc.

11. Explain the difference between anxiety and fear.

Answer: Fear is in response to a real external danger while anxiety is not.

12. Anxiety that is in response to an object or situation in the environment is often said to be a "phobia" of the particular object or situation. What is the term for anxiety that is experienced in the absence of any external stimuli?

Answer: Free-floating anxiety.

13. What are some of the physiologic changes that are characteristic in anxiety?

Answer: A rapid heart rate, rapid breathing, trembling and shaking, a sinking or sick feeling in the pit of the stomach, and a wish to empty the bladder.

14. Explain avoidance behavior.

Answer: Avoidance behavior is what we call the characteristic behavior of a person who is afraid of something, who takes action to avoid what he is afraid of.

15. Explain panic. What is a panic attack?

Answer: Panic is an extreme state of anxiety.

A panic attack is an episode of an extreme state of anxiety with intense affect and intense physiologic responses.

chapter 13

Emotion, Part 2

PANIC ATTACKS

Panic attacks are episodes of panic.

Panic is extreme anxiety. In panic attacks patients have intense anxious affect and intense physiological manifestations. The physiologic manifestations of anxiety are principally rapid heart rate, rapid respiration, trembling and shaking, dryness of the mouth, a sinking feeling in the pit of the stomach, and an urge to empty the bladder.

When anxiety is intense and physiologic responses are correspondingly severe, the physiologic changes due to anxiety exert direct effect on the body. This causes further signs and symptoms that are seen in the extreme states of anxiety termed panic.

The patient frequently experiences rapid heart rate as *palpitations* which are noticeable and sometimes unpleasant sensations of a pounding and rapid heartbeat. The patient's rapid respiration may be felt by him or her as a shortness of breath or as a difficulty in breathing.

The rapid heart beat together with the rapid respiration can be experienced by a patient with panic *as a discomfort in the chest or as chest pains*. Most chest pain in most panic attacks represent the patient's unpleasant experiences of palpitation or of the rapid deep breathing, or both, and does not mean that anything is "wrong" with their heart or lungs. In rare instances, there can be a different kind of chest pain caused by heart disease that is being brought out by the extreme state of anxiety. (Panic states are not good for patients who have insufficient blood supply to the heart. The demand on the heart for work is not matched by an adequate supply of blood. Such patients may experience chest pain that is a direct effect of lack of oxygen to the heart. Some patients have had heart attacks (myocardial infarctions) as a consequence of panic. That is one reason why patients who have had a heart attack are removed from their usual environmet during the early period of observation, as efforts are made to minimize the chance that they could become upset or excited, and develop rapid heart beat that would tax the already damaged heart.)

The rapid breathing in panic presents the body with a problem, by causing characteristic physiological changes of its own which we will discuss in a moment.

The rapid breathing creates, for the patient, a sensation of "having difficulty breathing" that can itself frighten the patient further.

What commonly frightens such patients is their inability to master and bring under control the rapid respiration by taking deeper breaths, and they may report that they have sensations of "choking" or "smothering". These sensations related to the rapid respiration can scare patients further.

Hyperventilation

It is a well established fact that rapid deep breathing, termed *hyperventilation,* creates characteristic physiologic changes by reducing the carbon dioxide concentration of the blood ("blowing off CO_2"), that upsets the chemistry of the blood, and will result in characteristic sensations of tingling in the hands and feet, or sensations of tingling around the mouth, together with feelings of dizziness and feelings that one is going to faint. These sensations of tingling in the hands and feet and around the mouth, and/or the feelings of dizziness and faintness, further increase the patient's fear that something terrible is going to happen to him or her. Thus, commonly, panic attacks are accompanied by a strong sense of impending doom, impending death, or where the feeling that one has lost control of his or her emotions and body; this may be experienced as the feeling of "going crazy".

The patient may feel that he is going to do something as a result of his intense distress that would be uncontrolled, such as shouting out in public, screaming, or fainting. The worry that he is going crazy or that he is going to do something as a result of his inner distress that would be uncontrolled, further intensifies his anxiety, and intensifies all of the physiologic responses that are characteristic of anxiety.

These feelings of being out of control of one's self can be experienced as a feeling of unreality related to one's identity, that may sound a bit like depersonalization when the patient describes it. In some cases, actual depersonalization can accompany these other major manifestations of mental disorder.

We are now going to group together the cardinal manifestations we have discussed under the heading of panic attack, to make a definition of Panic

Attack that will be used throughout the rest of this book.

A panic attack is an episode of intense apprehension, or fear, of terror, usually associated with feelings of impending doom, where at least four of the following symptoms appear:

1. dyspnea (shortness of breath or difficulty breathing)
2. palpitations
3. chest pain or discomfort in the chest
4. choking or smothering sensations
5. dizziness, vertigo (a sensation that the room or the environment is spinning), or unsteady feelings
6. feelings of unreality
7. parasthesias (sensation of tingling in hands or feet or around the mouth)
8. hot and cold flashes
9. sweating
10. faintness
11. trembling or shaking
12. fear of dying, going crazy, or doing something uncontrolled during and attack

GENERALIZED ANXIETY

When the intensity of anxiety takes a sudden jump to an extreme level of severity we speak of panic attack. What of the case where a continual level of increased anxiety is present for an extended period of time, perhaps several weeks to a month, without panic attack?

In such a case there are *signs of motor tension,* in the form of shakiness, jitteriness, jumpiness, trembling, tension, muscle aches, fatigability and inability to relax, twitching of the eyelids, furrowed brow, strained face, fidgeting, restlessness, and easy startling.

There is *autonomic hyperactivity,* with the symptoms of which we are already familiar. They include sweating, pounding or racing heart beat, cold clammy hands, dry mouth, dizziness, light-headedness, paresthesias, upset stomach, hot or cold spells, frequent urination, diarrhea, discomfort in the pit of the stomach, lump in the throat, flushing, pallor, high resting pulse, and high resting respiration rate.

It includes *apprehensive expectation,* meaning that the patient has anxiety, worry, fear rumination (a brooding and preoccupation with thoughts and feelings), and anticipation of misfortune to self or to others.

And it includes *vigilance and scanning* which is hyperattentiveness which results in distractability, difficulty concentrating, insomnia, feeling "on edge", irritability, and impatience.

When three of these four manifestations are present (motor tension, autonomic hyperactivity, apprehensive expectation, vigilance or scanning) the patient has the cardinal manifestation of *generalized anxiety.*

PHOBIAS

A phobia is an irrational fear of, and avoidance of, a specific object or situation.

Agoraphobia

Agoraphobia is a marked fear of and avoidance of being alone in public places from which escape might be difficult, or help not available in case of sudden incapacitation, such as in crowds, tunnels, bridges, or public transportation.

This is a cardinal manifestation of mental disorder.

Social Phobia

Social Phobia is a persistent irrational fear of and compelling desire to avoid, a situation in which the individual is exposed to possible scrutiny by others, and fears that he or she may act in a way that will be humiliating or embarrassing. Some patients may experience significant distress because of this problem, yet recognize that their fear is excessive or unreasonable.

Such specific fears of certain social situations could involve the situation of eating in public, where the patients worry that they will embarrass or humiliate themselves by doing something like spilling food or committing a breach of etiquette. Another such social phobia is a fear of public speaking where patients are afraid that they will act foolishly in front of an audience and either be ridiculed or otherwise feel embarrassed and humiliated. Some persons avoid writing while being watched by another person, fearing that they will be humiliated by making an error.

Such specific fears (that differ, by the way, from the ordinary anxiety of most normal individuals about successful performance in situations that are important to them) are often the result of previous panic attacks in social situations, where the individuals now are worried that a panic attack in the social situation will be noticed by others, and will humiliate or embarrass them, or fear that the panic attack will so impair their performance that they will be humiliated.

Similarly, patients with agoraphobia may have experienced panic attacks while in the situations they are afraid of, and therefore avoid these situations fearing that if they experienced another panic attack, they would be unable to escape, or if they were alone, they would have no one to aid them.

Simple phobia is the cardinal manifestation where an individual is afraid of some object or situation other than agoraphobia and social phobia. It includes specific fears like being afraid of dogs and snakes.

SEPARATION ANXIETY

An *attachment figure* is a person toward whom a child forms a deep affectionate bond. A *major attachment figure* is a person toward whom a child has formed their deepest and most important affectionate bond. Major attachment figures are usually parents, but in some cases can be other persons close to the child.

Separation anxiety in children, adolescents, or adults consists of unrealistic worries about harm befalling major attachment figures, or fears that the major attachment figure will leave and not return.

It includes unrealistic worries that a catastrophic event will separate the child from a major attachment figure, such as fears that the child will be lost, kidnapped, killed, or be the victim of an accident. A child who has such unrealistic worries shows a cardinal manifestation of mental disorder.

Excessive distress upon separation or when anticipating separation from a major attachment figure, shown by temper tantrums, crying, or pleading with attachment figures not to leave, is a cardinal manifestation of mental disorder. (To consider this a manifestation of a problem in children under the age of six, the distress shown by the child must be of panic proportions.)

OVERANXIOUSNESS

Generalized and persistent worrying about the future, about the appropriateness of the individual's behavior in the past, about competence in a variety of areas such as academic, athletic, and social areas, are each cardinal manifestations of mental disorder.

The need for excessive reassurance about *a variety* of worries also is a cardinal manifestation.

SELF-STUDY QUESTIONS, CHAPTER 13

1. Describe the physiologic changes that occur in panic attack.

2. What physiologic change in panic attack, by its effect on body chemistry, can insensify a patient's experience of unpleasant bodily sensations?

Answer: Rapid deep breathing or hyperventilation.

3. Discuss some of the ways that this rapid deep breathing can produce specific changes that could be felt as unpleasant by the patient. What are some of these unpleasant changes?

Answer: Dizziness, lightheadedness, tingling in the hands and feet or around the mouth, sensations of not being able to breathe sufficiently, unsteady feelings, chest discomfort.

4. What are four manifestations of generalized persistent anxiety (not panic attacks)?

Answer: Motor tension, autonomic hyperactivity, apprehensive expectation, vigilance and scanning.

5. Give some examples of motor tension.

Answer: Jitteriness, jumpiness, inability to relax, fidgeting, and so on.

6. What is meant by autonomic hyperactivity? Give examples.

Answer: These are similar to the physiologic changes associated with anxiety and fear in general. They are a pounding or racing heart beat, dry mouth, dizziness, lightheadedness, upset stomach, frequent urination, and so on.

7. What is meant by paresthesias?

Answer: A sensation of tingling, or pins and needles, in the hands, feet, or around the mouth.

8. What is meant by apprehensive expectation? Give examples.

Answer: Anxiety, worry, fear, anticipating misfortune befalling one's self or other people.

9. What is meant by rumination?

Answer: Preoccupation with a thought or a worry, excessive brooding. The word rumination refers to chewing, so when applied to thought, it means chewing the same thought over and over.

10. What is vigilance and scanning?

Answer: It is being excessively alert and looking around, or paying excessively close attention to what is happening. It can result in difficulty in concentration, difficulty in going to sleep, feeling "on edge", being irritable, and being impatient.

11. What is a phobia?

Answer: An irrational fear of a situation or thing.

12. Give some examples of phobias.

13. What is Agoraphobia?

Answer: An irrational fear of, and avoidance of, situations in which a person fears he will become incapacitated in some place from which he will not be able to escape *or* a fear of being alone in such places where the person fears they will become incapacitated.

14. Give some examples of situations that might be related to a person's agoraphobia.

Answer: Being afraid to enter tunnels, being afraid to drive on bridges, being afraid to ride on buses, being afraid to be in the middle of a large crowd, especially if by themselves.

15. What is a social phobia?

Answer: It is a specific fear of a specific social situation, such as eating in public, or writing while being watched by other people.

16. What is meant by simple phobia?

Answer: All of the other kinds of phobias we could imagine that are not agoraphobia or social phobias.

17. Give examples of simple phobias.

Answer: Fear of dogs, fear of snakes, fear of bugs, fear of mice, etc.

18. Once again, explain panic.

Answer: Panic is an extreme state of anxiety.

19. Explain panic attack.

Answer: A panic attack is an episode of extreme anxiety with an intense anxious affect and intense physiologic manifestations of anxiety.

20. Enumerate some of the prominent physiologic changes that occur as part of a panic attack.

Answer: If you don't remember, please go back to the text and look over the list.

21. Discuss separation anxiety. What is an "attachment figure"? What is a major attachment figure? What are some of the worries of the child or adult who has separation anxiety?

22. When children under six are thought of as having problems with separation anxiety, what special form of anxiety must be demonstrated?

Answer: The concern over separation from an attachment figure in children under six must be of panic proportions in order to consider them as manifesting a mental disorder.

chapter 14

Physiologic Changes and Physical Complaints, Part 1

Physiologic changes that occur during anxious moods, panic attacks, depressed mood, and manic mood have been discussed. Changes that occur in depressed and manic mood have involved mainly sleep habits, appetite and weight change, overall level of physical activity, and apparent physical endurance.

SLEEP

Sleep disturbances are cardinal manifestations of mental disorder.

A night's sleep is one of life's necessities. Like needing food and water, people must sleep. People vary tremendously in their individual requirements for sleep. Here we shall be concerned with difficulties in going to sleep, staying asleep, and ways that sleep can be disturbed.

Dreams and REM sleep

Dreaming accompanies sleep and occurs during a phase of sleeping called REM sleep. REM sleep is a period that occurs as a normal and essential part of every night's sleep, in which the eyes move rapidly and, if the person is awakened, he or she will be able to report dreams.

The electroencephalogram (EEG) is an instrument for observing the electrical activity of the brain and has shown that a normal night's sleep consists of several distinct phases, each with its own signature on the EEG. REM sleep is such a phase. All of the phases of sleep that are not REM sleep are called *non-REM sleep (NREM)*.

Insomnia

Insomnia is a term that means both difficulty going to sleep and difficulty remaining asleep.

There are three kinds of insomnia: *initial insomnia* which is difficulty going to sleep; *middle insomnia* where after persons have gone to sleep, they wake up in the middle of the night and have some difficulty going back to sleep (but eventually do); and *terminal insomnia,* also called *"early morning awakening"*, where persons awaken several hours before the time they customarily wake up and cannot return to sleep.

Insomnia is characterized by difficulty sleeping in spite of a wish to sleep. Patient's who cannot fall asleep frequently complain that they wish that they could go to sleep, and often ask for help with this problem. This can be contrasted with the decreased need for sleep in mania, where the lively wide-awake patient has no wish to sleep and may remain active and awake for days.

The patient with early morning awakening frequently complains bitterly about it, and expresses the desire to return to sleep after awakening so unusually early.

When DSM-III disucssed insomnia, and uses that term without further qualification, apparently it is referring to any one of the three varieties.

There are places in DSM-III where terminal insomnia, or early morning awakening, is specifically singled out.

Each of the three kinds of insomnia is a cardinal manifestation of mental disorder.

We need to look in addition at the actual quantity of sleep that a person usually receives each night, together with the patient's apparent need for sleep.

Some patients have a genuine decreased need for sleep, so that their customary sleep habits undergo change. This is a cardinal manifestation of mental disorder. We mentioned it as occurring as one of the physiologic changes in *manic mood.*

Some patients have an increased need for sleep, and the actual quantity of sleep each night may increase. This too, as a change from customary habits, represents a cardinal manifestation of mental disorder.

Decreased sleeping or increased sleeping are *both* cardinal signs of mental disorder.

Insomnia, as a term, does not single out any particular cause for the sleep problem. Some patients who cannot fall asleep may have "things on their mind" that they worry about and keep them awake; other patients may not.

Types of Insomnia

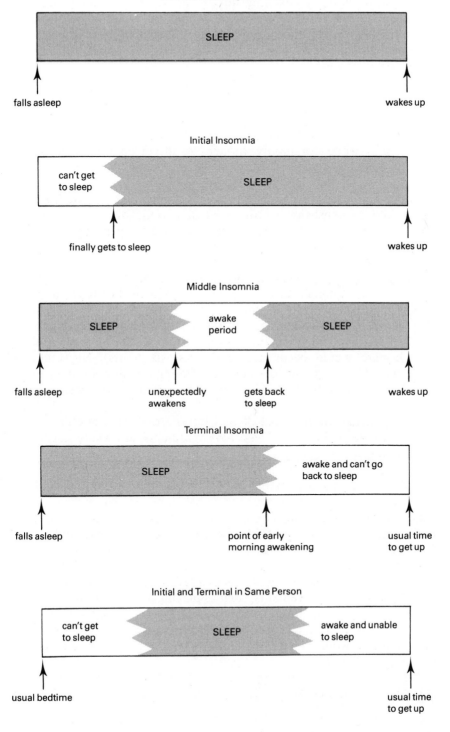

Patients who awaken early in the morning may or may not complain of thoughts or feelings that occupy them during the time that they were unable to return to bed.

Middle insomnia, awakening during the night and falling back to sleep, is commonly discussed in a way that does not involve the disturbance of sleep by nightmares, sleep terrors, or sleepwalking, but refers only to an unexplained episode of waking from sleep with eventual return to bed after some period of time.

Nightmares, Sleep terrors, and Sleepwalking

Nightmares, sleep terrors, and sleepwalking, disturb sleep once it has begun, and while commonly thought to affect children, may disturb the sleep of adults as well.

Three Periods of Sleep. We can think of the eight or nine hours of sleep of a child as consisting of three equal periods of time; for the sake of convenience, let us assume that a child's nine-hour period of sleep is divided into an *early,* a *middle* and a *late period,* each consisting of three hours.

Nightmares. Nightmares are distinctly unpleasant dreams that can awaken the sleeper, who can recall the unpleasant events of the dream in detail.

Nightmares can occur in persons of all ages. When they interrupt sleep, they can be distinctly recalled at that time. Nightmares occur in the middle and last thirds of sleep (so that in the case of a child who slept nine hours, a nightmare would occur during the last six hours). Nightmares always occur in REM sleep, and the person suffering a nightmare does not scream out during their sleep. Nightmares are not marked by a panicky scream.

Sleep Terrors. Sleep terror ("night terror", or "pavor nocturnus") is often confused with nightmares. *Sleep terrors* are episodes where sleeping persons are awakened from sleep and apparently have had a distinctly unpleasant experience which they cannot recall. They may appear dazed, as though they are still half asleep, are unable to give an account of the details of any kind of nightmare, and for some period of time appear extremely anxious, displaying prominant physiologic changes associated with anxiety, such as rapid heart rate, rapid breathing, sweating, dialated pupils, and piloerection (an erection of the hairs of the body—their hair stands on end).

The experience of a sleep terror is characterized by individuals being almost always confused and disoriented; they may perform repetitive meaningless motor movements, such as picking at their pillow.

Sleep terror is commonly accompanied by a panicky scream, invariably occurs in the first third of a night's sleep (so that in a child who slept for nine hours it would occur in the first three hours of the night), and never occurs in REM sleep.

Nightmares and sleep terrors are different. Sleep terrors are a cardinal manifestation of mental disorder.

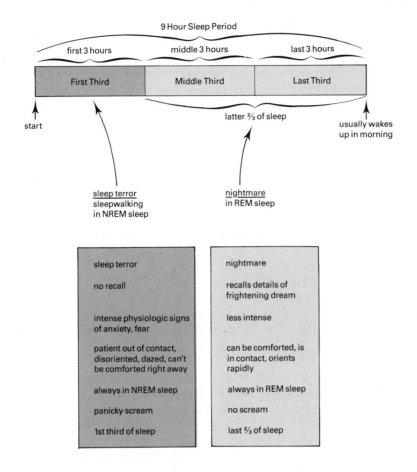

Recurring Unpleasant Dreams. Persons who have suffered through catastrophic life experiences may have recurring unpleasant dreams of the event. This is a cardinal manifestation of mental disorder that would be coded as "7-Catastrophic" on Axis IV.

Sleep Problems From Separation Anxiety. Children who have *repeated nightmares involving themes of separation* have a cardinal manifestation of mental disorder.

Children who persistently refuse to go to sleep or show persistent reluctance to go to bed without being next to a major attachment figure, or to go to sleep away from home, show a cardinal manifestation of mental disorder. These particular sleep problems of children are said to be manifestations of separation anxiety (see page 116).

Hyperactivity. Excessive movements during sleep are considered a cardinal manifestation of mental disorder and are mentioned again below under the subject of hyperactive behavior (see page 151).

Sleepwalking. Sleepwalking refers to repeated episodes, after falling asleep, of either sitting up in bed, or getting up out of bed and walking around. The term sleepwalking includes several varieties of the problem. Persons may not actually get out of bed and walk, they may only sit up in bed, perhaps performing some purposeless movement such as repeated picking at their pillow. Other individuals may actually get out of bed and walk, perhaps go to the bathroom, get dressed, and walk about the house. During such episodes they are apparently able to see where they are going, but usually appear to be in a kind of trance, and to have not fully awakened from sleep. Such patients may either wake up in the midst of such activity, or return to bed and go back to sleep without ever fully gaining consciousness. They usually have no memory for what they did after arising from sleep, whether they return to bed or not, they commonly have a blank staring face, and are usually not responsive to the efforts of other people to communicate with them or to influence them, and it is commonly difficult to wake them up during one of these episodes.

It is a misconception that sleepwalking is harmless to sleepwalkers and that during the episode they will take care somehow not to hurt themselves. This is not so. Sleepwalkers don't know what they are doing, are in a trance, and may accidently go out windows, fall down stairs or fire escapes, and be severely injured.

Sleepwalking occurs in the first one third of a night sleep. A child who slept usually for nine hours would most likely sleepwalk during the first three. Sleepwalking occurs in NREM sleep.

Sleepwalking is a cardinal manifestation of mental disorder.

Disturbance of Sleep-wake Cycle. Research on sleep has shown that individuals typically develop an internal rhythm to their periods of waking and sleeping. When this internal rhythm changes, or is upset, it is a cardinal manifestation of mental disorder when no physical disease is responsible for it. Such individuals might be up during the night (when they would customarily be in bed and asleep) and would either be drowsy or nap during the day (where they had previously spent their daylight hours being alert and awake).

Daytime drowsiness, with or without insomnia, represents a disturbance in the sleep-wake cycle and is a cardinal manifestation of mental disorder.

EATING DISTURBANCES, APPETITE, AND RELATED CHANGES IN BODY WEIGHT

Decreased appetite and increased appetite have been discussed as disturbances that are part of the physiologic changes associated with depressed moods.

Decreased appetite, called *anorexia,* is a common symptom of many *physical illnesses.*

Anorexia, when sustained, leads to weight loss. Weight loss and weight gain are other physiologic changes we have discussed in connection with depressed mood. Weight loss is also a physiologic change associated with many physical diseases. It is assumed, in this discussion, that anorexia and weight loss (as well as increased appetite and weight gain) are cardinal manifestations of mental disorder only after their significance as cardinal manifestations of physical disease has been investigated.

EATING DISTURBANCES

Weight Loss Through Diets and Fasts and Fears of Fatness

Persons who refuse to eat tend to lose weight.

Many persons in our society are preoccupied with being slim and with not becoming fat (obese). When such persons do gain some weight, they may exhibit concern, go on a diet, and then become less and less concerned as their weight approaches what they consider to be their ideal weight.

The large majority of people who behave in this fashion have the goal of reaching what is the physically normal weight for their height and stature.

This needs to be distinguished from persons whose goal of an ideal weight is considerably below what ordinary persons, or what physicians, would consider to be normal for their height, age, and stature.

Persons whose concern and preoccupation with being fat is excessive after an episode of gaining weight, then dieting and going down to their normal weight, and whose fear of fatness does not diminish as normal weight is approached, are showing a cardinal manifestation of mental disorder.

Persons who refuse to maintain their body weight only a small amount (a few pounds) above what is considered their normal weight for age and height, are also exhibiting a cardinal manifestation of mental disorder.

So are individuals who "feel fat" when they are underweight, not perceiving what others can often see: namely that they are too thin and below what would be normal weight for their age, height, and stature.

When not due to physical disease, a weight loss of at least 25% of the original body weight is a cardinal manifestation of mental disorder and is a serious sign.

All of the above manifestations are characteristics of *anorexia nervosa.*

Weight Losses in Children and Failure to Make Expected Weight Gains

Weight loss in children is likewise significant.

Children grow and need to grow.

For children of every age, there are norms for height, weight, and head circumference.

It can be determined from such tables of average weights how many pounds a child of say, 7 years old should be expected to gain by the time he is nine. Failure to make expected gains in weight that match accepted norms for age, and height, is a cardinal sign of mental disorder when it is not directly related to physical disease.

Since we can take the weight of a child of a given age, and determine how much weight the child should gain by the time he or she reaches any future age, we can determine what is called *projected weight gain* in passing from one age to another.

A child's loss of weight from his or her original body weight at a particular age, plus the projected weight gain that would be expected from these growth charts, may be combined to determine the overall effect of weight loss and failure to make projected weight gain; this is called *combined weight loss.*

Let us discuss this further. The average twelve year old girl weighs about ninety pounds. The average fourteen year old girl weighs about one hundred and eight pounds (these are the fiftieth percentiles). Thus, for a twelve year old girl, the projected weight gain in going from twelve years of age to fourteen years of age would be eighteen pounds (108 - 90 = 18). A twelve year old girl who weighs about ninety pounds, who *remains* at ninety pounds from age twelve to age fourteen has failed to make a projected weight gain of eighteen pounds.

Suppose that at age twelve she went on a diet, and stayed on it, so that while twelve, she dropped from her usual ninety pounds to seventy pounds, and weighed seventy pounds at age fourteen. Her original weight loss would be added to her failure to make the eighteen pound projected weight gain to give a combined total of thirty eight pounds.

If we looked only at how much weight she lost at age twelve by going from ninety pounds to seventy pounds, we would compute that she lost twenty two percent of her total body weight at age twelve. But by age fourteen, by maintaining her weight at seventy pounds, and failing to make the necessary projected weight gain of an additional eighteen pounds, we would calculate that her combined weight loss of thirtyeight pounds is actually a thirty five percent weight loss off the weight of a normal fourteen-year-old girl.

It is not necessary for a child to actually lose twenty five percent of his or her body weight at a particular age in order to have a cardinal manifestation of mental disorder.

What is necessary in the case of a child who is still growing, is that when we add together the failure to make a projected weight gain and the amount of weight that was lost off the original weight, *the total should be more than twenty five percent* of what a normal child would be expected to weigh.

Binges and Bulimia

Certain kinds of binge eating (the rapid consumption of a large amount of food in a discrete period of time, usually less than two hours) are a cardinal manifestation of mental disorder.

Fasting and binge eating may occur in the same person. When alternating binges and fasts produce frequent weight fluctuations greater than ten pounds, this is a cardinal manifestation of mental disorder.

A person who attempts to lose weight by severely restrictive diets, self-induced vomiting, or use of laxatives to induce diarrhea, or who take diuretics (water-loss pills), is exhibiting a cardinal manifestation of mental disorder.

Binge eaters who eat in secret for fear that others will see or know about their binges are also showing a cardinal sign.

Another sign is the consumption of high-calorie, easily indigested food during a binge.

A cardinal sign is shown by the patients who cannot stop eating voluntarily, or who fear that they cannot stop eating voluntarily, while being aware that their eating pattern is abnormal.

Cardinal manifestations involving such binge eating are called "Bulimia".

Pica

A patient who eats a non-nutritive substance such as hair or plaster persistently, is exhibiting the cardinal manifestation of the mental disorder known as *pica.* Some infants with pica may eat plaster, cloth, or hair. Children who are older may eat sand, mud, pebbles, or insects. Some children in schools are known to ingest large quantities of paste.

In such children there is no aversion to eating ordinary food, but there is persistent eating of these strange non-nutritive substances.

Such behavior is to be distinguished from the unusual diets of some children who refuse to try new foods, or who will eat foods of only certain textures (commonly seen in children with infantile autism).

Food Fads, Food Preferences, Peculiar Food Aversions

Some children have truly unusual food preferences and food aversions. These food fads or food aversions become important when they represent a child's resistance to change, as in the case of small children who have peculiar diets because they refuse to accept the eating of new foods. One such four-year-old child would eat only Rice Krispies that had been pulverized by his mother to a fine powder, and then mixed with water (not milk) and made into a thick sludge. The child refused other foods.

While certain food fads (vegetarianism) and food aversions ("eggs make me sick") have been pointed to by psychiatrists, psychoanalysts, and psychologists as indications of mental disorder DSM-III does not recognize that kind of behavior with food as significant, unless it falls under the category of bizarre behavior, represents resistance to change (as we discussed above), or occurs in association with one of the cardinal manifestations of mental disorder.

In this regard judgment has to be used. For example, a child who refused to eat eggs in any form and became panicky when confronted with eggs or with the prospect of having to eat them, and who avoided eggs because she was completely convinced that she would become pregnant if she ate one, would need to be carefully approached to determine how pervasive the idea was, how shakable the idea was, how closely it was related to ideas held by members of her family, and how it might have been related to stories she had been told that she swallowed whole and uncritically, before the examiner decides that this is part of a pattern of bizarre behavior or represents bizarre ideas or delusions in a child.

Similarly, an adult who behaved the same way towards eggs, believing that they would make her pregnant, would have to be questioned to determine whether this was a false belief that was unshakable and not explainable by her social or cultural background, in order to assess whether it represented a delusion.

Vomiting and Rumination

Vomiting is a cardinal manifestation of *physical* disease.

Self-induced vomiting for the purpose of losing weight is a cardinal manifestation of mental disorder.

When infants self-induce vomiting, it is a cardinal manifestation of mental disorder. Such infants bring up the contents of their stomach and may either eject it from their mouths, chew the contents and reswallow them or allow it to dribble out of their mouths. This problem in infants is called *rumination,* and comes from the chewing or swishing around in the mouth of the regurgitated stomach contents that some of these infants appear to enjoy. (It has nothing to do with rumination as discussed under disorders of thought, where an individual "chews" a thought over and over in his or her mind).

Any infant who cannot retain feedings suffers from a serious problem.

When regurgitation in infants cannot be shown to be vomiting due to a physical disorder, then rumination needs to be considered.

Grief

Patients with *uncomplicated bereavement* may not eat. This is not a cardinal manifestation of mental disorder as we have discussed under uncomplicated bereavement. (See page 106).

Significant *weight loss* that occurred in an individual following the death of a close relative, due to disinterest in food and poor appetite, would represent a complication of the bereavement. The bereavement would no longer be uncomplicated, since now it would have the complication of significant serious loss of weight.

In such individuals, other cardinal manifestations of mental disorder should be looked for.

SELF-STUDY QUESTIONS, CHAPTER 14

1. Define insomnia.

   Answer: It is a disturbance in falling asleep or remaining asleep.

2. What are the names of the three kinds of insomnia? Explain each one.

   Answer: There are three kinds of insomnia: initial, middle, and terminal. Initial insomnia is difficulty falling asleep. Middle insomnia is waking up during the night, being up for a time, and then going back to sleep. Terminal insomnia is waking up several hours before one's customary time to awaken, and being unable to return to sleep.

3. What is early morning awakening? How is it related to terminal insomnia?

   Answer: Early morning awakening is waking up several hours before one's customary time and being unable to return to sleep. Early morning awakening and terminal insomnia are two names for the same problem.

4. What is meant by the sleep-wake cycle? If a person usually slept at night and was awake during the day, what might we expect to result from a disturbance in their sleep-waking cycle?

   Answer: The sleep-wake cycle is the patients' usual rhythm or pattern to their periods of sleeping and waking. Patients who usually slept at night and were awake during the day would show a disturbance in their sleep-wake cycle if they were up at night and slept during the day—such individuals might show daytime drowsiness with or without insomnia.

5. What is important about REM sleep?

   Answer: REM sleep is the period or phase of sleep where dreaming occurs.

6. What is a nightmare?

   Answer: A nightmare is an unpleasant dream that may arouse the dreamer from sleep.

7. What are the important characteristics of nightmares?

8. Discuss sleep terror.

9. In what phase of sleep (REM or NREM) do nightmares occur?

   Answer: Nightmares occur during REM sleep.

10. In what phase of sleep do sleep terrors occur?

    Answer: NREM sleep.

11. Of what significance is a panicky cry in distinguishing a nightmare from a sleep terror?

    Answer: A sleep terror is usually accompanied by a panicky cry, whereas a nightmare is not.

12. Of what significance is the patient's being able to recall a dream that was unpleasant and aroused him or her from sleep?

    Answer: If he or she can recall a dream in detail that was unpleasant and aroused him or her from sleep, it is probably a nightmare. Sleep terrors are not accompanied by such capacity to recall.

13. If a child slept usually nine hours each night, in what part of his sleep period would we expect a nightmare to occur? In what part would we expect a sleep terror to occur? In what period would we expect a sleepwalking episode to occur?

    Answer: A nightmare would occur in the last six hours. A sleep terror in the first three hours. A sleep walking episode would occur in the first three hours.

14. Describe sleep walking. Do sleep walkers go back to bed? What of a child who sat up in bed during the night, appeared to be in a daze and then lay down and went back to sleep?

15. What sleep disturbances are associated with quantity of sleep?

    Answer: Sleeping too much or sleeping too little. Note: *hypersomnia* is the term used to describe sleeping too much.

16. What emotion or mood has insomnia as one of the physiologic changes?

    Answer: Depression (generalized anxiety can manifest insomnia also).

17. A person who had a decreased need for sleep differs how from the patients with insomnia?

    Answer: Patients with insomnia usually complain that they would like to be able to sleep but have trouble or that they want to go back to bed but are woken up prematurely in the morning for some unexplained reason.

18. What is pica? Give examples of things that children with pica might eat.

19. How much weight does a person have to lose off of their original body weight in order for us to consider their weight loss to be serious and a major manifestation of a mental disorder if it has no physical cause?

    Answer: Twenty-five percent or more.

20. In growing children who lost weight at a particular age, how would we determine the significance of their weight one year later if they still weighed considerably less than other children of that age?

    Answer: Determine from standard tables what the expected weight gain would be in growing over that one year period, and add it to the amount of weight they had lost at the beginning of the one year period. The combined amount in pounds is the amount that would be figured against what they should weigh a year later in order to determine the percentage of combined weight loss.

21. In doing such a problem, what percentage off the current weight (taking into consideration original weight loss and failure to make projected weight gain) would be significant.

Answer: A weight difference of twenty-five percent or more.

22. Why would anorexia not be considered a major sign of mental disorder in uncomplicated bereavement? What additional bodily change would be necessary in order for us to consider that something serious had occurred?

    Answer: Disinterest in food or lack of appetite commonly accompanies grief. Significant weight loss during the period of bereavement would be a complication.

23. Explain rumination in infants.

24. Discuss some behaviors in relation to dieting, fasting, weight loss, and being fat that are cardinal manifestations of mental disorder.

25. *Psychomotor epilepsy always* needs to be distinguished from sleep terror. Some EEG Labs in Children's Hospitals test a large number of children every year just for this. *Psychomotor epilepsy* may be a sign of more serious trouble, and psychomotor epilepsy has a special treatment that is different from the treatment of sleep terror, (which is not a sign of neurological problems as is epilepsy). Therefore the two conditions often need to be distinguished.

    In sleep terror there is a panicky cry or scream. This is not usually the case with psychomotor epilepsy. Psychomotor epilepsy occurring at night also needs to be distinguished from sleep walking. In sleep walking patients very often return to bed and go to sleep without waking up. This is not the case with psychomotor epilepsy. In psychomotor epilepsy patients usually do not get out of bed but may only sit up in bed and go through some repetitive meaningless movements. But if they do get out of bed, they rarely, if ever, return on their own.

26. *Case Study*

    A seven-year-old girl was found severely injured one morning outside of her house beside a tree in the backyard. For some months before that, the family had had problems with the patient getting out of bed and walking around the house during the night, apparently in a daze. The family had even locked the doors every night to keep her from walking out of the house and going out into the street.

    What do you think was the matter with this girl?

    Answer: Probably sleep walking, since the behavior was so complex. Psychomotor epilepsy usually involves sitting up in bed and making repeated steretoyped movements and doesn't usually result in the patient getting out of bed and walking around. This was a case that could be called *"sleep-climbing"* because the girl had gone out of the house and climbed the tree as part of a sleepwalking episode, and then fallen out of it and injured herself seriously. Naturally you would need to know much more about the girl, her history, and maybe have some EEG studies taken during the night in order to make a firm diagnosis of sleep walking versus psychomotor epilepsy.

27. What two disturbances of going to sleep and of sleep are manifestations of separation anxiety?

    Answer: Persistent reluctance to go to sleep without being next to a major attachment figure, or similar refusal to go to sleep away from home, as well as having sleep disturbed repeatedly with nightmares that have themes of separation from parents.

chapter 15

Physiologic Changes and Physical Complaints, Part 2

Increased Energy

Increased energy, described earlier as a physiologic change in the discussion of manic mood, is a cardinal manifestation of mental disorder. Such patients may say that they have unusually large amounts of energy, or it may be inferred by observing that they perform large amounts of work, being quite productive, while suffering no fatigue or feelings of tiredness.

Decreased Energy

Decreased energy may be a complaint by the patient or it may be inferred because the patient seems less able to perform his usual everyday tasks without tiredness. Lack of energy and easy fatigability can be a cardinal manifestation of *physical disorder*. Taken by itself, decreased energy and easy fatigability is a manifestation of mental disorder only when physical disorders are ruled out.

It might be supposed that individuals who go on prolonged fasts and lose more than twenty-five percent of their body weight as a result might be tired. This is not the case. Most such individuals have normal activity levels, or are more active than normal (hyperactive). This is one of the ways we distinguish such a weight loss (on the basis of overall activity level) from similiar weight loss resulting from serious physical illness. (Weight loss from physical illness is *usually* accompanied by a drop in activity level, but not always - for example in cases of hyperthyroidism (overactive thyroid gland).

In addition, the use of certain drugs, or withdrawal from drugs, can result either in increased activity (such as in people who drink large amounts of coffee with apparent inexhaustability), or patients can seem extremely and easily fatigued.

PHYSIOLOGIC CHANGES ASSOCIATED WITH
DRUG INTOXICATION, AND DRUG WITHDRAWAL

The changes that we are going to discuss here we will discuss only briefly. Each is a physiologic change that is an important manifestation of the mental disorders that relate to *intoxication from, and withdrawal from drugs,* but any one of them can occur in specific physical diseases as well.

They include effects on speech, such as slurring, and effects on overall coordination and ability to walk, such as incoordination and an unsteady gait (ataxia).

They include effects on the eyes, including dilated pupils, constricted pupils, and rapid side-to-side movements of the eyes known as *"nystagmus".*

They may include nausea and vomiting. Changes in blood pressure may occur, either increased blood pressure or a tendency of the blood pressure to fall severely when individuals go from a lying or seated position to an erect posture: in such cases they may actually feel faint and dizzy (orthostatic hypotention). They may include lacrimation (watering of the eyes); they may include some of the changes that we saw under *autonomic hyperactivity* (See above page 114) including rapid heart beat, piloerection, sweating, dry mouth, and so on.

Fever may occur; redness of the eyes may occur (conjunctival injection). Other changes involving the body, such as coarse tremor of hands, tongue, and eyelids; irregular heart beat (cardiac arrhythmia), diarrhea, blurring of vision, flushing of the face, are all physiologic changes that may accompany either drug overuse or the drug withdrawal (withdrawal refers to a person who has been using a drug for some time who either reduces his usual dosage or stops using it completely).

These physiologic changes are cardinal manifestations of mental disorder for DSM-III when their significance as signs and symptoms of other physical illnesses has been ruled out.

PSYCHOLOGICAL FACTORS AFFECTING
PHYSICAL CONDITION

Here there is a demonstrable physical illness that produces structural damage to the body, such as peptic ulcer disease, or rheumatoid arthritis (peptic ulcer disease produces changes in the lining of the gastrointestinal tract that can be seen on x-rays and by other tests; rheumatoid arthritis produces structural damage to joints), but some psychological factor is related to the onset, the causation, the worsening, or to the reappearance of episodes of the physical illness.

Case Illustration

A nineteen-year-old college student who suffered from diagnosed peptic ulcer disease was referred for psychiatric treatment by the college health service because he experienced severe symptoms of his disease each time he had to take an examination in his college courses.

The distinctive relationship of reappearance of serious symptoms of ulcer disease to stress on the patient (taking exams) is an example of a psychological factor affecting a physical condition.

Major life changes and major life stresses are psychological factors affecting physical condition that are of great importance, and research has shown that they can be associated with the onset and worsening of major physical illnesses such as heart disease, stroke, and cancer. Some research has shown that in the case of the death of a spouse, the death rate of the surviving spouse in the first year after the death is six to seven times higher than that of the general population of the same age, where this is a death rate from *all* causes of death.

A situation where a psychological factor is related to the onset or the worsening of a real physical illness is a cardinal manifestation of mental disorder.

PHYSICAL COMPLAINTS NOT ASSOCIATED WITH REAL PHYSICAL DISEASE

Whenever patients complain about their health, or have specific complaints of physical symptoms, or complaints that sound referable to a physical illness, but where no physical illness can be demonstrated by competent medical studies, then a cardinal manifestation of mental disorder is present.

This includes the cases where some physical disorder can be demonstrated, but where the physical disorder is insufficient to account for the degree of trouble that the patient experiences or reports.

There have been numerous studies that suggest that each year about one third of the patients who see their family doctor have no real physical illness that underlies their complaints or symptoms, and that in another one third, disease is found but it cannot fully explain the complaints and symptoms that these patients have. Thus in about two thirds of all persons who consult a physician about physical complaints and symptoms, something is happening that cannot be explained on the basis of physical disease of the body.

Because of the importance of these problems to medicine and to psychiatry, and because it always seems hard for persons to understand this area of mental disorder, we shall try to give a careful explanation of these cardinal manifestations.

Whenever a patient appears to have a loss of physical functioning, or an alteration in physical functioning that suggests a physical disorder but which instead is shown not to be due to a physical disorder, then a cardinal manifestation of mental disorder is present.

These complaints by patients often suggest disease of the nervous system, such as paralysis, seizures, weakness of an arm, a leg, or a hand, blindness, loss of sensation on the hand, foot, or other part of the body, apparent disturbance of coordination, unsteadiness of gait, tunnel vision (a problem where the patient complains that he can only see what is in the very center of what would be his normal field of vision—as though he were looking at things through a long tunnel or tube), inability to smell, or sensations such as pins and needles, or sensations of electric shocks.

Vomiting without any basis in physical illness can occur. Vomiting is a condition usually associated with serious physical illness, but can also occur in response to psychological factors.

A devoutly Jewish woman attended a banquet where, unknown to her, pork was served; the woman said the meal was delicious but when she was told in the parking lot of the restaurant that she had eaten pork, she instantly suffered prolonged and violent vomiting. Here, bodily function, such as vomiting, is strongly and instantly affected by a psychological factor.

Vomiting that is not explainable by physical illness and is a predominant complaint, or part of a pattern of other complaints about physical illness, for which no basis can be found, is a cardinal manifestation of mental disorder.

Pseudocyesis is a condition where some or all of the signs of pregnancy appear in a woman who is not pregnant. These signs can include vomiting and nausea (simulating morning sickness); it can include an enlargement of the abdomen (in such cases usually due to the swallowing of air and its retention in the gastrointestinal tract); and importantly, it can involve amenorrhea (no mentrual periods). The picture of pregnancy is closely simulated; these signs of apparent pregnancy occur involuntarily, leading the patient to conclude that she is pregnant and to seek medical attention.

The appearance of "blindness" in soldiers witnessing horrors of combat, where medical examination of the eyes and the nerve pathways of vision demonstrate that no physical abnormalities exist, have been common enough.

A complete loss of the voice with inability to utter even a sound, when vocal chords and nerve pathways to the larynx (voice-box) are intact, is another example. Such loss of the voice would be called *aphonia*.

A story is often told of a famous psychoanalyst who was visited by an equally renowned opera singer who had suddenly lost her voice and was seeking emergency treatment so she could perform that night on stage. After learning the facts of her case as told by others and as written down by her (remember, she was unable to talk), he concluded that she had lost her voice the previous night after a date with her fiance who insisted that she engage in fellatio and threatened never to see her again if she refused. It is reported that the renowned psychoanalyst excused himself from the office and went across the street to a delicatessen where he purchased a frankfurter. He returned to the office keeping the frankfurter hidden behind his back and suddenly surprised her by sticking it directly in front of her mouth, whereupon she let out a loud scream, was cured, and was able to perform on stage that night.

The opera star who lost her voice and the soldier on the battle field who lost his eyesight were both patients who had no physical abnormality of the organs involved, but had clear loss of function of a part of the body, apparently related to a psychological stress.

We have just discussed how psychological factors might be related to the cause or worsening of *real physical illnesses.* What we are speaking of now is psychological factors related to something that *sounds like* (and can look like) a physical illness where no physical illness can be demonstrated. Furthermore, we are not talking about conditions that are faked. These patients, the opera star and the combat soldier, experienced their symptoms as something that they could not voluntarily overcome. The appearance and persistence of the loss of function (loss of voice or loss of eyesight) was not intentional—it was not related to the conscious intention of the patient—the loss of physical functioning was involuntary, while nevertheless being related to a psychological factor that was judged to be causally related to the symptom.

In the case of the opera singer, *her distress over having to choose* between performing a sexual act distasteful to her or suffering the painful loss of her fiance, was the apparent psychological factor.

The battlefield soldier, who went blind after seeing close friends killed in a mutilating explosion, lost the use of his eyes in relation to a psychological factor.

We judge that a psychological factor is related to the appearance of the symptom when there is a relationship among something that happens in the environment, a psychological conflict or need, and the beginning or worsening of the symptom.

In such cases we also conclude that a cardinal manifestation of mental disorder is present: a loss or alteration of physical functioning has occurred not due to a physical illness.

Let us look at an example. Study this carefully as it is important to distinguish these manifestations of mental disorder from instances where loss of physical function is *deliberately faked* (consciously and deliberately produced by the patient - not loss of function that arises apparently *involuntarily* as we have been discussing).

Case Illustration

An unassertive and timid right-handed man became involved in an argument with his wife and became intensely angry. He then got drunk and threatened to hit her. She told him if he "laid a hand on her" she would "call the police" and moreover, said she would "leave him". He immediately suffered severe anxiety. He withdrew from this confrontation with his wife into another room of the house whereupon he discovered that his right arm was paralyzed. The arm remained paralyzed, and necessitated visits to a neurologist and other medical specialists who could not explain the sudden loss of function on the basis of any physical disorder. All findings on every possible medical test and examination showed that his right arm should have functioned normally.

This man who was faced with the *conflict* over whether or not to beat his wife, suffered *severe anxiety* as a result. His right arm, by becoming paralyzed, solved the conflict, and allowed him to avoid an activity that was noxious to him—namely hitting his wife, together with the likely result that he would be confronted with police and probably be divorced by his wife.

Physical loss or alteration of function of part of the body apparently due to physical illness (but which can not be explained by physical illness) that arises and is maintained involuntarily and is related to a psychological factor that appears to cause it, was once thought to be due to a converting of emotional problems into physical ones. In this theory the "energy" involved in the psychological conflict became "converted" into a physical loss of function, usually involving a part of the body that had a symbolic relationship to some feature of the conflict.

In this theory we would say that "the energy" involved in the man's conflict over whether to beat or not to beat his wife "had been converted" and turned into the physical loss of function of the right arm which has a "symbolic" relationship to the nature of the conflict, namely the beating of his wife. (He was right-handed and would have hit her with his right hand.)

Although the symptom arises involuntarily, the loss of function of part of the body may additionally allow the patient to receive support from his environment that he might not otherwise get. People may feel sorry for him because they believe that he is physically ill, so that persons who lose function of part of the body involuntarily as part of avoiding a noxious activity may gain something more in addition.

The old theory that describe these kinds of problems as a "converting" of an "emotional energy" into a physical problem supplies the name for this cardinal manifestation of mental disorder; we call all such cardinal manifestations *conversion symptoms*.

PAIN

Our discussion of conversion symptoms focused on loss or alteration of function of part of the body that could appear to be caused by a physical illness but which really wasn't. When severe and prolonged pain is the apparent physical problem, and where the pain has all of the features of conversion symptom we have already discussed, we refer to it as *psychogenic pain*. It is a cardinal manifestation of mental disorder.

These are prolonged and severe pains that, like conversion symptoms, have either a relationship to an event or stimulus in the environment that is related to a psychological conflict or need, and which is related to the onset or worsening of the pain. The appearance of the pain enables the individual to avoid some activity that is noxious to him or her, or enables the individual to get support from the environment that might not otherwise be forthcoming. Such pain is shown by thorough medical studies not to be due to any real physical disorder, or if a real physical disorder is present, the pain is grossly in excess of what would be expected from the findings of the physical disease that is present.

Thus, in the case above of the man who lost the function of his right arm, if he instead developed an excruciating severe pain in his right arm after he withdrew from the confrontation with his wife, where the pain persisted, requiring the same kind of extensive medical investigation that turned up no physical illness, the man would have the manifestation of psychogenic pain.

Here again, the pain would be related to the *conflict* over whether to hit or not to hit his wife, the conflict would be solved by the severe pain, and he would escape from an activity that would have been noxious to him (hitting his wife).

If the man whose arm became paralyzed, or whose arm was in severe pain, stopped going to work while he went from doctor to doctor seeking help for the apparent physical problem, and began to collect disability payments while undergoing medical studies for his unexplained and incapacitating physical complaints, he would have gained something in addition—being able to collect money without going to work. Although the symptoms of paralysis or pain would continue to be involuntarily maintained, something in addition would be gained from the environment over and above escaping from the original conflict of whether to hit or not to hit the wife at the time of the argument.

What the person gains from the original appearance of the symptom is often referred to as the *"primary gain"*. The primary gain for the man who couldn't decide whether or not to hit his wife was an escape from that unpleasant conflict.

The protracted period of being able to collect disability and not work that came to him, in addition, as a result of having the physical problem, was his *"secondary gain"*.

It is important to distinguish conversion symptom and psychogenic pain from situations where individuals *fake* loss of function, perhaps claiming to have pains solely for the purpose of staying out of work and collecting insurance. In the case of conversion symptoms and psychogenic pain, the apparent physical problem arises *involuntarily* and the maintenance of it is *not under the conscious control of the patient*. He cannot make it stop on his own. Patients who fake pains or disabilities are different. Fakers may be manifesting behavior that is nevertheless a major manifestation of mental disorder, if it is part of a pattern of dishonesty, or if the faking, or excuse-making through complaints about physical illness, is part of other problems in occupational functioning as we discussed above under the subject of the *antisocial work manifestation* (see page 36). Fakers who have a *recognizable goal,* such as not having to work while being supported by insurance, avoiding jury duty, avoiding military service, or avoiding trial for a crime by simulating complaints of physical illness, are called "malingerers".

Some persons fake the complaints or the signs of physical illness *without such a recognizable goal,* doing it only to assume the role of being patients in a hospital. Patients who fake the signs of symptoms of illness without any clear recognizable goal and who do it only to become patients in a hospital and receive various kinds of medical treatment that they do not need have a cardinal manifestation of mental disorder called the *factitious manifestation.*

Persons who fake symptoms who are in pursuit of a goal that is obviously recognizable when the person's circumstances are understood, such as a narcotic addict who complains of serious pain and asks the doctor to prescribe pain medication, hoping to receive a narcotic, is said to be *malingering.* Malingering is not a cardinal manifestation of mental disorder. *Malingering, factitious manifestation, conversion symptom, and psychogenic pain, all need to be distinguished from one another.*

HEADACHE

Headaches receive special treatment from DSM-III now that it has been shown that tension of the muscles of the head (of the forehead, of the sides of the head and of the back of the 'neck—frontal, temporal, masseter, occipital, and nuchal muscle groups) is a demonstrable physical cause of headaches in patients where a psychological factor is related to the headache.

Since the muscle spasm is a known physical cause, such cases would not be regarded as instances of psychogenic pain (psychogenic pain is defined as not having a demonstrable physical cause). Tension headaches are an instance of psychological factors affecting physical condition rather than of psychogenic pain.

There is no way, on the basis of how the human body is put together, or on the basis of what is known about the functioning of the human body, to explain the production of pain or the loss of function in patients with conversion symptom or psychogenic pain.

PERSONS WITH MULTIPLE AND RECURRING COMPLAINTS ABOUT PHYSICAL PROBLEMS OF SEVERAL YEARS DURATION: SOMATIZATION

Some patients display a cardinal manifestation of mental disorder of having multiple and recurrent physical complaints of several years duration.

Such patients complain not about one problem, and not about two or three, but about a large number of different kinds of complaints, none of which can be adequately explained by a physical disorder or physical injury, and none of which are side effects of medicine, drugs, or alcohol.

To be said to have this manifestation of mental disorder, a patient would need to have taken some action about the physical complaint or symptoms, such as taking medicine other than aspirin, altering their life style, or consulting a doctor.

This is the manifestation which we will call *somatization*.

HYPOCHONDRIASIS

Patients who have unreasonable fear that they have a serious illness after medical evidence to the contrary has been gently and carefully explained to them, suffer the cardinal manifestation of mental disorder called *hypochondriasis*.

Hypochondriacal delusions were discussed above (page 86), and differ from hypochondriasis in that the patient with hypochondriasis can entertain the possibility that the disease they are afraid to have may not be present, while the patient who has a hypochondriacal delusion is unable to do this.

Persons who interpret physical sensations within their own bodies as signs of physical illness, where these sensations are really only what ordinary people might experience if they paid attention to what their body is doing, are also said to manifest *hypochondriasis* when their interpretation of, or close attention to bodily events and sensations are evidence to them that they suffer from a serious disease.

Everyone's heart beats. When a person's heart stops beating, the person dies. A person's heart beats all day and all night, whether they are at rest or whether they are exerting themselves. Most ordinary people pay little attention to the beating of their own heart.

But some persons pay particularly close attention to the beating of their heart, perhaps taking their pulse frequently, and becoming alarmed when their heart speeds up and slows down as part of its daily work. Such a person who claimed that "there is something wrong with me" would be exhibiting this variety of hypochondriasis.

Certain aches and pains are part of everyday life. Even the greatest athletes, when they overexert themselves, may experience aches and pains either in the process of overexertion or afterwards. Paying unusually close attention to one's aches and pains and interpreting them as signs of serious illness, when these are judged by competent medical examination and history-taking to lie within the realm of degrees of discomfort that are normal under the patient's circumstances, is a cardinal manifestation of mental disorder, and it is also called hypochondriasis.

Some Physiologic Changes and Physical Complaints as Cardinal
Manifestations of Mental Disorder that are Discussed in this Section

	Type of Problem	Physical Illness Responsible?	Arises How	Gain Derived
Psychological Factor Affecting Physical Condition	physical symptoms	yes	psychological factor influences real disease	
Conversion Symptom	loss of, or alteration of function of part of body	no	involuntary	may allow person to escape from noxious situation or receive support from environment not otherwise forthcoming
Psychogenic Pain	pain	no	involuntary	may allow person to escape from noxious situation or receive support from environment not otherwise forthcoming
Somatization	over the years many, many, physical complaints	no	involuntary	
Malingering	any physical complaint	no	faked	recognizable goal exists
Factitious Manifestation	any physical complaint	no	faked	no recognizable goal other than being a patient
Hypochondriasis	fear of serious illness	no	involuntary	

SEXUAL DYSFUNCTIONS

When we talk about the relationship between the body and the mind, a subject of philosophers for centuries, there is probably no better example of the interaction between mental and physical than sexual function.

Sexual excitement is an emotion with an internal subjective experience of excitement (affect), characteristic physiologic changes, and characteristic behavior.

Persons can cause themselves to be sexually aroused by thinking about images or other sensory stimuli that they consider arousing, and then can develop corresponding physiologic changes indicative of sexual excitement, such as erection of the penis in the male, and erection of the clitoris and nipples in the female, without there being any external stimulus. A person can be "turned on" by just a thought.

Similarly individuals who become sexually aroused can diminish their sexual arousal ("turn themselves off") by thinking about something else, perhaps something repugnant or anxiety provoking.

Indeed, the only aphrodisiac that has ever been discovered is the mind.

Physical diseases can affect the desire to have sexual relationships and can impair performance, in spite of desire, by preventing the physiologic manifestations that are essential to performing sexual activities. Certain drugs and diseases may impair erection of the penis and prevent coitus, in spite of a person's wish to have sexual intercourse. Certain diseases in the male can prevent ejaculation, and therefore prevent orgasm. Corresponding drug effects and effects of physical disease occur in women.

But the influence of the mind in normal sexual functioning is striking. Some persons can become sexually aroused and even achieve orgasm without any physical contact whatsoever—from only a thought.

In the absence of physical disease, the influence of the mind as the cause of various sexual difficulties is equally striking. The impairments of sexual functioning and performance specifically related to the effects of the mind are cardinal manifestations of mental disorder; they are called *psychosexual dysfunctions.* They are distinguished from a different group of problems in sexual relations known as *paraphilias,* that do not involve impaired performance, but deal with unique varieties of sexual preference for certain activities or situations in sexual activity. An example of a paraphilia known as zoophilia, is a person whose preferred mode of sexual excitement leading to orgasm involves animals.

The psychosexual dysfunctions that are cardinal manifestations of mental disorder do not concern the patient's preferred mode of achieving sexual excitement leading to orgasm, but rather grant that when the person is indulging in their preferred mode, they experience inhibited sexual excitement, or have inhibited sexual desire, or that they are unable to achieve orgasm or achieve orgasm prematurely. The descriptions of psychosexual dysfunctions in DSM-III do seem to presume, for the most part, that the person does at least have a living human sex partner.

Inhibited sexual desire is a cardinal manifestation of mental disorder. It is a persistent and pervasive inhibition of sexual desire, taking into account the person's age, sex, health, and intensity and frequency of sexual desire, and the social and cultural context of the individual's life.

Inhibited sexual excitement is recurrent and persistent inhibition of sexual excitement during sexual activity. In males it is shown by partial or complete failure to attain or maintain erection until completion of the sexual act. In women it is shown by a partial or complete failure to attain or maintain the lubrication - swelling response of sexual excitement until completion of the sexual act.

Problems in inhibited sexual excitement require that a judgment be made that the individual does engage in sexual activity that is adequate in its focus, intensity, and duration, so that ordinary persons would be expected to achieve or maintain the physiological responses affected.

Inhibited female orgasm is a cardinal manifestation of mental disorder involving recurrent and persistent inhibition of female orgasm, as manifested by a delay in, or the absence of, orgasm following a normal sexual excitement phase during sexual activity that is judged by the examiner to be adequate in its focus, intensity, and duration.

Inhibited male orgasm is a cardinal manifestation of mental disorder. It is recurrent and persistent inhibition of male orgasm as manifested by a delay in, or absence of, ejaculation following an adequate phase of sexual excitement.

Premature ejaculation is a cardinal manifestation of mental disorder where ejaculation occurs before the individual wishes it, because of recurrent and persistent absence of reasonable voluntary control of ejaculation and orgasm during sexual activity.

Here a judgment of "reasonable control" is made by taking into account factors that affect duration of the excitement phase of sexual activity, such as age, novelty of the sexual partner, and the frequency and duration of sexual intercourse.

Functional Dyspareunia is a complaint of pain, experienced during the act of coitus, in either men or women, where the pain is recurrent and persistent and where it interferes with sexual relations.

Functional Vaginismus is a recurrent and persistent involuntary spasm of the muscles of the outer third of the vagina that interferes with coitus. Some women can voluntarily contract the muscles of the vagina. Functional Vaginismus is an involuntary spasm and creates an interference with the sex act.

HUMAN SEXUAL RESPONSE — THE FOUR STAGES

Our current understanding of the physiological changes that occur during sexual excitement leading to orgasm customarily discuss four phases of sexual activity.

Excitement – First Stage

The first phase, called the *excitement phase,* is brought on by the stimulation of the presence of a sex partner, or by fantasy, or by physical stimulation of kissing, or by touching, or any combination of these. In men erection occurs, and in women vaginal lubrication takes place, usually occurring within ten seconds of whatever constitutes effective stimulation. In both sexes the nipples usually become erect, and in women the clitoris becomes hard. In women the labia majora and labia minora become observably thicker as the result of engorgement by venous blood. An excitement phase of sex can last only a few minutes, or it can last up to several hours.

Plateau – Second Stage

If stimulation continues, other physiologic changes occur in a second stage leading to orgasm, called the *plateau phase.* During the plateau phase, other physiologic changes occur in women. Breast size increases twenty-five percent, the clitoris lifts up and retracts under the bony part of the pelvis that lies across the lower abdomen (known as the symphysis pubis) and the clitoris is then no longer accessible. The outer third of the vagina constricts, a change which is called the orgasmic platform.

In men, as part of the plateau phase, the testes become fifty percent larger and move closer to the body within the scrotal sac.

The duration of the plateau phase between excitement and orgasm varies from time to time, and from person to person, and can last anywhere from half a minute to several minutes. (The plateau phase is short and goes rapidly to orgasm—it is the excitement (first) phase that is highly variable and can be very long (hours) or too short before plateau begins).

Orgasm – Third Stage

When orgasm occurs the third phase of sexual activity is reached and has characteristic physiologic changes that have been studied. In men orgasm involves four to five rhythmic spasms of the prostate gland, the semenal vesicles, the vas deferens, and the urethra, and has characteristic sensations for the man, and is accompanied by a spurt of semen from the penis.

Orgasm in women involves anywhere from three to twelve involuntary contractions of the muscles that form the orgasmic platform of the vagina. In both men and women, involuntary contractions of the external and internal anal sphincter occurs. In both men and women heart rate becomes rapid and blood pressure increases.

Resolution – Fourth Stage

In the fourth phase of sexual relations known as resolution, there is a reduction in, and disappearance of, the physiologic changes that have characterized the previous three phases. In men, blood that had engorged the penis, and in women blood that had engorged the labia and clitoris, now leaves those organs gradually as processes of erection and engorgement diminish. The body returns to the state it was in before sexual excitement.

Persons in the health profession who wish to use DSM-III should familiarize themselves with the physiologic and psychological changes accompanying normal sexual relationships, perhaps by reading a book like "Human Sexual Response" by W. H. Masters and V. E. Johnson, Little Brown, Boston, 1966. Here, we can only give the briefest of descriptions of this important area of concern in mental health and social relationships.

It is emphasized once more that the psychosexual dysfunctions are a cardinal manifestation of mental disorder so long as there is *no physical disease* or drug related problem that accounts for them.

PHYSICAL ILLNESS CONSIDERED AS A LIFE STRESS

In all cases where there is definite physical disease or definite physical injury, the presence of the physical problem may act as a stress on the patient and be associated with other manifestations of mental disorder, over and beyond whatever effect could be created by the physical illness or injury itself, or by the specific treatments used to manage the physical disease or the injury.

SELF-STUDY QUESTIONS, CHAPTER 15

1. Discuss conversion symptom. What are three manifestations of mental disorder involving a conversion symptom?

   Answer: A conversion symptom is a loss or change in the function of part of the body, not explainable by a real physical illness or injury after competent medical examinations have been done. Conversion symptoms can arise when there is an environmental stimulus that is judged to be causally related to the onset or worsening of the loss or change in function of the body part, where the conversion symptom allows the person to escape from an otherwise noxious situation *or* where the conversion symptom allows the person to obtain support from the environment that would otherwise not be forthcoming.

2. Discuss psychogenic pain. How is it related to a conversion symptom?

   Answer: The concept is virtually identical, but instead of loss or change of function, there is a complaint of pain.

3. What kind of pain, even if it seems psychogenic, should not be thought of immediately as a psychogenic pain until pain from muscle tension is excluded?

Answer: Headache—muscle tension headaches need to be excluded.

4. Explain somatization as a manifestation of mental disorder.

Answer: Somatization is a history of several years of frequent complaints about a variety of physical problems, none of which are explainable by the presence of a real physical disorder, and about which the individual took some action in each case, such as taking medicine other than aspirin, changing his or her life style or habits, or consulting a physician.

5. Explain complaints about physical illness that are said to be factitious.

Answer: Factitious complaints are faked but they are done purely for the purpose of assuming the role of a patient and have no clearly recognizable goal other than that, when the patient's social background and cultural circumstances are taken into account.

6. How are conversion symptoms and psychogenic pain different from faking?

Answer: The loss of function or change in function of a part of the body in conversion symptom, and the pain in psychogenic pain, arises *involuntarily* and continues against the apparent conscious wishes of the individual - this differs from faking where the person *deliberately* tries to give people the impression that he has a physical illness either by complaining of a symptom or by creating circumstances that lead other people to believe that he is sick, such as holding a thermometer under a hot water faucet to give people the impression that he has a fever.

7. Explain hypochondriasis.

Answer: Hypochondriasis is an unreasonable fear of having a serious illness, and includes instances where persons overemphasize or become alarmed about bodily sensations and processes as part of their attempt to look for evidence that they suffer from a serious disease.

8. How does hypochondriasis differ from hypochondriacal delusions?

Answer: In hypochondriacal delusions, the patient has an unshakable false belief that he or she suffers from a serious disease. In hypochondriasis the patient can at least entertain the possibility that he or she may be wrong.

9. Name four specific neurological difficulties that while indicating real physical disorder, are cardinal signs of mental illness, in that DSM-III uses them as part of a specific disease category cluster.

Answer: Aphasia, apraxia, agnosia, and constructional difficulty.

10. Give a brief explanation of aphasia, apraxia, agnosia, and constructional difficulty.

11. How are psychological factors affecting physical condition different from conversion symptom?

Answer: Conversion symptoms are loss or change in functioning of a part of the body that has no explanation in terms of real physical disease. Whereas *psychological factors affecting physical condition* do affect a real physical illness that is present in the patient.

12. What is malingering? Is malingering a cardinal manifestation of mental disorder?

Answer: Malingering is pretending to have an illness for the purpose of achieving some goal that is clearly understandable when one takes into account a person's life circumstances. An example is pretending to be sick so that one does not have to go to work. Malingering is not considered a cardinal manifestation of mental disorder by DSM-III.

13. What is the only aphrodisiac that has ever been discovered?

Answer: The mind.

14. What are the four phases of a sexual encounter that begins with excitement?

Answer: Stage one, excitement, stage two, plateau, stage three, orgasm, stage four, resolution.

15. Review the four stages and try to describe in your own words what happens in each stage in both men and women.

16. What is a paraphilia? What is a psychosexual dysfunction?

Answer: A paraphilia is a cardinal manifestation of a mental disorder involving sexual behavior where a person has a preferred mode of obtaining sexual excitement and orgasm not involving coitus with a live, consenting, human sexual partner.

A psychosexual dysfunction usually presumes the existence of a live, human, consenting sex partner of either sex, but focuses on difficulties in sexual desire, sexual excitement, and orgasm in sexual relations with a partner, usually revolving around a coital act.

17. Name the seven kinds of cardinal manifestations of mental disorder that are included under psychosexual dysfunction. Explain each one in your own words.

Answer: The seven kinds are: inhibited sexual desire, inhibited sexual excitement, inhibited male orgasm, inhibited female orgasm, premature ejaculation, functional dyspareunia, and functional vaginismus.

18. Which of the seven occur only in males?

Answer: Premature ejaculation and inhibited male orgasm.

A twenty-year-old boy living at home with his mother, his aunt, and his ten-year-old brother was seen by a psychiatrist because of chronic complaints, occurring every four days, of severe abdominal pain, with indigestion, nausea, and occasional vomiting when eating a variety of foods. He had been worked up in several renowned medical centers over the previous four years, but thorough medical studies were unable to demonstrate a physical illness that could explain the patient's complaints.

During periods of distress the patient would stay home from school, and was completely free of any responsibility, because the family felt that he was too sick to take on any chores or household obligations. He spent his time watching television and doing whatever he liked.

19. What are some of the possibilities you would consider in this case?

Answer: The patient has complaints about physical illness with no physical disorder to explain them. Assuming that he doesn't have a delusion, he might be either faking or he might be suffering from psychogenic pain, or he might have conversion symptoms relating to the gastrointestinal tract involving indigestion, nausea, vomiting, and diarrhea.

20. If you know that the patient "hates hospitals and doctors," and complains that "I would like to be well." What would that rule out?

Answer: It would rule out factitious manifestations in that the patient was not interested in assuming the role of a patient under the care of hospitals or doctors.

21. When considering conversion symptoms and psychogenic pain, which one of the three kinds of situations associated with those manifestations does this patient exhibit?

Answer: Receiving support from the environment that might not otherwise be forthcoming, in that he is allowed to stay home and do whatever he likes, and not have to carry the obligations of school performance or performing household chores and obligations. Also, if going to school turns out, for him, to be a noxious situation, he has avoided it for the better part of four years by having a bellyache.

We do not yet have enough information to point out a specific environmental stimulus that is related to the onset or worsening of the patient's complaints - (if his pain got worse everytime he tried to go to school, that would be an example of a connection with the environment.)

22. In this case, as in all cases, on what crucial point does the issue of malingering versus psychogenic pain hinge?

Answer: It hinges on the question of whether the pain is something he complains about but really doesn't have, or whether when he says he experiences such pain, it does come upon him as an *involuntary* phenomenon.

23. If he complained vigorously that he feared he had a serious illness, such as cancer, refusing to accept the medical evidence, and paid unusually close attention to his bodily functioning and processes, what additional things would you think of?

Answer: Hypochondriasis or hypochondriacal delusions.

24. What would make the difference in deciding between those two possibilities?

Answer: If he could entertain the idea that perhaps he had no physical illness such as he feared, he would not have a delusion.

Case Study

A married couple in their early thirties come to see a doctor because of problems in their sexual relationship that have been going on for a year. The wife complains that whenever she has sexual intercourse with her husband, she experiences severe pain, and wants to terminate the sex act as soon as possible. She says she *does* become sexually aroused before beginning to participate in sexual relations with her husband. The husband says that he doesn't understand the reasons for his wife's problem, but during the past year, because she has had such pain during coitus, he has tried to, "get in and get out as soon as possible," and now says in private to the doctor that whenever he tries to have sex, he ejaculates almost immediately. He says that he thinks that part of his wife's problem is that he doesn't provide her with sufficient stimulation or give her a satisfying sexual experience as a result of his own difficulty. The wife sticks to her complaint about having severe pain and is sent to a gynecologist who does numerous studies: x-rays and examinations and laboratory tests, and is unable to explain her complaint of pain during sexual relations by any physical disease.

25. What cardinal manifestation of mental disorder is being shown by the husband? By the wife?

   Answer: The husband shows the manifestation of premature ejaculation. The wife shows functional dyspareunia.

chapter 16

Disturbances in Behavior

Behavior can be looked at in terms of its quantity. Is there too much behavior or too little behavior? Here we are looking once again at the overall activity level of the patient. Is the behavior overactive or is there underactivity?

We can look at the quantity of behavior on a spectrum. At one end of the spectrum, there is almost no behavior, with the patient sitting withdrawn and motionless, exhibiting no movements and no facial expressions for long periods of time. At the other end of the spectrum are extremely active patients who never seem to stop moving; they move quickly, rapidly, perhaps going from one thing to another so quickly with much movement of the body and so much animation of the face for such long periods of time, perhaps without needing to sleep, that the quantity of behavior displayed is enormous.

Psychomotor retardation and *psychomotor agitation* have been discussed above under the respective categories of depressed and manic mood (see pages 103 to 105).

Underactive behavior is both a physiological and behavioral change associated with *depressed mood.* Likewise extreme overactivity with seeming unlimited energy is a physiologic and behavioral change associated with *manic mood.*

Patients who have the emotion of anxiety may shake and tremble with fear, and may seem active. We discussed how patients who manifest generalized anxiety may seem jittery, nervous, unable to sit still, unable to relax and may otherwise appear to exhibit an overabundance of behavior.

150

HYPERACTIVITY OF CHILDREN

In the case of children, hyperactivity can mean excessive running about or climbing on things as well as having difficulty sitting still or fidgeting excessively. Children may have difficulty remaining seated, they may move excessively during sleep, and may always seem "on the go" or act "as if driven by a motor".

IMPATIENT OR IMPULSIVE BEHAVIOR

Impatience may be a cardinal manifestation of mental disorder; it is being unable to wait one's turn in a group activity, whether it is a game, an academic activity, an occupational situation, or a social interaction. In the case of children it is a cardinal manifestation of mental disorder.

Impulsivity implies acting before thinking. Perhaps not being able to think ahead and forsee the consequences of one's act. The person commits acts that bring an untoward reaction by the environment that the person didn't want and didn't expect, and that could have been avoided if he had foreseen the consequences of his action.

Children are said to be impulsive when they shift from one activity to another excessively, when they act before thinking, when they have difficulty organizing their work (that is not related to an impairment in intellectual ability), where they need a lot of supervision, when they frequently call out in class, and when they have difficulty waiting their turn at games or in group situations.

Impulsive behavior can be seen in patients with overactivity, such as we have described in manic mood, where patients can have excessive involvement in pleasurable activities, together with a lack of concern for whatever potential there may be for painful consequences. Such persons can spend a lot of money, make foolish business investments, or drive recklessly.

SPECIFIC DEVELOPMENTAL DISORDERS IN CHILDREN

Any time a child persistently fails to manifest behavior appropriate to the level of development of other children of his chronological age, or social and cultural background, that child shows a cardinal manifestation of mental disorder. Specific delays in development related to the acquisition of language skills which were discussed earlier (page 71). Children additionally can show specific delays in the acquisition of skills involving arithmetic alone, or skills in the pronunciation of words (articulation). These are characteristics of the Axis II disorder of children.

OTHER DISTURBANCES IN ADAPTIVE
BEHAVIOR IN CHILDREN

The reader is asked to recall now, or to review, the manifestations of mental disorder where children do not achieve adequate bowel or bladder training commensurate with their age (page 71), or where other problems in adaptive functioning in relation to behavior with family, peers, or school are a concern.

SELF-DESTRUCTIVE AND SUICIDAL BEHAVIOR

Impulsiveness and unpredictability can result in behavior that is potentially self-damaging, such as spending money, gambling, use of drugs, shoplifting, overeating, and frequent casual sexual involvements.

Individuals who indulge in any of these self-damaging activities in an impulsive or unpredictable way, as part of a pattern of behavior, show a cardinal manifestation of mental disorder.

Self-mutilation, where people may burn parts of their bodies with cigarettes, write their initials on their bodies with a sharp instrument, or attempt to amputate or otherwise destroy some part of their bodies is a cardinal manifestation of mental disorder.

Individuals who recurrently become involved in physical fights and individuals who have recurrent "accidents" (accident-proneness), show a major manifestation of mental disorder.

All persons who make attempts to kill themselves show a cardinal manifestation of mental disorder, as do individuals who announce to others that they intend to commit suicide.

VIOLENT AND OVERLY AGGRESSIVE BEHAVIOR

Persisting patterns of violent behavior towards others, as well as isolated outbursts of excessive violence, committed against persons or property are cardinal manifestations of mental illness.

A sudden outburst of violence in persons without a persisting pattern of violence, is termed an *explosive episode of violence*. Such explosive episodes of violence can be *isolated* catastrophically violent acts, or they can be *recurrent* incidents of assaults or destruction of property.

TICS

Tics are repetitive, seemingly purposeless movements of various muscle groups of the body. They are involuntary. They may involve the face, and appear as various kinds of "twitching" of facial muscles (brow, eyelids, or mouth). They may involve the trunk or limbs, appearing as a sudden but repetitive shrugging of the shoulders, or nodding of the head.

Such patients are sometimes able to voluntarily suppress such movements for a few minutes or for several hours. Tics tend to go away when the individual is more relaxed or asleep.

Vocal tics involving grunts, yelps, howls, and sometimes the shouting of obscene words can occur.

Multiple tics, including vocal tics, are characteristics of *Tourette's Disorder.*

INFANT BEHAVIOR

Some infant behavior is regarded by DSM-III as a cardinal manifestation of mental disorder. This would include a lack of visual tracking of eyes and faces by infants older than two months of age, lack of smiling and response to faces by an infant of more than two months of age, a lack of reciprocity of visual response in an infant who is older than two months, or a lack of vocalizing and response to the voice of the caretaker in an infant older than five months.

It would include a lack of alerting and turning toward a caretaker's voice in an infant older than two months, and a lack of spontaneous reaching for the mother by an infant of more than four months.

It would include a lack of anticipatory reaching when approached to be picked up in an infant over five months of age, or a lack of participation in playful games with the caretaker by an infant older than five months.

It may include a weak cry, excessive sleeping, lack of interest in the environment, underactivity, poor tone of the muscles, and weak grasping and rooting responses in attempts to feed the child.

Any of these behaviors in an infant is a cardinal manifestation of mental disorder.

("Rooting" is the reflex exhibited by infants younger than three months, where, after their cheek is stroked, the infants will turn their heads in that direction; *"grasping"* is the reflex in infants younger than six months of closing their hand when the palm is stroked.)

PARAPHILIAS

The paraphilias are a group of cardinal manifestations of mental disorder where the repeatedly preferred or exclusive method of achieving sexual excitement involves certain objects or acts.

Fetishism is the use of non-living objects (called fetishes) as a repeatedly preferred or exclusive method of achieving sexual excitement; the fetishes are not limited to articles of female clothing used in cross-dressing (transvestism) or to objects designed to be used for the purpose of sexual stimulation (such as a vibrator).

It is a cardinal manifestation of mental disorder.

Transvestism has been discussed above and involves cross-dressing for the purpose of sexual excitement, at least initially in the course of the problem.

Zoophilia is the *act or fantasy* of engaging in sexual activity with animals, as a preferred or exclusive method of achieving sexual excitement.

Pedophilia is the *act or fantasy* of engaging in sexual activity with a preadolescent children, as a repeatedly preferred or exclusive method of achieving sexual excitement.

Exhibitionism involves repetitive *acts* of exposing the genitals to an unsuspecting stranger for the purpose of achieving sexual excitement with no attempt at further sexual activity with the stranger.

Voyeurism is where the individual repeatedly observes unsuspecting people who are either naked, in the act of disrobing, or engaging in sexual activity, and where no sexual activity with the observed people is sought. This manifestation of mental disorder needs to be distinguished from the watching of pornography. Judgment must be used.

Sexual Masochism is where the preferred or exclusive mode of producing sexual excitement involves being humiliated, tied up, beaten, or otherwise made to suffer, or where the person has intentionally participated in an activity where he or she was physically harmed or his or her life was threatened, in order to produce sexual excitement. Sexual masochism focuses on acts that are *actually performed* and does not involve *fantasies* of such activities. Masochistic fantasies are not cardinal manifestations of mental disorder, but the acts described above are.

Sexual Sadism is a major manifestation of mental disorder and can involve either a consenting or a nonconsenting partner.

When involving a non-consenting partner, it is the repeated intentional infliction of psychological or physical suffering in order to produce sexual excitement.

When involving a consenting partner, it is where the preferred, or exclusive mode, or achieving sexual excitement of the individual combines humiliation with simulated or mildly injurious suffering on the consenting partner, or where bodily injury that is extensive, permanent, or possibly lethal is inflicted on a consenting partner in order to achieve sexual excitement.

Other Paraphilias

The above are the principle paraphilias that the reader should be familiar with. There are many others where feces (coprophilia), rubbing (frotteurism), enemas (klismaphilia), filth (mysophilia), corpses (necrophilia), making lewd remarks over the telephone (telephone scatologia), and urine (urophilia) are repeatedly involved in the preferred mode of producing sexual excitement for the individual.

Ego-dystonic sexual practices

Any sexual behavior or sexual practice that causes a person significant subjective distress is a cardinal manifestation of mental disorder. The term "ego" refers to those mental processes that are said to mediate the relationship between the mind and the outside world, and which are responsible for our integrated sense of ourselves and our identity. The term "ego-dystonic" implies something that is disagreeable to one's self and to one's sense of identity, with associated feelings of distress.

The paraphilias are cardinal manifestations of mental disorder that merely describe various preferred modes of achieving sexual excitement. Many persons who have paraphilias experience little or no subjective distress as part of their engaging in these sexual practices. In a paraphilia, the cardinal manifestation of mental disorder is contained completely in the description of what a person *does* and not how a person *feels about what they are doing,* or how they feel afterward.

Any person who experiences significant subjective distress related to a particular sexual activity has a cardinal manifestation of mental disorder.

Homosexuality

Homosexuality (sexual relations where the preferred mode of achieving sexual excitement leading to orgasm is with a sexual partner of one's own sex) is not a cardinal manifestation of mental disorder in DSM-III !

Whenever homosexual relations are associated with significant distress related to the homosexual acts, then a cardinal manifestation of mental disorder is present.

DISTURBANCES OF BEHAVIOR DISCUSSED IN EARLIER SECTIONS

The reader is advised now to look back over this chapter and familiarize himself with some of the terms we have already used in earlier sections.

We have discussed *dependent* behavior where individuals seek to establish with others a relationship in which they will be taken care of.

We have discussed *conduct manifestations* both aggressive and unaggressive where the rights of others were violated in various ways; we have discussed *antisocial work habits,* we have discussed *passive-aggressive styles* of dealing with people, and we have discussed the suspicious and pervasive mistrust of others involved in relating socially, as well as individuals who avoided others for various reasons, whether because they had no interest in social relationships or because they were afraid of humiliation or embarrassment.

We have discussed *avoidance behavior* in connection with *anxiety,* and with specific situations such as specific social occasions, specific objects, and the avoidance of situations where the individual feared that they might become incapacitated.

Children who are afraid to be separated from their parents may go to great lengths and exhibit much behavior such as temper tantrums, in order to avoid separation from those to whom they have a strong attachment.

We have discussed *bizarre behavior* that could result from having *delusions* or *hallucinations,* where the bizarreness of the behavior can reflect the bizarreness of the delusion.

We discussed *grossly illogical thought,* such as occurs in severe *loosening of associations* and *incoherence* when we discussed *formal thought disorder,* where the behavior, to the degree that it reflected the illogical thinking, made no sense. Examples were given of grossly disorganized behavior, such as the man who was rearranging the garbage and tracing designs on the brick wall of an alley.

Here are some further examples of Bizarre Behavior.

Case Illustration

A twenty-six-year-old man disappeared from his job and was found several months later by friends living alone in a filthy, roach-infested apartment that was covered from floor to ceiling with hundreds of empty milk cartons he had found in garbage cans and hoarded. The man ignored his friends when they entered and he stood, unwashed and unkempt, before a grimy mirror and smiled, made noises, and adjusted and readjusted the collar and buttons on his shirt. This seemingly meaningless activity absorbed him totally, and after being taken to a nearby hospital he continued to stand in front of mirrors, laughing and grimacing in a similar way for hours at a time.

This man's behavior is bizarre, is disorganized, and makes no sense.

CATATONIC BEHAVIOR

There are five kinds of catatonic behavior that are major manifestations of mental disorder.

Catatonic Stupor is a marked *decrease in activity,* including spontaneous movements, with perhaps mutism (no speech), or it is a marked *decrease in reactivity* to the environment, where the individual may appear to take no notice of what goes on about him or her. If both of these manifestations would occur together as part of a catatonic stupor, the individual might be seen to sit motionless, stare into space and take no notice of anything that was seen or heard.

Catatonic negativism is a resistence to all instructions or attempts to be moved that apparently has no motive. The negativism may be in the form of refusal of food, soiling of clothes or bed with urine and feces, active resistence to any requests such as to dress, to wash, or to leave the bed, and the muteness manifested by patients may also be thought of as a kind of negativism, where such patients may not respond to anything that is said to them until, perhaps, the examiner turns his back, when the patient will then answer or at least begin to answer a question.

Such patients may leave plates of food put in front of them untouched but then steal food from other patients' dishes.

Catatonic rigidity is the maintenance of a rigid posture against efforts to be moved. It can be thought of as another variety of negativism. In some cases individuals will become rigid only when touched or when attempts are made to move them, and the rigid posture and refusal to move may disappear when the patients are left by themselves.

Catatonic Excitement is a state of markedly excited physical activity that is apparently purposeless, and is not influenced by an external stimuli. Such patients, when seen, are dramatic in their presentation and they give the impression of "a person who has gone completely berserk". Such patients may be extremely dangerous and manifest tremendous strength.

Catatonic Posturing is the voluntary assumption of an inappropriate or bizarre posture.

An example of a patient who first manifested catatonic posturing together with catatonic negativism, rigidity and stupor, who then manifested catatonic excitement is described in the following case.

Case Illustration

A seventeen-year-old boy, after two weeks of basic training in the army, suddenly disappeared from his barracks, and after a day of searching the grounds, was found standing inside of a large closet with his arms outstretched, his feet together, and his head inclined toward his left shoulder. *(catatonic posturing.)* In this bizarre posture, the patient resembled the figure of Christ crucified on the cross.

Efforts to move him from the closet were difficult because of his rigid maintenance of his posture. *(catatonic rigidity.)*

Efforts to speak to him or to look into his eyes appeared to produce no response. One soldier passed his hand in front of the patient's eyes repeatedly but the patient stared straight ahead with a blank expression on his face. *(catatonic stupor.)*

The sergeant, the lieutenant, and then finally the colonel in charge of the base ordered the new recruit to leave the closet and get back to his barracks. All of these instructions were ignored and efforts to move him failed. At one point the soldiers walked several yards away from the patient and talked among themselves about what to do. At that point the patient seemed to move a little bit and make some noises. *(catatonic negativism.)*

Suddenly he became active, leaping about the barracks picking up foot lockers and hurling them through the window. He took a fire axe off the wall and quickly smashed a hole in the wall of the barracks. He hurled the fire axe at the soldiers and began running aimlessly. Occasionally he would stop and pick up objects such as crowbars and rifles and beat them against whatever was at hand.

Over twenty people were necessary to physically subdue this one adolescent who was a relatively slight build and was only 5'7" tall. In his state of extreme activity he was difficult to restrain and had to be chained to a stretcher.

Psychiatric personnel at the hospital did not believe the incredible story of the degree of activity and violence that was reported about this young boy, and made the error of removing him from his restraints. For about fifteen minutes he lay motionless on the stretcher, and then once again burst into a blur of purposeless and excited motor activity and destroyed a piano by ripping out every key with his bare hands before he was subdued once again. *(catatonic excitement.)*

This was an example of all five kinds of catatonic behavior occurring in the same individual. Any single one of the catatonic behaviors is a cardinal manifestation of mental disorder.

"PARANOID" BEHAVIOR

Behavior that is dominated by marked suspicion and distrust of others or behavior in response to delusions of persecution or jealousy or the grandiose delusions or to hallucinations with persecutory or grandiose content is called "paranoid".

DISORDERS OF BEHAVIOR INVOLVING THE USE OF SUBSTANCES

This includes a wide variety of problems with drugs. Here the focus is on patterns of use of a drug, where the individual is unable either to cut down or stop, where repeated efforts to control the use of the drug result in a variety of difficulties, where patients may go on binges where they remain intoxicated throughout the day, and where the pattern of use frequently involves the necessity to take increasing amounts of the drug in order to produce the effect that the patient feels is desirable.

It may include, in addition, patterns of behavior that are necessitated by the individual's need for the drug, and can involve criminal acts, violation of the rights of others, rule breaking, lying, taking advantage of other people, or using them for one's own purposes, or can involve a disruption of social relations and academic and/or occupational functioning as part of the maladaptive pattern of use.

SELF-STUDY QUESTIONS, CHAPTER 16

1. What are two kinds of manifestations of mental disorder related to the amount of behavior displayed by a person?

   Answer: Overactivity and underactivity.

2. In the case of children, what are five kinds of behaviors that would be considered hyperactive behavior?

   Answer: Excessively running around or climbing on things, having difficulty sitting still or fidgeting excessively, having difficulty remaining seated, moving around excessively during sleep, being always "on the go" or acting as if "driven by a motor".

3. Discuss overactive behavior in relation to people who have a manic mood. What particular manifestation of this kind of behavior is of concern?

Answer: Patients with manic mood display overactive behavior, motivated by apparent boundless energy, with over-involvement in a variety of activities: recreational, social, and occupational. Of particular concern is their tendency to be reckless and to become involved in activities with a high potential for self-harm, such as reckless driving, foolish spending and business investments, and poorly thought out social and sexual involvements.

4. Discuss the underactive behavior sometimes seen with depressed mood. What term might be used to describe it?

   Answer: Depressed mood has physiologic and behavioral accompaniments that can involve overall reduction in activity, sometimes to the degree that everyday activities seem to be a great effort to the patient. *Psychomotor retardation* is the term used to describe this kind of overall reduction and output of behavior when it is predominant or particularly striking.

5. Discuss impulsiveness and impatience. Give some instances of impulsivity in the case of children.

   Answer: Impulsiveness refers to unpredictability and acting without thinking about the consequences of one's act. Impatience refers to the inability to wait one's turn in a social, occupational, or academic situation. In the case of children, impulsivity can be said to be present where children often act before thinking, shift excessively from one activity to another, have difficulty organizing their work when this is not due to lack of ability, needing a lot of supervision, and when children frequently call out in class, or where they have difficulty awaiting their turn in games or group situations.

6. Discuss bizarre behavior. How can it be related to delusions?

7. What are five kinds of catatonic behavior?

   Answer: Catatonic stupor, catatonic negativism, catatonic rigidity, catatonic excitement, catatonic posturing.

8. Explain each of the above varieties of catatonic behavior.

   Answer: Catatonic stupor is a marked decrease in reactivity to the environment and/or reduction of spontaneous movements and activity, and/or mutism.
   Catatonic negativism is an apparently motiveless resistance to all instructions or attempts to be moved.
   Catatonic rigidity is maintenance of a rigid posture against efforts to be moved.
   Catatonic excitement is excited, apparently purposeless physical activity that is not influenced by external stimuli.
   Catatonic posturing is a voluntary assumption of an inappropriate or bizarre posture.

9. What is meant by the term "paranoid"?

   Answer: Behavior is accordance with, or resulting from excessive suspiciousness or mistrust of others, or behavior that is in response to delusions of persecution, delusions of jealousy, delusions of grandeur, or to hallucinations with persecutory and grandiose content.

10. Explain what paraphilias are.

    Answer: They are disorders of behavior involving use of certain objects or situations as the preferred and predominant mode of producing sexual excitement.

11. What are some paraphilias? Explain them.

12. What are tics?

    Answer: Stereotyped involuntary, apparently purposeless, motor movements such as twitching of the eyes, face, shrugging of the shoulder, nodding of the head, etc.

13. Describe the cardinal manifestations of mental disorder termed explosive acts of violence. What are the two kinds?

    Answer: They are episodes of violence that are unexpected in view of the individual's lack of a previous pattern of violent behavior; they are either episodic or isolated instances. The isolated instances, when they occur, usually involve catastrophic acts of violence against others.

14. What are some behaviors characteristic of separation anxiety?

    Answer: All behaviors related to, or resulting from an irrational fear of being separated from major attachment figures or the irrational fear that harm will come to major attachment figures, or that harm will come to one's self when one is separated from attachment figures. It may involve difficulty working, socializing, or sleeping away from the attachment figures.

15. What are some infant behaviors that are cardinal manifestations of mental disorder?

    Answer: Not showing adequate reciprocal gaze and eye contact, not showing adequate reciprocal vocalization with the caretaker, not showing adequate anticipatory response when a caretaker approaches the infant to pick them up, etc., where each one of these particular behaviors are not manifested when they are considered appropriate for the baby's age (measured in specific number of months after birth).

16. In your own words, give an explanation of grossly disorganized behavior.

17. Discuss some disorders of behavior that might be related to use of a drug.

    Answer: Inability to stop using the drug, making repeated unsuccessful efforts to stop, requiring more and more of the drug in order to produce the effect desired, difficulties in various areas of adaptive behavior owing to the patient's persistent use of the substance, etc.

18. Give examples of some areas where children and some adults may have problems related to delay in acquiring specific abilities usually required for successful performance in schools.

    Answer: Specific problems involving delay in acquiring skills with language, arithmetic pronunciation, and reading.

chapter 17

Psychosis

Psychosis is said to be present when *any one* of the following cardinal manifestations occur;

1. Delusions
2. Hallucinations
3. Loosening of associations or incoherence
4. Grossly disorganized or catatonic behavior

When any one of these cardinal manifestations of mental disorder occur, we can refer to the patient as "psychotic" or as having "a psychosis".

While only one of the four need be present in order to use the term "psychosis", psychosis is present also when more than one of the four cardinal manifestations of delusions, hallucinations, grossly disorganized or catatonic behavior, or loosening of associations or incoherence are present.

Psychosis is a cardinal manifestation of mental disorder.

When none of the four cardinal manifestations that are part of the definition of psychosis are present, we say that the patient is *not psychotic* and we refer to any other mental disorder present in the patient as *non-psychotic.*

Psychosis by itself, is not a mental disorder. Psychosis is a cardinal manifestation of mental disorder that is used at times to make a major division of mental disorders into two kinds: those where psychosis has occurred (psychotic), and those where psychosis has not occurred (non-psychotic).

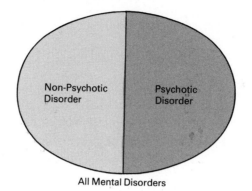

All Mental Disorders

REALITY TESTING

Reality testing is defined as the ability of a person to tell the difference between what is going on inside of his mind from what is going on in the real world.

Reality testing is what psychiatrists call the process by which we can distinguish reality from imagination and fantasy.

When a person's fantasy is treated by him as though it were reality, as manifested by his thought, feelings, or behavior, then reality testing is said to be "grossly impaired".

When delusions are present, reality testing is clearly impaired because the patient has an unshakable false belief that is out of keeping with his or her social or cultural background. It is on the point of the falseness of the belief that reality is challenged.

Hallucinations are likewise an impairment of reality testing. Here a false sensory experience not related to any external stimulus of a sense organ is perceived by the patient as though it were a real one. Here again, it is the falseness that is the point where reality is challenged, where the individual insists that he has seen, heard, or otherwise experienced something that was "real".

There is a certain relationship of one external event to another, and a certain logic about ways in which human beings can interact with their environment that makes sense. Looseness of associations, or incoherence, whether in thoughts alone, or reflected in grossly disorganized or catatonic behavior, reflect an idiosyncratic personal logic that challenges reality.

Behavior that is grossly disorganized or catatonic is behavior that so disrupts social, occupational, academic, recreation, or self-care functioning that it is out of keeping with the demands of reality, where the patient is "living in their own world", and it is on this issue that reality testing is said to be impaired. For this reason, some mental health professionals define psychosis as "impairment of reality testing".

You will encounter the concept again as you continue to deal with mental health professionals, and read further about mental disorders.

In this book and in the DSM-III diagnostic system, psychosis means specifically having at least one of the following four cardinal manifestations:

1. delusions
2. hallucinations
3. loosening of associations or incoherence
4. grossly disorganized behavior or catatonic behavior

SELF-STUDY QUESTIONS, CHAPTER 17

1. What is the definition of psychosis?

   Answer: It is having at least one of the following four cardinal manifestations of mental disorder: delusions, hallucinations, loose associations or incoherence, or grossly disorganized or catatonic behavior.

2. Discuss reality testing.

3. How do each of the four cardinal manifestations that are part of the definition of psychosis show that a person's reality testing is grossly impaired?

4. How is the cardinal manifestation of mental disorder called psychosis used to divide mental disorders into two categories?

   Answer: It divides them into psychotic disorders (disorders where psychosis is present) and disorders that are non-psychotic (disorders where no psychosis is present).

5. Is psychosis a mental disorder?

   Answer: No. Psychosis is a cardinal manifestation of mental disorder and by itself, like other cardinal manifestations of mental disorder we have discussed, it only points to the possibility of a mental disorder.

part III

Evolution of Views of Mental Illness:

DSM-III in Historical Perspective

Just as all mental disorders can be divided into psychotic and non-psychotic types, so can psychosis itself be divided into two kinds: Schizophrenic type and non-schizophrenic types. This is an extremely important distinction. It is part of what makes psychosis serious when we see it. One of the things that psychosis can mean is that the patient has schizophrenia, and that is a serious matter. Why is that? To understand, we have to discuss the history of the diagnosis of psychiatric disorders.

DSM-III is a step that was taken in a long tradition that has viewed the whole of mental disorder in definite ways. DSM-III in many respects is part of that tradition, and while incorporating important changes which we will discuss, it does continue as another chapter in the story of our understanding of what mental disorder is and what it is not.

In reading through Chapter II, you have been exposed to a large number of different kinds of symptoms that can be part of mental disorders. What to make of all of this is partly answered by what has been made of it in the past. The reader who is unfamiliar with the various mental disorders probably doesn't know what to make of the various symptoms and signs we have discussed as cardinal manifestations of mental disorder. The reader who has some familiarity with the field of mental health probably knows what was made of these things in the past, and would like to know what DSM-III makes of these now.

The central concept that ties everything together both now and historically is the idea of psychosis, and secondarily the idea of, and concepts surrounding schizophrenia.

INSANITY

In order to orient yourself in relationship to the subject of mental disorders, we need to go back to the basics. The layman has always thought of mental disorder in terms of the contrast between sanity and insanity. The word insane is not a word that psychiatrists use, certainly not in any official way, and it will never appear in a diagnosis in DSM-III. It never appeared in DSM-II either.

Sane and insane have always been important concepts. They are old concepts. We can do more in discussing what is the matter with someone who has one of the cardinal manifestations of mental disorder than merely classify them as sane or insane.

We have tried to discuss mental illness and mental disorder in various dimensions, the most important of which is adaptive functioning (social, occupational, self-care). We have also discussed mental illness in terms of subjective distress: the patient's own report of emotional hurt, analogous to the pains within the body that would cause persons to seek medical attention.

In the contrast of sanity to insanity, persons who are psychotic are clearly insane. Some persons would make a case that some other kinds of mental disorders should be included in these forms of insanity, such as severe depression, and severe manias where psychosis is not present.

It is interesting that in older classification systems, when psychosis as we have defined it (in terms of delusions and hallucinations and so on) was not present, *the severe mood disorders were still considered psychoses* because the breakdown in adaptive functioning that occurred as a result of the severe mood disorder was felt to be sufficiently severe to indicate that something extremely serious had happened in a person's relationship with his environment.

You will recall that we characterized psychosis *as a breakdown in reality testing,* meaning that a person was "living in his own world" and was not able to function. The severe mood disorders can also cause such problems.

AN HISTORICAL PERSPECTIVE

The perspective that we need to understand mental disorders is an historical one. It will explain mental disorder because it will trace our understanding of what mental disorder is, and it will trace our understanding of how people came to subdivide the various kinds of "insanity", and why they did that.

The whole progression from a simple description of people as falling into one of two classes, either sane or insane, there to what we have in 1980 as the diagnostic criteria of DSM-III, contains the whole of the story of what mental disorders are today in 1980, and will give you the understanding you need of the principles on which DSM-III is organized and its role in being *the next step* in a logical progression of efforts to understand more about mental disorder.

It is first of all important to understand that the split between sane versus insane people is a very old one. And while people recognized that not all insane people were alike, we know now today that persons were lumped together in the past who really had relatively different disorders.

Tertiary syphilis can cause a form of insanity which was relatively common throughout the history of man before the advent of modern antibiotics that gave us a treatment for syphilis in the early stages. Tertiary syphilis is an *organic mental disorder.* But we know now that many persons with this problem were grouped together with persons who had what we today call functional mental disorders, which are a very different matter from Tertiary Syphilis.

MIND VERSUS BODY

The division between the mind and the body has been an important area for philosophers down through the ages, and has created another duality, namely, the division between mental disorders and physical disorders, which is still carried on in DSM-III as we mentioned in Chapter I.

As twentieth century scientists, mental health professionals accept that all behavior, all emotion, all thought, and even many features of sensory perception, arise in, and are determined by, events that take place in the brain. The distinction that is made by the rest of medicine of dividing disorders into physical and mental (not just by the rest of medicine, but by the way most people tend to conceptualize themselves as a composite of mind and a body) is carried on in psychiatry itself through the distinction between *organic* versus *functional.*

Historically, it was a tremendously important discovery that some mental disorders could be shown to be based on identifiable structural damage, or traceable to chemical disturbances that arose in the brain, where these changes arose in such a way that they were gross enough so that they could be picked up by the customary methods of medical examination and laboratory studies.

Thus the insane were then divided into two groups, those who were thought to have an "organic insanity" and those where something different seemed to be taking place that defied the efforts of scientists, and pathologists, and doctors everywhere to come up with an adequate explanation of what was wrong with these people.

Of all the cardinal manifestations of mental disorder, probably the one which is the greatest in seriousness and stands out as so much more important than the rest is the whole category of psychosis.

It has always been important historically because psychosis as a concept, while variously defined by various investigators, nevertheless corresponds closest in many ways to what the layman really tried to encompass with the term "insanity". While perhaps, from the layman's point of view, not all insane people would be psychotic, it is certainly true that all psychotic people are insane.

THREE GROUPS: THE MIDDLE ZONE

From the layman's simplified concept of insanity versus sanity, psychiatry moved into making three divisions.

All people were divided into three groups: psychotic persons, sane persons, and persons who occupied a middle zone; they were not psychotic, but they were not sane in the layman's sense of being free of impairment in adaptive functioning, or free of significant subjective distress, owing to their having one or more cardinal manifestations of mental disorder of the kind we have discussed already.

This intermediate zone, or intermediate category, which contains a very important group of people, has problems that are significantly different from the problems encountered by psychotic persons, or persons who have disorders where there is recurrent psychosis or where psychosis occurs and seems to subside but enters some kind of chronic phase of residual impairment.

MORAL INSANITY

Lying somewhere in this group was a condition that was called moral insanity where individuals were not psychotic and maybe did not even suffer significant subjective distress, but where behavior toward others and toward authority involving criminality, dishonesty, rule breaking, and the kinds of things that we have discussed under conduct disorder manifestations already, began to distinguish them as a separate group.

PSYCHOSIS IS DIVIDED

The next step that took place, or the next logical subdivision of disorders came with a subdivision of functional psychosis. It was discovered that some persons with psychosis seemed to have recurrent attacks, and to get worse and deteriorate after each one so that they followed a kind of downhill course all of their lives beginning with their very first attack of acute psychosis, whereas other people seemed to have repeated attacks of psychosis, but then they would really get better and seem to function fairly well in between attacks, and not have the kind of downhill deteriorating course that was noticed in some persons.

SCHIZOPHRENIA IS DISCOVERED

The case of the downhill course with repeated episodes of psychosis was called *schizophrenia* and was characterized by certain fundamental signs by the original persons who described and studied it. The word schizophrenia, which means splitting of the mind, has nothing to do with multiple personalities as we described it earlier in the book. In schizophrenia the splitting that is referred to in the name doesn't refer to two separate personalities being present in the same person, but it refers to a disorganization that takes place on various levels of the mind, where the person seems to have a peculiar mixture of abnormal and normal characteristics. The typical picture of this problem would be seen in the case of a person who at one moment would seem to be making sense, and would be someone that one could deal with, who suddenly and without warning would begin to talk illogically or behave in a nonsensical or mysterious fashion, or who would begin to have hallucinations and lose contact with the real person with whom they were talking, and who then would be able, even for a brief time, to seem to be in contact with reality.

It was this peculiar mixture of logical versus illogical, of appropriate versus inappropriate, of sensible versus nonsensical, that gave rise to the concept of a mind that was split.

MANIC-DEPRESSIVE PSYCHOSIS IS DISCOVERED

The other type of insanity that had acute attacks but which seemed to get better, and had recurrent attacks without a downhill course, was grouped under the term *manic-depressive psychosis*. In these persons it was noticed that mood disturbances were a prominent feature even when psychosis was present. Thus two streams developed, and two categories.

DISORDER OF THOUGHT VS. DISORDERS OF AFFECT

In the meantime work was being done on the middle zone, work was being done on moral insanity, and more importantly work was being done on a whole group of problems that seemed to be related to anxiety as a principal organizing concept beginning with the work of Freud and the other psychoanalysts who subdivided problems into the middle zone and gave us some of the categories that have come down to us today in DSM-III.

Now in looking at the whole subject of psychosis and of schizophrenia, which was being distinguished at that time from the possibility of organic mental disorder that caused a variety of symptom clusters that could be confused with schizophrenia or with manic depressive psychosis, the original investigators who brought schizophrenia to the attention of medicine as a disease in its own right and as a principal form of insanity, characterized it in terms of what we have been calling *looseness of associations and incoherence*, seeing that as somehow the fundamental problem. Also described at that time was *the blunted, flat, or inappropriate affect*, a *tendency to withdraw from social relations* into a world of one's own, something that was called *"autism"*, and as part of the notion of splitting, characteristics that we haven't even mentioned in DSM-III but which seemed important at the time, (ie., ambivalence which was a tendency to feel different ways about the same thing, but not in the way that ordinary people have mixed feelings).

Hallucinations, delusions, bizarre behavior, and catatonic behavior were looked upon as *secondary symptoms,* while the disorders of thought and of flat, inappropriate affect and so on were considered *primary,* and *defining characteristics of the condition.*

There is a long historical tradition involving these concepts and their being taught to generation after generation of mental health professionals.

Schizophrenia was believed to have, at its core, a disorder of thought, emotion, and social relating, where the disorder of thought was believed to be the principal problem. Schizophrenia, as a form of psychosis and as a form of insanity, came to be known and conceptualized as a *disorder of thought,* and was contrasted with the manic-depressive psychosis, where severe manic moods and severe depressed moods occurred, sometimes with hallucinations and delusions, and where manic depressive psychosis was considered *a disorder of affect.*

Thus, there were then two kinds of functional psychosis, schizophrenia, a disorder of thought that ran a progressively downhill course throughout the life of the patient, and the manic-depressive psychosis of affect, which, while equally serious, and taking its place beside schizophrenia as a form of insanity, was held up in sharp contrast to schizophrenia, based on this fundamental concept that schizophrenia was a disorder of one kind of mental sphere, namely of thought and of the logic that connected one thought to another, while affective disorder was a disorder of whatever controlled the level of mood and made it either depressed or elated.

The third kind of psychosis or insanity was the organic kind, and it began to be recognized as medicine advanced, that various medical disorders that were being discovered and learned about and further described, could cause what we have described as cardinal manifestations of mental disorder—disturbances in adaptive functioning, together with considerable subjective distress—and could even look like problems that were either common to schizophrenia or could look like mood problems.

Thus insanity had been divided into really four kinds: organic, schizophrenic, manic depressive, and moral insanity.

And then there was the middle zone which historically was never held to represent as serious a problem as the four kinds of insanity.

THE MIDDLE ZONE

This middle group lying somewhere between the pole of insanity and the pole of normalcy was nevertheless felt to represent the variety of abnormal mental life but just as we have distinguished organic versus functional as a basic division, at this point in the understanding of psychiatric disorders, the middle zone was considered minor in comparison with the other forms of insanity as we have discussed them.

Furthermore, at the time, it was held and reported that *problems in the middle zone had a cure.* They could be treated with psychoanalysis and in some cases by hypnosis, whereas disorders like schizophrenia, manic depressive psychosis, organic psychosis, and moral insanity had no treatment—there didn't seem to be anything that could be done that made much of a difference in the course of the illness. Humane methods of treatment of affected persons were found to sometimes modify the reaction of such patients to a hospital or institutional setting, but the influence of just tender love and care on the overall course of the disease, in the majority of affected individuals was insignificant.

REACTION

Through all of this work was the overriding issue of *reaction,* which means that in some cases it seemed that some people developed whatever problem they had: a psychosis of one kind or another, except for the organic, in response to the things that were happening to them or that had happened in the past, and the role of environmental stress and of reaction to environmental stress was a subject of great interest.

It had been learned, especially in treating disorders in the middle zone, that childhood experiences seemed to make an impact on the onset or worsening of the symptoms in the middle zone, known as neurotic disorders, and related as we said principally to problems of anxiety (such as we have already discussed under phobic manifestations, generalized anxiety manifestations, free floating anxiety, obsessions, and compulsions).

MAJOR VERSUS "MINOR"

Thus you see how we have a historical basis for looking at some mental illness as *major* and other mental illness as *minor.* (There is some mental illness that doesn't seem to fit in either the major or the minor category, in some cases it is very bad, in others it isn't, but it isn't consistently major or minor.)

MORAL INSANITY RECONSIDERED

The moral insanity, which later became known as *antisocial behavior,* sociopathic behavior, or psychopathic behavior, didn't seem to fit anywhere on the spectrum of functional disorders and was not a problem characterized by a definite onset of a symptom or an episode of illness as was the case in psychosis, or as in the case of a neurotic symptom, such as panic attacks or of phobias, or of conversion reactions (which at that time were problems in the middle zone and felt to be related to anxiety).

Problems with the antisocial personality didn't seem to have a definite onset or a definite cause. This seemed to be a pervasive life-long problem that did not seem to respond to pressure from the environment, but seemed to consist of deeply pervasive aspects of the individual's personality, enduring through the years, and having a pervasive effect on the individual's relationships with other people, occupational relationships, and relations to authority.

Thus a new division was born, and there evolved now a concept that there was psychosis, neurosis, and there was personality disorder.

ADJUSTMENT DISORDERS

There were also some short term disturbances which weren't as bad as neuroses, and certainly never as bad as psychoses (although in some cases brief psychosis could occur), that were definite reactions to environmental stress. These were reactions, later called adjustment reactions, and now in DSM-III called *adjustment disorders.*

You can now see some of the things that have happened. The personality disorders on Axis II are outgrowths of the difficulty of what to do with problems such as moral insanity and other styles and clusters of enduring personality traits that were discovered as people were studied more and more closely. Axis II is the heir to this group of life long, pervasive, enduring problems that cause impairment in adaptive functioning and at times subjective distress.

Psychosis, as far as it consists of the three major causes, organic, schizophrenic, and major mood problems, has also found its way into DSM-III, but with some very important changes.

ORGANIC DISORDERS

The organic disorders in DSM-III have under gone a very careful and really rather good characteriziation into a variety of nine different kinds, of which there are two principal pictures, *dementia* and *delirium.*

Delirium is characterized by a clouding of consciousness, disturbance of memory, together with a group of associated problems, but the principal feature of delirium is the clouding of counsciousness and the disturbance of memory and orientation. Psychosis can occur apparently as a secondary phenomenon, and be part of the delirious picture: hallucinations and delusions can occur.

Dementia is a different picture, characterized by a progressive loss of intellectual ability, together with memory impairment and poor judgment, and perhaps a group of definite neurological findings indicating that something is going wrong with the nervous system on a structural level.

Delirium

Differential diagnosis. Schizophrenia, Schizophreniform Disorder, other psychotic disorders, Dementia, Factitious Disorder with Psychological Symptoms.

Diagnostic criteria.

A. Clouding of consciousness (reduced clarity of awareness of environment), with reduced capacity to shift, focus, and sustain attention to environmental stimuli.

B. At least two of the following:

(1) perceptual disturbance: misinterpretations, illusions, or hallucinations
(2) speech that is at times incoherent
(3) disturbance of sleep-wakefulness cycle with insomnia or daytime drowsiness
(4) increased or decreased psychomotor activity

C. Disorientation and memory impairment (if testable).

D. Clinical features that develop over a short period of time (usually hours to days) and tend to fluctuate over the course of a day.

E. Evidence, from the history, physical examination, or laboratory tests, of a specific organic factor judged to be etiologically related to the disturbance.

A page from *Quick Reference to the Diagnostic Criteria from DSM-III,* available from The American Psychiatric Association, 1700 18th St. N.W., Washington, D.C. 20009. A recommended reference to all DSM-III disorders and their diagnostic criteria (what we have called "cardinal manifestations of mental illness").

The other organic mental disorders that DSM-III created were disorders that appeared with *no clouding of consciousness* and were definitely distinguished from delirium and dementia, but where because of some definite physical factor, either disease or a drug, hallucinations occurred, delusions occurred, affective disorder occurred, or there was a particular kind of personality change involving rapidly changing mood, suspiciousness, and so on.

DSM-III also included two special categories called intoxication and withdrawal to encompass the effects of drugs that couldn't be included in these other descriptions of organic mental disorders.

Organic mental disorder in DSM-III, then, is divided into the picture of delirium, the picture of dementia, and psychotic or mood disorder disturbances that occur on an organic basis.

PSYCHOSIS, SCHIZOPHRENIA, AND MOOD DISORDERS

A great change, though, has taken place in what happened to the functional mental disorders that were considered psychotic, and here is where DSM-III parts company with tradition and tries to reflect some of the research and directions of progress that have been taken by psychiatry most recently.

This has to do first of all with schizophrenia, and with psychosis, and with the relative place of mood disorders in the scheme of what was originally called insanity.

The idea that schizophrenia had a core problem with a disorder of thought has been de-emphasized in DSM-III, and what for decades were considered secondary problems in schizophrenia of hallucinations and delusions, have now been elevated to symptoms of principal importance.

Schizophrenia is now definitely *redefined* as involving characteristic delusions, characteristic hallucinations, together with, during the acute phase of psychosis, a kind of deterioration from a previous level of functioning that is always understood to occur, and where the role of thought disorder—a "formal thought disorder", with incoherence and loosening of associations—has been de-emphasized and is now only treated as a criterion of schizophrenia on its own if it occurs together with the blunt, flat, or inappropriate affect, or if it occurs with some kind of delusion or hallucination, or if it occurs together with some grossly disorganized or catatonic behavior.

Catatonic behavior, which is usually seen exclusively in schizophrenia, almost never being described in the history of psychiatry in any way occurring with any other condition, remains characteristic of schizophrenia. A tradition developed, historically, of separating schizophrenia from a group of disorders known as *paranoid disorders,* which were felt to represent a different condition, essentially because they had a different age of onset and a different course.

Schizophrenia tended to be a disease of younger people, and to make its first appearance in young adulthood so that there was a clustering of cases in relatively younger people.

Paranoid disorders, however, did not make their first appearance in younger people, but seemed to appear in persons relatively older, in their 40's, and although delusions occurred which were predominantly jealous delusions or persecutory delusions, they seemed to be much better organized (systematized delusions).

The thought of these people was not marked by the disorganization that was so evident to the early describers of schizophrenia, and so another class of psychosis was created historically to contain individuals who had this particular clustering of symptoms; the category of paranoid disorder continues into DSM-III.

Not only has schizophrenia undergone a revision as to what defines it in terms of symptoms, but great changes occurred in our understanding of the difference between affective disorder and schizophrenic disorder.

It became apparent when it was discovered that lithium could be used to treat manic mood and to stabilize the condition, so that further mood shifts were prevented, that there were quite a lot of people who were originally diagnosed as having schizophrenia because they had delusions and hallucinations, and whose thought seemed rather loose, who turned out on a number of measures to be suffering from a form of affective disorder, either severe depression or severe mania.

One of the important changes in DSM-III is that schizophrenia, once considered a category into which almost all severe psychosis belonged that was not of organic origin (and therefore what the layman and the psychiatrist alike would consider the worst kind of insanity), now became a category that shrank in number.

The group of patients called functionally psychotic, who could be basically classified into either affective disorder or schizophrenic disorder, were now shifted and reshuffled, and the membership of affective disorder grew at the expense of the membership of schizophrenia which has become a more restricted and more carefully delineated category.

The schizophrenic disorders were considered the most severe because of their progressive downhill course over a lifetime. The patient fell into a state of disorganization of thought and behavior with delusions and hallucinations that impaired adaptive functioning so severely that the only life possible for such persons was in institutions for the insane. Psychiatrists clearly recognized at that time that it was a condition for which there was no hope.

It was noticed that psychoses occurred that did, after a time, get better, and were characterized by prominent disturbances of mood such as manic mood or depressed mood. Because some individuals with severe mood problems were also psychotic (having delusions or hallucinations, or whose racing thoughts of mania were so severe that the associations were loose), these mood disorders with psychosis were regarded as serious. When persons developed severe mood problems without psychosis, it was a logical step to group them with the mood disorders that did have psychosis because of the potential that existed for the display of psychotic symptoms.

IMMEDIATE VERSUS RETROSPECTIVE DIAGNOSIS

At this point it is important to make a distinction between two different kinds of diagnosis. There is the diagnosis that is made at the time the person is sick and is brought in for help, and is based on observations of the person that are made at that particular time, together with some account of how he or she happened to develop the problem. A different kind of diagnosis can be made in retrospect after an illness has been present for some considerable period of time and then undergoes changes, becoming either worse or better.

The retrospective diagnosis does not serve to help the patients at the time that they present their acute illness, but it does serve to advance medical knowledge when it takes relatively large groups of people who have suffered from disease, and looks back over all of the things that have happened, and looks over all of the things that were observed, with a view to making comparisons and finding similarities between certain groups and subgroups.

While this serves to advance medical knowledge by looking at the lifetime course of various diseases, it can only serve to help the individual doctor if it provides him with information that would allow him to tell one disease from another when he sees a patient in the acute phase of an illness.

In the practical situation where a patient with an acute psychosis is brought for help, the diagnosis of the patient cannot be based at that time on what is yet to be the lifetime course of the patient's disorder, but can only be based upon characteristics and features of the acute phase of the illness that might allow the various severe mental disorders to be distinguished from one another.

Now that we have entered into an era where some specific treatments are available that appear to make a significant difference in the overall outcome of these major conditions, where drugs are available that appear to work in some of the cases of severe disorder but not in others, and where in some of those other cases a different drug would produce an overall better result, the decision about what diagnosis applies to a particular patient becomes a very important and practical point.

Furthermore, some of the drugs that are helpful in certain kinds of severe mental disorder, when given to patients with other severe mental disorder will make them worse.

We are at a point now in psychiatry that is very different from where the field was in the first quarter of this century. When you look back upon that situation, you see that the psychotic disorders, and the very severe depressions and manias that occurred without psychosis, had no effective treatment.

What had at least been discovered at that time was that some severe psychoses did run a chronic downhill course, while other severe psychoses could spontaneously get better, allowing the patient to resume a reasonably adequate level of adaptive functioning.

The only practical aspect of distinguishing between these two kinds of severe disorder at that period in the history of psychiatry would have been to distinguish the truly hopeful case from the patient who stood a chance of "coming out of it".

At that period of time in psychiatry there were no specific treatments available for these severe mental disorders. Little more could be done than to place them in asylums for the insane.

The reader can appreciate what a difficult problem it was to manage an acutely psychotic patient in that era, where for the most part there were no drugs available to relieve the suffering patient's experiencing of the intense anxiety that can result from hallucinations or delusions, or where there were no drugs to calm the intense and reckless overactive manic patient whose behavior was often dangerous to himself or to others, and where there were no effective methods for coping with the suicidal preoccupations of the severely depressed person.

Much medical knowledge today about the treatment of specific physical illnesses that is often taken for granted was unavailable at that period of history. Patients with organic mental disorders that today are treatable, and in some cases reversable conditions, such as the organic mental disorders caused by vitamin B12 deficiency, could likewise receive no effective care; there really was no hope for the patient who had such a condition.

In the case of patients who made spontaneous recovery from these severe mental disorders, it was even known at that time that such conditions could recur without warning, and there were no methods, such as we have today, that can prevent patients from having further problems with their disease.

The outlook for these patients was bleak.

Efforts were being made by dedicated doctors to study these severe conditions and attempt to discover common characteristics among groups of patients in an effort to understand these ailments. But the knowledge that was being gained from such work, and the categories that were being created, did not appear at the time to be of much practical value in knowing what to do for an individual patient who suffered from one of these severe problems.

HELP COMES TO THE MIDDLE ZONE

By contrast, the success that was being made in treating the disorders of the middle zone, which were problems with anxiety, conversion symptoms, phobias, and so on, by using the methods of psychoanalysis and hypnosis, was to have a far-reaching influence on the development of psychiatry.

Psychoanalysis is a method of treating mental disorders where the patient is encouraged to freely talk about whatever is on his or her mind, where the patient makes a kind of self-exploration of his or her own mental processes with some special coaching from the doctor.

The psychoanalysts did a very good job of categorizing the kinds of disorders that they were treating which they described under the general term of *"neurosis"*, and they created theories about these disorders that were interesting and elaborate systems that tried to explain how the mind worked, and how the person with the neurosis came to develop their "neurotic symptom", and that explained how the methods of hypnosis and psychoanalysis were able to help patients get better. The success that the psychoanalysts were having gave rise to a number of developments.

The psychoanalysts had discovered that the problem of moral insanity or antisocial behavior was not something that they had success at treating. It became clear that the antisocial personality really represented a different kind of mental disorder than neurosis.

So that now we had gone from a classification of persons into sane versus insane to a classification where the most severe cases were called "psychotic", where there was a middle zone, which was the grouping of neurotic illnesses, and there was another category that was different from both of these and that was described as a "personality disorder".

Keep in mind that the category of psychosis which included the very severe mood disturbances, included schizophrenia, paranoid disorders and included the very important group of organic psychosis and organic mental disorder where physical causes were starting to be discovered for those conditions.

Neurotic disorders included conditions that are characterizable by the cardinal manifestations that we've discussed in Chapter II under Problems with Anxiety and also under Problems with Conversion Symptoms and, in addition, included less severe depressions, where it was thought that these less severe (and therefore "minor") mood problems represented another form of the kind of disorder that the psychoanalysts were characterizing as neurotic.

CONSCIOUS AND UNCONSCIOUS

The psychoanalysts' concepts essentially revolved around the idea that there were at least two levels to the mind: a conscious level and an unconscious level. The conscious level included everything that persons usually thought of as "my own mind". The unconscious level included thoughts, feelings, and strong urges that person had no awareness of, and also included important memories that were protected from any effort to remember them by powerful forces in the unconscious mind.

This concept of mental disorder involved the idea that strong urges existed in the unconscious mind that were trying to express themselves and that the rest of the mind, on the unconscious level, was trying to keep under control.

These processes were conceptualized as being driven by a kind of "energy", as were also the forces on the unconscious level of the mind whose purpose was both to keep the urge from being expressed and also to keep it out of conscious awareness.

In these theories, it was the conflict between the urge that was trying to be expressed and the other forces of the mind that were trying to keep the urge under control that was believed to be the basis of neurosis. When one of these unconscious urges was extremely strong and the force in the mind that was supposed to keep the urge under control was almost at the point of giving way, then *anxiety* was created that acted as a signal to the rest of the mind that this type of internal problem was occurring.

What happened to the anxiety after that determined what kind of neurotic symptom would result. There could be free-floating anxiety, which would produce manifestations such as what we had discussed in terms of generalized anxiety manifestations (see page 114) and could also produce unexplained panic attacks (page 112). Anxiety could become "bound" instead of being free-floating and could become "bound" in the form of a conversion symptom, such as the man we discussed on page 136, who had a conflict over whether to beat his wife or not to beat her and developed a paralyzed arm. It was thought that when anxiety became bound in this fashion, that the kind of symptom that developed had some symbolic relationship to the essential aspects of the conflict that was occurring on the unconscious level of the mind.

In the case described earlier of the man who developed a paralyzed right arm, the kind of symptom he developed "symbolized" or "represented" the rough outline of the kind of conflict that was occurring in his mind: his symptom was an inability to use the arm that would have administered a beating to his wife.

It was also thought that anxiety could become bound to specific objects or situations and give rise to phobias, where the object or situation about which the patient had an irrational fear was also something that had a symbolic relationship to the underlying conflict on the unconscious level of the mind.

It was also thought that minor mood disturbances such as mild depression and hypomania could be similarly explained. However, it turned out that the explanations for these mood disturbances were somewhat different, and the treatment of mood disturbances with psychoanalysis was somewhat less successful, overall, than the success with the other so-called neurotic conditions.

KINDS OF NEUROSIS

Each of these different kinds of neurosis was given a name. The ones that predominantly involved free-floating anxiety or unexplained panic attacks were called *anxiety neurosis.*

The ones that involved phobias were called *phobic neurosis.* The minor depressions were called *depressive neurosis,* while conversion symptoms became associated with a form of neurosis that was called *hysteria.*

Just as the energy involved in an unconscious conflict was thought to be convertible into a physical symptom, it was likewise thought that psychological processes in the mind could be effected in a similar way. So that instead of an arm becoming paralyzed, a psychological process like memory, or a person's sense of identity would be the faculty that would be affected. And, it was thought that conditions such as fugue, multiple personality, and problems involving depersonalization and amnesia, were being caused by problems in the binding of this internal "energy" in a way that was supposed to be similar to what happened in conversion symptoms.

Fugue, multiple personality, minor problems with depersonalization or depersonalization that involved anxiety or panic attacks, and the kinds of psychogenic amnesia that we discussed on page 55 were called dissociative symptoms. Conversion symptoms and dissociative symptoms were considered different forms of the neurosis called hysteria.

Some psychoanalysts thought that psychosis could be treated with methods of psychoanalysis and theories about psychosis were created using concepts similiar to those involved in theories about neurosis. Psychoanalysis was for the most part a lengthy treatment involving considerable expense together with a commitment and dedication of the patient to see it through.

But the success that the psychoanalysts were having in treating some of the conditions they worked with offered hope. It was hoped that something new had been discovered that could possibly benefit patients with other forms of mental disorder if only the new method could be adapted to treating these other kinds of patients. And it stimulated much inquiry and study because the theories created by the psychoanalysts had given us a new way to try to understand both normal and abnormal mental functioning.

Psychoanalysts put particular importance on the influence of both forgotten childhood memories as well as on emotional conflicts occurring during childhood that could set up in the early years of a person's life the kind of conflict on the unconscious level of the mind that was believed to have a potential for the development of neurosis and other kinds of mental disorders.

This stimulated much research and study into the family backgrounds of persons with all varities of mental disorder.

The psychoanalysts for the most part did not have much success treating the psychotic disorders but psychiatrists learned to modify some of the techniques used in psychoanalysis and to use them in similar sessions and encounters with patients that were held less frequently and that were less intense than that which was used by the psychoanalysts. This new development became known as psychotherapy.

STRESS

While this was going on, other medical specialties such as internal medicine and gynecology were becoming aware that physical illnesses could arise and be made worse by the events in the patient's environment that caused distress, either because such situations were ones that would be difficult for almost anyone to deal with or because an individual patient had some particular trouble in some area of adaptive functioning.

Work began on the subject of *stress* and its role in the causation of bodily disease. This was enormously important in helping all health care professionals to form a bridge between the mental life of patients and the events in their bodies.

Thus, the psychotic disturbances remained essentially incurable conditions. The psychoanalysts and psychotherapists put much effort into trying to treat them in with little success. But there was great hope for the disorders that occupied the middle zone.

The reader will notice that we have been talking almost exclusively about adults and have had very little to say about the problems of children except in mentioning the psychoanalysts' theories that adult psychiatric disturbances were rooted in childhood experiences. For the time being we will leave out the story of children and the disorders associated with childhood. But the reader needs to understand that during these times, when psychoanalysis and psychotherapy opened an avenue for treatment of some mental disorders, some psychoanalysts did begin to turn to attempts to understand various kinds of problems that appeared in children. We will discuss more of this later.

RECLASSIFYING INSANITY AND THE MIDDLE ZONE

Psychiatry thus went from a kind of classification of people into sane versus insane to a classification consisting of severe disorders—major disorders, most of which were psychotic or involved severe mood disturbance—neurotic disorders which were of lesser severity and were in a middle area between sanity and insanity, and personality disorders about which by now it seemed not much could be done but where the cardinal manifestations seen in psychosis did not appear and where there was not the kind of subjective distress for the most part that occurred in neurosis. These personality disorders largely dealt with various kinds of difficulties in relating with people that seemed to be characteristics or traits of the personality that stayed pretty much the same throughout the life of the individual. They made their first appearance during a person's childhood and continued throughout life.

The classification of mental disorders at this point included also what were called *psychosomatic disorders*, meaning the physical disorders that were either caused or worsened by psychological factors or by a person's reaction to external stress. It also included a group of disorders called adjustment reactions, or transient situational disturbances, which were relatively less severe conditions where some cardinal manifestations of mental disorder were displayed in response to recent life stress, and where individuals could often, by rather brief treatment with psychotherapy, overcome the difficulty or achieve a new adaptation to stress based on finding a more effective way to cope with it.

Also included were a group of disorders that involved sexual practices such as we've discussed under the paraphilias, which were an interesting group of problems because the psychoanalyst who originally had been very interested in sexual urges as being among the important ones that caused problems on the unconscious level of the mind, understandably became interested in treating these kinds of difficulties; however, it turned out that many of these paraphilias were extremely difficult to treat and were by and large at that time rather hopeless conditions.

The conditions that we have called disturbances of sexual response such as *inhibited sexual excitement, premature ejaculation,* and so on (see page 143) were conditions that were treated by psychoanalysts with psychotherapy with mixed success. That were essentially the way things stood around 1950. The most serious functional disorders—the psychotic disorders—and the severe mood disturbances, had been subdivided, based on study of affected patients, into several groups. Progress in the fields of neurology, endocrinology, internal medicine, and surgery together with a greater understanding of the side effects of medication on behavior had continued to expand our knowledge of the organic mental disorders and had even given us the knowledge and the technique to reverse some of them or to prevent other kinds from getting worse.

SCHIZOPHRENIA SUBDIVIDED

In the case of the severe functional mental disorders: these had been classified into schizophrenia, into a condition called manic-depressive psychosis, into certain other kinds of severe depression, and into paranoid disorders. At that time, schizophrenia was thought to consist of several subtypes which were really described mostly on the basis of the patient's predominant cardinal manifestation.

There was controversy about what was the core problem in schizophrenia, that is, what were the characteristics that schizophrenic patients all had in common that allowed us to group them together as though they were suffering from the same illness. One school of thought believed that the basic problem lay within an impairment in the ability to associate one thought logically with another. What we refer to as formal thought disorder together with a disorganization of the ability to have an appropriate emotional response to a situation, combined with a tendency to withdraw from others, was the central problem that all schizophrenic patients shared; all other problems they had were an outgrowth of these. These other problems were considered, as we mentioned before, secondary symptoms that were used to sub-divide persons with schizophrenia merely on the basis of whether a particular cardinal manifestation of mental disorder was the predominant secondary symptom. Schizophrenic patients who displayed mostly catatonic behavior were called (and still are) the catatonic type. Patients who suffer from predominant delusions of persecution, delusions of jealousy, and grandiose delusions, and who had hallucinations of voices were called the paranoid type (and DSM-III still does). Patients who had mostly a flat, inappropriate, or silly affect, whose behavior was grossly disorganized and accompanied by prominent loosening of association or incoherence were called the hebephrenic type (in DSM-III this is called the disorganized type).

There was also described a type called the simple type which was different from all of the others and seemed to be characterized mostly by a social withdrawal and a disinterest in associating with people, but which was not characterized by the other kinds of symptoms we have mentioned for schizophrenia. Such persons seem to become lifelong drifters and loners who keep by themselves, but who nevertheless seem to be able to exist and live out their lives with this problem.

The simple type sometimes seemed to contain two groups of people, though: those who had the social withdrawal and social isolation and a disinterest in social relations as a kind of continuous enduring lifelong problem where they were nevertheless able to find some way to function as a drifter or loner, people who had some of the same features but who from time to time would develop some of the other symptoms of schizophrenia, such as the loosening of associations, peculiar ideas, peculiar behavior, disorganized behavior, or hallucinations and delusions.

Then there was a type called the undifferentiated type which was enough of a mixture of the cardinal manifestation of some of the other types (catatonic, paranoid and so on,) that it couldn't be classified as specifically any one of them (this continues in DSM-III).

Schizophrenia was then conceived of as a disorder that could come on relatively suddenly, or could begin with a prodromal period before the active phase of the disease. In the prodromal period, the person, over a period of time, showed increasing social withdrawal, peculiar ideas, peculiar behavior, speech that was starting to sound vague, difficult to understand (as thought it were the beginning of loosening of associations), where affect became either blunt, flat, or inappropriate, where unusual experiences or illusions would occur (see page 64), or persons would have some of the unusual perceptual experiences we described on page 65, where they would sense the presence of a person who was not really there or they would sense the presence of a force. In the prodromal period, a decline could begin in personal hygiene and self-care and some impairment could be noticed in the individual's ability to function at their occupation or in school or in relations with other people.

And, as had been noticed decades before, whether or not there was a prodromal period where the disease crept up slowly on the individual, there was a downhill course that was a discouraging and tragic aspect of the condition. Once the psychosis actually set in as an acute and active phase of the disease, it continued on without any improvement, or it got a little better and remained at that level, perhaps to worsen again at some later time. Even when an episode of psychosis seemed to go away, the person seemed always to be left with some kind of residual problem that was much like the kind of cardinal manifestations that would occur in a prodromal period of the disease and where such cardinal manifestations would usually continue as a chronic phase of the disease.

These symptoms of the prodromal period had also been noticed in some patients who seemed to have them as a lifelong problem without ever getting the acute phase of the illness. It was also seen in persons who had various kinds of unstable emotional behavior, unstable and sometimes unrealistic social relationships, and who had various problems related to their sense of identity, being unable to tolerate being alone, and who sometimes committed self-destructive or self-mutilatory acts. It seemed as though exposure to certain stressful situations made some individuals psychotic for brief periods of time (sometimes a few hours to a couple of days), whereupon the psychosis would then suddenly go away, such individuals did not seem to suffer any residual impairment or any downhill course.

When psychoanalysts had treated such persons, they were often patients who came with various kinds of subjective distress and often had a mixture of the kinds of problems that neurotic people seemed to have; however their manifestations of those types of problems were a changing picture, as opposed to the kind of symptom that the psychoanalysts had been used to treating (such as a person who had a phobia or who had panic attacks and who had the problem consistently unless he got treatment). This other group had symptoms that seemed to change. They had too many neurotic symptoms to fit into one clean category, together with some of the things that from time to time suggested psychotic ideas or psychotic behavior which never lasted long enough to constitute a problem that needed to become a focus of management or treatment.

Such individuals were referred to as *"borderline schizophrenia"*. It was thought that in the division of all people into three kinds, insane, middle zone, and sane, that on the borderline between the middle zone and the psychotic group were these borderline people.

Psychiatrists and psychoanalysts really didn't know where to put them, just as they didn't know where to put some of the personality disorders that had been discovered up to that time which seemed to lie in a category all of their own.

Another problem with schizophrenia was that there were some individuals who did seem to develop definite signs of schizophrenia for considerable periods of time, perhaps several months, who got better and who didn't seem to have any residual problems. These persons were also felt to have some form of schizophrenia, although psychiatrists could not understand why some persons with schizophrenia continued to suffer from it all of their life in some way, and why other individuals who had schizophrenia got completely well.

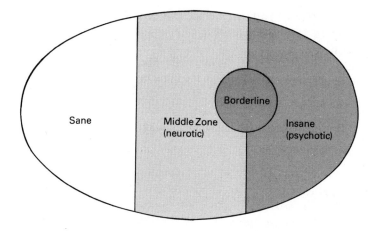

MOOD DISORDERS

By this time, there also had been distinguished a group of major affective disorders involving severe depression or severe manic mood which were recurrent, where persons would suffer from an extreme depression and after six to nine months of proper care would recover, returning to a better level of functioning, perhaps to become depressed again in a similiar way at another time in their life perhaps equally or seriously as before.

Likewise there were patients with severe manic mood who, if they could be contained and treated during their period of overactivity, racing thoughts, boundless energy, and tendency to become involved in reckless and self-injurious pursuits, could after three to six months occasionally get better, returning to a level of mood that had been their usual level or a normal level, only to have the same problem recur at a later time in their life, perhaps with the same degree of severity.

It was also noticed that some individuals who developed such severe manic moods could also develop severe depressions as well. A problem with abnormally elevated mood could be preceded or followed by a problem with a very low and depressed mood, where all the characteristics that we have discussed for depressed mood on page 103, and for manic mood on page 103, could be part of the picture and extremely severe, and where some patients in severe manic mood or severe depressed mood could be psychotic, with delusions and hallucinations.

Experience with the retrospective kind of examination of the life history of patients with these kinds of problems revealed a significant number of cases where the level of mood went up and down, way above and way below normal many times in the life of the individual. There were even some cases where the level of mood would swing back and forth between severe mania and severe depression every few days.

It was clear from studying these patients that they seemed to form a distinct group of their own, and it seemed as though whatever it was in the brain that controlled the level of mood was malfunctioning.

It was also noted that, in many patients, the depressions or the manic episodes did not seem to begin in response to any stress in the environment. The mood level changes seemed to have their origin in something that was wrong inside of the patient.

ECT

The progress that psychiatry had made up until about the fifties saw the discovery of an important method of treatment that could be applied very successfully to some of the patients who had severe depressions. This was "electric shock treatment" or "electroconvulsive therapy" (ECT).

Someone noticed that depressed persons who had epilepsy were less depressed after they had an epileptic seizure (convulsion). This led to research on whether artificial induction of a convulsion could help depressed people.

Severely depressed patients are not merely patients who suffer severe distress from their mood and who cannot function, becoming severely withdrawn and apathetic. In some cases they commit suicide.

Today, in 1980, major depression remains a highly lethal condition, despite our improved methods of treatment. In a variety of follow-up studies, the death rate of patients from suicide over a lifetime of major depressive illness is about fifteen percent, and that's with the methods of treatment we have today.

Back in the thirties when these discoveries about the relationship between convulsions and depression were discovered, there was *no* effective treatment for major depression!

But, through trial and error, a way was found to reliably induce a convulsion artificially in patients by passing a mild electric current through the brain, and that after a series of such treatments, a substantial number of severely depressed patients improved.

As with psychoanalysis, which had found a way to treat the disorders of the middle zone, and which was seized upon as a possible answer to other forms of mental disorder, so electric shock treatment began to be used in a wide variety of the different kinds of mental disorders we have already discussed.

Several decades of experience with the new treatment showed that it was highly effective in major depression, and particularly in major depressions where the physiologic and behavioral changes were intense, and where the dysphoric mood was of a special and distinctly unpleasant kind known as *melancholia.*

It was also of significant benefit in the kinds of severe depressions that occurred in those patients who had, or were likely to have, episodes of severe mania.

Interestingly, administering electric shock treatments to some of these patients threw them into mania, and while this was not of benefit to such patients, this observation suggested that there was something that controlled the level of mood (and that low mood and elevated mood were related) in some deeper level of the brain.

Electric shock treatment was discovered after these several decades to be of only limited benefit in the other mental disorders, and impact made by ECT was not significant when we look at the fate of the majority of these patients.

It seemed to be of *no* benefit whatsoever in the disorders of the middle zone and of only limited benefit in schizophrenia, except in the case of catatonic excitement where it was possible to terminate such a wild episode of purposeless physical activity with sometimes only one electric shock treatment.

ECT was of no benefit in the personality disorders, or in any of the other conditions we have mentioned.

But it was of significant benefit in major depressions much of the time, and much good came of it. Psychiatry had found another tool.

This is essentially where we stood in the fifties before the next step. It was a giant step, a leap forward that put psychiatry on a new course and changed completely the concepts and attitudes of mental health professionals toward the care of the severely mentally ill. A way was found to alter the course of schizophrenia.

THE MAJOR TRANQUILIZERS

This occurred with the introduction of the first of the drugs known as the major tranquilizers. These are drugs very different from what most laymen mean by the "tranquilizers" that are often perscribed by physicians for states of minor anxiety. The major tranquilizers are drugs which, for the most part, are not effective in that kind of minor anxiety. They are different.

Major tranquilizers can change the course of schizophrenia! It was discovered that a patient in the active phase of schizophrenia who received adequate treatment with sufficient doses of major tranquilizers could experience a relatively rapid relief of many features of the psychosis.

Patients were then able to become somewhat better organized, and it was found that patients who suffered from delusions and hallucinations had problems related to a special kind of anxiety associated with the schizophrenic process that major tranquilizers seemed to help.

In some cases patients actually lost their delusions and hallucinations, and the patients who continued to have delusions and hallucinations appeared much less concerned about them and less preoccupied with them.

While it wasn't a cure (although in some patients its effect was almost miraculous), the overall effect of such drugs on the majority of schizophrenic patients was to significantly reduce the severity of the symptoms and in many cases allow them to return to some maintainable level of adaptive functioning. This was an achievement that only a decade before, would have been held to be impossible; for many patients schizophrenia would have meant the prospect of a lifetime in a mental institution.

The use of this medicine over the next couple of decades changed the way psychiatry viewed schizophrenia. It was no longer viewed as a completely hopeless condition.

Unlike the doctors of 1910, we no longer see in the patient who has an acute schizophrenia, a person who faces a virtual certainty of a lifetime of hardship and incarceration.

What we see instead is someone who has a reasonable chance of achieving some relief, perhaps significant relief, from the symptoms of the illness and who after a period of time will most likely not have to spend much of their life in a hospital.

From the standpoint of classifying the insane, the use of the major tranquilizers was very important. For one thing it was noticed that while some individuals did extremely well, extremely rapidly on these drugs, being able almost to return completely to a previous level of functioning, other individuals did not do as well and continued either to have the residual symptoms of the disease after some relief of the acute phase. The use of the major tranquilizers seemed to make much difference in some patients, but in others, aside from making them easier for nurses and hospital technicians to deal with, the drug did little to make an impact on the psychotic symptoms. Did such persons have a different disease, or did they just have "a bad case" of the same disease?

A DRUG FOR MANIA AND NEW ONES FOR DEPRESSION

It was also found that the major tranquilizers were valuable in the treatment of mania. Acutely manic patients, when heavily medicated with major tranquilizers, could have their manic behavior brought under control. However they usually remained ill for the typical three to six months and then the mania went away.

The use of the drug dampened the mania and made them manageable during the period of time that had to elapse before the symptoms disappeared on their own.

A problem developed in psychiatric diagnosis as a result of the availability of the major tranquilizers.

There was now a drug that could be used for schizophrenia which was a psychotic condition, and could also be used in mania, which often presented delusions and hallucinations. Therefore, the need to make a fine distinction between those two groups was, in a practical sense, no longer necessary.

It was also found that the major tranquilizers, suprisingly, made a difference in some cases of acute depression.

But another tremendously important discovery was yet to come that would force us to make a sharper distinction among persons who were both depressed and psychotic.

That was the appearance of *the anti-depressant medicines*. These were medicines that, when administered to patients with severe depression, within two to four weeks produced a significant reduction in symptoms, and that were able to produce a result virtually equivalent to the use of electro-convulsive therapy.

It now became important to distinguish patients who had schizophrenia with depressive symptoms—that is, with aspects of depressed mood—from patients who had major depression with psychosis.

It was found that in some patients who were really suffering from schizophrenia, who had secondary symptoms of depression, that the use of anti-depressant drugs *made them worse* and brought the schizophrenia out as a more prominent problem.

Anti-depressant medication could not be indiscriminantly used for any patient who was both depressed and psychotic.

It was also quite clear that while the major tranquilizers could be of benefit in depressed patients, many depressed patients did somewhat better with anti-depressant medication, particularly if they had the symptoms of melancholia (rather more pronounced physiologic and behavioral changes).

There was now a reason to look carefully at depressed persons to determine whether they were really suffering from schizophrenia, and to look very carefully at patients who seemed to be suffering from schizophrenia because they were psychotic and wonder whether they were suffering from a form of depression that was accompanied by psychosis.

DISCOVERY OF LITHIUM BRINGS CHANGES

Then in the sixties came an advance in the treatment of the mentally ill that ranks among the greatest discoveries in the history of medicine: the introduction of lithium as a specific treatment of mania.

The effect of lithium on mania is miraculous. When administered to a patient suffering from severe manic mood, in seven to ten days the mania can be brought under control; the mood is then stabilized, and by taking maintenance doses (somewhat lower doses) of the drug, further recurrences of manic mood can be prevented.

The relief of mania by lithium is much more complete and much more specific in the sense of being a "cure" than is the "relief" of schizophrenic symptoms by major tranquilizers.

Experience with lithium showed that a significant number of patients who were once thought to be schizophrenic were in fact suffering from mania. This was diagnosis in retrospect through the use of lithium on various kinds of patients.

It was discovered that many patients who had been previously classified as suffering from schizophrenia could be quickly and specifically treated with the new anti-manic drug, and that other patients who superficially appeared to have similiar symptoms did not improve when given lithium but instead showed relatively better improvement with a major tranquilizer.

This was a tremendous discovery and it has led to a great shift in our thinking about mental disorder today.

The success that was had with the treatment of mood disorders, both through the use of anti-depressants and through the use of lithium, led to extensive study and research in an effort to allow us to better distinguish between the patients with mood disorder who were psychotic and the patients who were psychotic but had schizophrenia (the disease with the steady downhill course). The pattern of disease in the relatives of patients, when taken together with the patient's own response to treatment, and the kinds of symptoms that the patient had (immediately before the acute phase of illness, during the acute phase, and afterward) made it rather clear that the category of schizophrenia would have to shrink, and the category of affective disease would have to be enlarged.

In the most recent previous official classification system, DSM-II, a category of disease existed known as *schizoaffective disorder*. It was, at that time, appreciated that there were patients who had such a thorough mixture of schizophrenic symptoms—either depressive or manic—that it was impossible to classify them as belonging to the group of schizophrenic patients or to the group of affective disorder patients. It was additionally noticed that the schizoaffective disorder patients (the ones who were put into that category) did seem to have a different course, and that they didn't seem to have, as a rule, the steady downhill progression that had been always pointed to as the characteristic signature of schizophrenia.

Here too, DSM-III has made a significant change. Schizoaffective disorder has been relegated to a smaller residual category.

What has happened is this. The functional psychotic disorders, once considered the most serious of the functional mental disorders, because of their utter hopelessness, now have good treatments that do not involve psychotherapy or psychoanalysis, but involve a direct assault on the disease by means of drugs.

The essence of the disease today is conceptualized as a biochemical disturbance in the brain which is understood at the present time as a disturbance of the process that allows nerve impulses in the brain to pass from one nerve to another.

THE NEUROTRANSMITTER THEORY

This theory is principally based on our knowledge of depression and schizophrenia. It doesn't solve all the questions about why the anti-depressant drugs and the major tranquilizers are effective, but it is a guideline in psychiatry for the moment.

The theory is simply this: a nerve carries a kind of electrical impulse. When that impulse flows down a nerve from one end to another, the way it is passed on to the next nerve is not by an electrical impulse that jumps across a gap like a spark. Although the impulse does not jump across the gap like a spark, it does cause a release at the end of the nerve of chemicals that flow across the gap between the first nerve and the second. The chemicals, when they reach the second nerve, excite it, and cause it to generate its own electrical impulse, and thus to continue the chain.

It is currently believed that certain nerves that are involved in parts of the brain related to level of mood and in parts of the brain related to the kinds of problems that are seen as physiologic and behavioral changes of depression have *a deficiency* of the chemical that is supposed to flow across the gap and to allow one nerve to pass its impulse successfully to the next. The overall effect of this deficiency is to lower the activity level of the brain in these particular nerve pathways. Drugs such as reserpine which are notorious for causing severe depression cause a deficiency of the transmitter chemical.

It is believed that the antidepressant drugs work by preventing the nerve cell from removing the transmitter chemical from the gap between the nerves once the transmitter has been released. The overall effect of such a blockade is to make more of the transmitter chemical available at the gap, so that small changes will make a bigger difference. In mania it is believed that the opposite problem of an over-activity occurs in these same nerve pathways, and that lithium can act to stabilize this. Similar theories have been advanced for the success of the major tranquilizers in treating schizophrenia tying them to other transmitter chemicals in other nerve pathways where it is thought that an over-abundance of a nerve-transmitter chemical called dopamine can have its effects blocked by the major tranquilizers, resulting in an improvement in the psychosis.

Whether our current theory is correct or not, we do have effective treatment today. These serious illnesses, functional affective disorders, and functional psychoses have been reclassified and redefined to reflect not only what we know, but also what we can do to help afflicted individuals.

MAJOR DEPRESSION AND BIPOLAR DISORDER

What has happened to the classification is this.

There are now recognized two kinds of major affective disorder: *major depression* and *bipolar disorder*. Bipolar disorder exists when a person has had, or is having an episode of mania. The name of the disease, "bipolar disorder", was intended to imply that there is a swing back and forth between the two opposite poles of mood. *Major depression* is the category used for patients who have severe depressions that meet the criteria for a major depressive episode in DSM-III, but have never had a manic episode. Their mood seems to swing *down* from normal to a low level, and then back again to normal, repeatedly. A person who is having their first such episode is said to have *major depression, single episode,* and a person who develops another episode of major depression after having already had one is said to have *major depression, recurrent.*

DSM-III teaches that when mania has occurred even once, a patient has *bipolar disorder.* When a patient is currently sick, the kind of bipolar disorder they are said to have is based on whether they currently have a manic episode, whether they currently have a depressed episode, or whether they have the peculiar mixed type where the full manic and the full depressed picture alternate back and forth every few days (the depression periods must last at least a day).

Thus, if a person has bipolar disorder, and they currently have a depressed episode, their diagnosis at the moment is bipolar disorder, depressed. The term *"bipolar disorder"* carries the name of the basic disease, while the qualifying word, "depressed" (or "manic" if it happened to be a manic episode) describes the nature of the current episode of mood disturbance.

Research that was done using the new drugs has caused a great shift in our thinking. The category and the concept of affective disorder has been expanded to include almost all disturbances of depressed mood and elevated mood, whether major or minor.

The concept of affective disorder is no longer split up as it was decades ago, when patients with severe mania or severe depression, perhaps with psychosis, were put into the category of the most serious or the most insane, while patients with less severe depressions or elevated mood found their way into the middle zone to be treated by psychoanalysts and by psychotherapists.

Except for certain rather special varieties of less severe, self-limiting depressed moods that occur in direct response to environmental psychosocial stressors, all the major and all the minor mood disorders have been combined into one large class. These less severe moods in response to stress, which are self-limiting—where the disorder occurs within three months of the psychosocial stressor, and where the response is not part of a general reaction to stress, or part of a larger pattern of fluctuating mood—describes the condition called "adjustment reaction with depressed mood". Except for this special case, major affective disorder and so called minor affective disorder are now viewed to be in the same family.

This shift in concepts is reflected in the definition of bipolar disorder. Bipolar disorder has a mood level that goes up and down between mania and either normal or depressed mood. Bipolar disorder is considered an affective disorder that is distinct from major depression. While both are serious, *they are not the same disease.*

There are many particular features of the people who have recurrent major depressions without mania and the people who have bipolar disorder that provide the reasons for separating them into these two broad groups. To see how DSM-III has embraced some minor mood disturbances as part of a larger concept of affective disorder, we can note in DSM-III that when a person with bipolar disorder has had one manic episode, DSM-III does not require the full, serious picture of manic episode again in order to have it counted as a recurrence.

Similarly if a person with bipolar disorder has had one severe depression, then becomes depressed again, but not so severely as to be a major depressive episode, DSM-III still counts it as a recurrence of the bipolar disorder. It is felt that in such patients the mood fluctuation itself is the disease, and "minor" mood fluctuations are indications that the disease is smoldering.

MAJOR AFFECTIVE DISORDER VERSUS SCHIZOPHRENIA

The second major change was to delineate these two very serious conditions, major affective disorder and schizophrenia, from one another. This is done partly through the device of the distinction we made once between mood congruent and mood-incongruent delusions or hallucinations (see page 106).

An affective disorder with psychosis must not have preoccupation with a mood-incongruent delusion or hallucination, and must not have bizarre behavior during any stage where a full affective syndrome is not present. Those would be characteristics not consistent with the affective picture. In affective disorder, when delusions or hallucinations occur, they are cosistent with the tone of the patient's mood in most instances.

Furthermore in the case of schizophrenia, when the full picture of schizophrenia is present with characteristic delusions and hallucinations, if a patient also has, or develops, a full-severe-manic or full-severe-depressed picture, it must have developed *after* any psychotic symptoms in order to make the diagnosis of schizophrenia.

If a significant mood problem developed before the appearance of the psychosis, then DSM-III believes that the patient really has an affective disorder.

If the psychosis and the severe mood picture develop at the same time, schizophrenia can now only be diagnosed when the mood picture is relatively brief in duration compared with the duration of the psychotic symptoms.

It can be seen how extensively schizophrenia is being whittled down.

Patients previously classified as schizophrenic merely on the basis of the presence of delusions or hallucinations now must have the content of their delusions and hallucinations looked at more carefully, and the onset and the course of the illness in relation to both mood and psychotic symptoms has to be carefully examined to determine whether the patient belongs in the affective disorder category.

SCHIZOPHRENIA AND SCHIZOPHRENIFORM DISORDER

Schizophrenia has been further redefined to draw attention to its chronic downhill course, and to separate schizophrenia as a distinct disease from the schizophrenia-like disorders in patients who develop severe psychosis but who get better relatively quickly. Such fortunate patients, by a variety of measures, seem to have a different disease. Follow-up studies of patients who develop a psychosis that looks like the acute phase of schizophrenia, but who get better relatively quickly, give the impression that they are suffering from a different illness than the patients who develop a schizophrenic picture and who either maintain it in its acute form or who have had a prodromal period that when taken together with the duration of the acute psychosis, gives a relatively longer total period of illness, or who after the acute phase subsides maintain a lengthy period of residual symptoms.

No person will now be called schizophrenic unless they maintain a continuous period of illness for at least six months.

Any patient who develops an acute psychosis that matches the description for schizophrenia but has their disorder for less than six months, cannot receive the diagnosis of schizophrenia.

Only patients who maintain that condition for longer than six months will receive the diagnosis of schizophrenia.

Any patient who develops a schizophrenia-like picture that lasts longer than two weeks but less than six months, and then goes away, has had what DSM-III calls a *schizophreniform disorder.*

Apparently the six month cut-off point, on the basis of statistical studies of the two groups of patients (those who have a lengthy course of illness and those who get better quickly), seems to be the most reliable basis on which to break these disorders into two groups.

DSM-III further wants to distinguish the psychosis of schizophreniform disorder from certain very brief psychoses that may last less than two weeks. There are two kinds of very brief psychotic illnesses.

Brief Reactive Psychosis is a short psychosis lasting less than two weeks, and occurs as a direct response to an environmental psychosocial stressor that would be expected to produce a significant degree of stress in almost anybody (although not necessarily produce a psychosis)

Atypical Psychosis is the name that will be given to any psychosis that lasts less than two weeks but developed without an identifiable psychosocial stressor that was related to it.

DSM-III includes any prodromal period as part of the total duration of illness, so that in making a determination of how long a person has been suffering from symptoms of schizophrenia, if the length of time of prodromal period plus length of time of the active phase is greater than six months, or if prodrome plus active period plus some period of residual phase is greater than six months, then the diagnosis of schizophrenia *can* be made. It not, such a disease would be called schizophreniform disorder (when it has lasted longer than two weeks).

Persons who have no history of a prodromal period who really have schizophrenia, are going to have their diagnosis changed twice. When they appear acutely ill without a history of a prodromal period, the first diagnosis they will receive will be either Atypical Psychosis or Brief Reactive

Psychosis. This will be done with the understanding that it is too early to make a diagnosis of either schizophrenia or schizophreniform disorder, and there is still the possibility that the psychosis might go away in less than two weeks. If the occurrence of the illness has a relationship to a recent psychosocial stressor, then the patients will receive the diagnosis of Brief Reactive Psychosis. If not, the diagnosis will be Atypical Psychosis.

If they then remain sick for longer than two weeks, their diagnosis will be changed to Schizophreniform Psychosis. It is still too early to know whether they suffer from schizophrenia or not because the patient may yet get better, and would statistically have a different chance of successful return to a previous level of adaptive functioning.

If they remain sick for longer than six months, or if they get a little better but maintain some residual symptoms that carry them across the six month mark, then and only then do they receive the diagnosis of schizophrenia.

Schizophrenia remains the most serious of all the psychotic disorders because of its tendency to be chronic.

What has happened is that our knowledge grew; we discovered that not all schizophrenic-like psychosis is schizophrenia, even when it shares a great many of the cardinal manifestations.

We have also learned that much of what we thought was schizophrenia is, in fact, a form of affective disorder with psychosis and responds specifically to the special treatments for severe affective disorder.

The enlargement of the category of affective disorder at the expense of the category of schizophrenia also threw out the category of schizoaffective illness as a diagnosis in its own right. Schizoaffective disorder in DSM-III is intended to be used only as a residual category, when, after a genuine effort, it is truly impossible in the case of a particular patient to make a distinction between affective disorder and schizophrenia. The intent of DSM-III is that this effort should always be made, and when the examiner cannot make the distinction from his direct interview with the patient, and his sifting of the patient's history or onset of illness, the examiner might even question the family members to determine whether there is a history in the family of affective disorders that might tilt the decision in favor of affective disease.

Affective disease has a specific treatment. When properly used, the majority of patients have significant improvement and can receive medicine to prevent a recurrence.

Schizophrenia as defined in DSM-III remains a disease with a steady downhill course, and patients who develop acute episodes and then appear to recover always have residual symptoms. The principle underlying the classification of schizophrenia is that if the patient really does get better, and is truly symptom-free, then the patient probably did not have schizophrenia, but had another disorder and the diagnosis of schizophrenia was made in error.

Furthermore, schizophrenia is still thought of as a serious disease of younger people. DSM-III says that the diagnosis will not be made in the case of patients who are over the age of forty-five at the time their illness begins (taking the point of onset of the prodromal period as the point of true onset of the illness). Cases that begin after forty-five that fit all the criteria for schizophrenia, including the duration of illness restriction that the condition be present continuously for six months, will receive a diagnosis of Atypical Psychosis and will not receive a diagnosis of schizophrenia.

This circumscribes even further the population of persons having schizophrenia.

Schizophrenia is further cut off from the paranoid disorders by insisting that if a patient has delusions that have a predominantly persecutory or jealous content that they must suffer some sort of hallucination as well, and not a delusion alone.

Paranoid disorders are the group that are characterized by systematized delusions of persecution and jealousy without hallucinations.

GIANT STEPS

Thus when we look back and take an historical perspective, we can see the change that has taken place in how psychiatrists view these psychotic disorders.

Once a condition for which there was no hope, schizophrenia remains a chronic disease, but it is no longer a disease that requires hospitalization for a lifetime. Major tranquilizers have made it possible for schizophrenic persons to experience significant reduction in severity of symptoms, and in some cases to attain and maintain significant levels of adaptive functioning in spite of the ongoing disease process.

Psychiatry has made giant steps.

WHAT HAPPENED TO NEUROSIS?

We see that great progress had been made in treating the serious mental disorders.

What of the disorders in the middle zone?

Great changes have occurred here too, because a door has opened to the future.

The term neurosis is being abandoned. In the original drafts of DSM-III the term was dropped entirely. When the final version of DSM-III was adopted by the psychiatric profession, it was agreed that there were some individuals who really knew how to use the term neurosis correctly, and that the term could continue in relation to certain disorders.

The old group of neuroses, consisting of anxiety neurosis, phobic neurosis, and hysteria (conversion neurosis and dissociative neurosis) have been renamed. They don't even appear in the same section together.

What happened to neurosis, and why was this done?

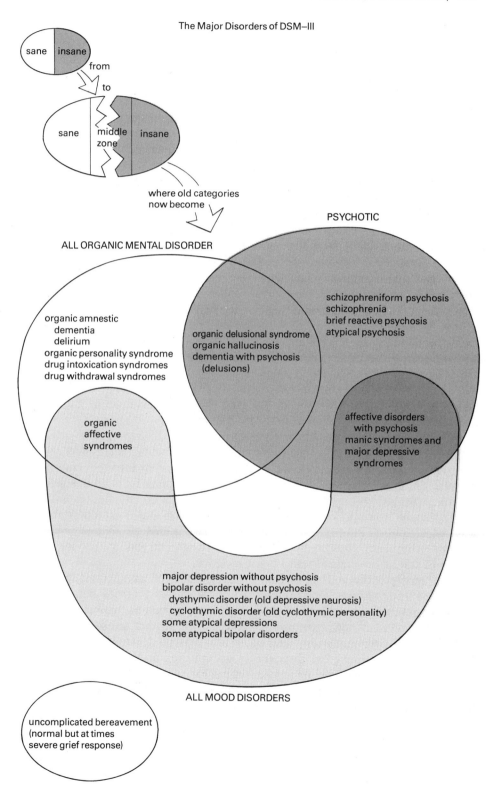

The Major Disorders of DSM–III

sane | insane

from

to

sane | middle zone | insane

where old categories now become

ALL ORGANIC MENTAL DISORDER

PSYCHOTIC

organic amnestic
   dementia
   delirium
organic personality syndrome
drug intoxication syndromes
drug withdrawal syndromes

organic delusional syndrome
organic hallucinosis
dementia with psychosis
   (delusions)

schizophreniform psychosis
schizophrenia
brief reactive psychosis
atypical psychosis

organic
affective
syndromes

affective disorders
with psychosis
manic syndromes and
major depressive
syndromes

major depression without psychosis
bipolar disorder without psychosis
   dysthymic disorder (old depressive neurosis)
   cyclothymic disorder (old cyclothymic personality)
some atypical depressions
some atypical bipolar disorders

ALL MOOD DISORDERS

uncomplicated bereavement
(normal but at times
severe grief response)

Many decades ago, when the major mental disorders were tragically hopeless conditions, the persons who were treating the "neurotic" disorders in the middle zone were the ones who gave psychiatry hope.

As you recall, neurosis was a group of diseases in the middle zone that dealt predominantly with anxiety, where patients either experienced the anxiety openly as generalized anxiety, or as attacks of panic, or where anxiety was bound to a particular object or thing, as in the case of a phobia.

Elaborate theories were created to describe how anxiety could be created within the mind as a result of conflicts occurring between opposing mental forces.

Neurosis as a concept goes hand in hand with those theories. A diagnosis of neurosis is not just a description of symptoms, but implies understanding the symptoms and conceptualizing the patient's problem and the focus of treatment along the lines of the theories of psychoanalysis.

One of the reasons that the term neurosis was abandoned was to make the new language of psychiatry free of a close tie to psychoanalytic theories.

But there are other reasons why the term *neurosis* was dropped. There are very important reasons that also explain the appearance of certain new terms in DSM-III that rest on new knowledge about mental disorders.

AGORAPHOBIA AND IMIPRAMINE

The cardinal manifestation of mental disorder that we called agoraphobia (see page 115) had often been considered as a manifestation of the kind of anxiety that was at the basis of neurotic disturbances.

Furthermore, the condition in children, called *"separation anxiety"*, which was felt to be the basis of what child psychiatrists called *"school phobia"*, where children refused to go to school—not to be truant—but because in most cases they suffered from irrational fears that something terrible was going to happen to their major attachment figure, and they wanted to be home in order to be certain that the major attachment figure was safe. School Phobia and Truancy are two kinds of *school refusal*—in *truancy,* the child goes with friends or roams the streets. In *school phobia* the child stays home and doesn't want to leave.

Both agoraphobia and separation anxiety were for psychoanalytic theory important touchstones as examples of what those theories believed were major mental processes that lay at the bottom of much normal and abnormal human behavior. When agoraphobia and school phobia are severe they can be highly disabling conditions, and often are difficult to treat.

Now came another great discovery: agoraphobia and school phobia could be treated by a drug used in severe depression. One of the most important drugs for treating major depression is imipramine. Many persons have been helped back to a useful life because of it, and it is a drug that any new antidepressant medicine will be compared with. Imipramine is a benchmark in the treatment of depression. It has recently been found that there may be two categories of depression that differ from one another chemically, where imipramine is more successful in the treatment of the one, and another drug called amitriptyline is more effective in treating the other.

Agoraphobia with panic attacks is a disorder in which there are two kinds of fear and two kinds of anxiety. There is the fear of going out into public places for fear of being incapacitated without help, or without ability to escape, as is characteristic of agoraphobia in general. When confronted with that particular situation away from home, the individual does experience panic attacks. The second kind of anxiety that the patient has is an *anticipatory fear* that if he should leave the home, and go to one of those public places, that he will have a panic attack.

It was discovered that imipramine could treat this kind of agoraphobia. And while agoraphobia is not a depression, and while these patients did not match the criteria in DSM-III for the depressive disorders, imipramine was nevertheless successful in quickly ending the panic attacks. When anticipatory anxiety was then treated with minor tranquilizers (like valium) individuals who had been virtually incapacitated by severe agoraphobia now became able to leave their homes and mingle once again with people.

It was found that in the case of agoraphobia without panic attacks, this kind of treatment with imipramine was not successful, and so DSM-III begins its discussion of anxiety disorders with a description of agoraphobia with and without panic attacks.

Agoraphobia is a "neurosis" that is now treatable with a drug. The need for long months, possibly years, of psychoanalysis or psychotherapy for patients who have benefited from drug therapy is today not necessary.

Another reason why the term was dropped came from dealing with the related issue of separation anxiety in children. After the success of treating agoraphobia with imipramine, the related condition where children are reluctant to leave their major attachment figure, or leave the home, became the next focus. The condition of school phobia had often required difficult, sometimes fruitless, battles to get children to return to school when the children were insistent upon staying home, because of their desperate fears about their attachment figures.

These children often required long psychotherapy and sometimes psychoanalysis to produce relief from their problem. A large number of these children were helped by imipramine, sometimes in a matter of a few days. Children were able to quickly leave their home and return to school without suffering the intense fears, without the temper tantrums, and without the uneasiness that caused them to suffer, and had complicated the treatment of this condition for decades.

Imipramine, which was thought of as a drug for depression, now became a specific treatment as well for these two conditions.

Why these two problems related to anxiety, problems of the middle zone, have responded to treatment with a drug used to treat the most serious forms of depression is a mystery.

What the anxiety in separation anxiety, and the anxiety and panic attacks in agoraphobia have to do with depression, and how they are linked deep within the processes of the mind is a question future research will answer.

Finally, depressive neurosis, which was a chronic but "minor" depression, consisting of at least a couple of years of significant periods of depressed mood, sometimes punctuated with periods of normal mood that never reached the severity of a major depressive episode, was taken out of the category of the middle zone and made part of the family of affective disorder.

The disturbance in mood in depressive neurosis, which is now called *"dysthymic disorder"* is chronic, troublesome, and persistent. Dysthymic Disorder is now held to be the same kind of problem as the disturbance in the chemistry of the brain that causes major depression. Dysthymic disorder, while consisting of prolonged periods of depression, none of which are severe enough to reach the intensity of a major depressive episode, nevertheless can give rise to suicidal thoughts and possibly suicidal attempts, and has never been a disease to be trifled with. It has never fitted in well with other neuroses, which never had suicide as a complication.

These three steps, growing out of the progress in mood disorder, have elevated mood disorder even more as a central area of psychiatric research. But mood disorder has enlarged by diminishing the category of neurosis. The middle zone has shrunk.

These three things: being able to treat agoraphobia with panic attacks using the mood disorder drug imipramine to specifically treat the panic, the use of imipramine to treat separation anxiety and repair the problem of school phobia in children, and the removal of depressive neurosis altogether from the neurotic category, seeing it as another version of biochemical disturbance of mood, are among the reasons that the new language of psychiatry no longer includes the term neurosis.

This is not to diminish the theory, or the accomplishments, of the psychoanalysts who helped so many patients who suffered from the middle zone disorders. The psychoanalysts have contributed much to the field of psychiatry and the understanding of human behavior.

But something new has happened and another door is open now to the future, because two "neurotic" problems can now derive relatively quick relief from a medicine used to treat depression.

DSM-III allows the use of the term *phobic neurosis* to cover any *phobia* and lists the three phobias as: agoraphobia, with and without panic attacks; *social phobia,* which is a specific fear of a specific social situation, such as eating, writing or speaking in public; and simple phobia, which is the residual category for all of the phobias that are not agoraphobia or social phobia.

Simple phobia would include the kinds of common phobias such as fear of dogs, fear of snakes, fear of mice, and so on. *Social phobia* apparently was distinguished as a separate category of its own largely because it makes its appearance in a different way than that of simple phobia and probably represents a different disease process.

Simple phobia tends to arise fairly early in childhood. Persons who have simple phobias have "had them all their life". Social phobias are circumscribed phobias related to a particular social situation and tend to arise somewhat later in the life of a patient.

Neurotic problems with free-floating anxiety have continued on in DSM-III in two forms. The first is panic disorder, which is repeated panic attacks which are not tied to a specific situation, as in the case of agoraphobia. The second is *generalized anxiety disorder* which we have already discussed on page 114 as a cardinal manifestation of mental disorder, which is a continuous unremitting level of over-anxiousness, worry, and nervousness, with physiologic and behavioral accompaniments of anxiety that don't seem tied to any particular fear of a particular object or situation.

Obsessive-compulsive neurosis comes down to us in DSM-III as obsessive compulsive disorder, a condition where there are obsessions and/or compulsions.

The other important disorder of the middle zone, hysteria, is a disorder involving conversion symptoms or dissociative symptoms and has also passed into history. The disorder that presents the conversion symptom is now called *conversion disorder.*

The four dissociative symptoms have each become disorders: psychogenic fugue, psychogenic amnesia, multiple personality, and depersonalization disorder.

Hypochondriacal neurosis was a middle zone disorder that appeared in DSM-II and has become hypochondriasis, while somatization, which we dicussed as a cardinal manifestation of mental disorder on page 139 is a disorder in DSM-III, and a new one that was not present in older classifications.

A new category of anxiety disorder called *post-traumatic stress disorder* appears in DSM-III as a reaction to unusually severe stress, and is another addition to our vocabulary in the new language of psychiatry, describing the untoward reactions of some individuals after undergoing extreme stress.

THE AXIS II DISORDERS

In the history of psychiatry in this century, we traced the evolution of classification of the group of psychoses, which were severe disorders, the neuroses, which were less severe, and various other disorders that didn't seem to fit either of those two categories.

Antisocial personality is one such condition which originally stuck out like a sore thumb under the name of "moral insanity".

The Redistribution of Functional Mental Illness in DSM–III

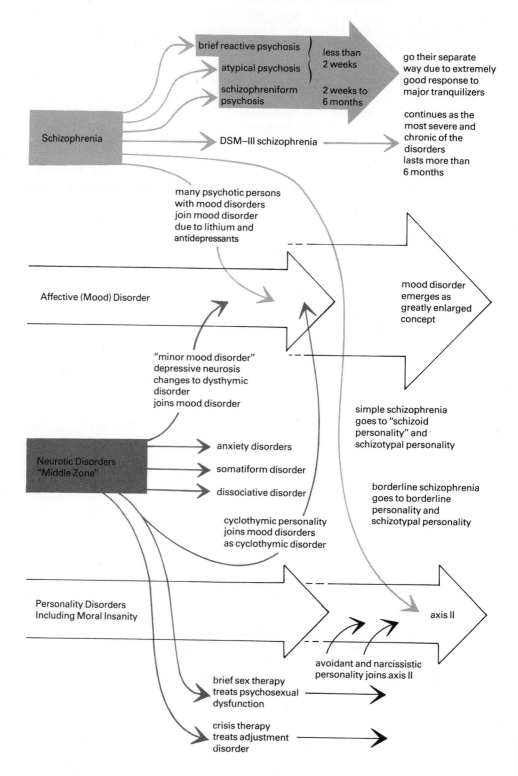

brief reactive psychosis

atypical psychosis

less than 2 weeks

schizophreniform psychosis

2 weeks to 6 months

go their separate way due to extremely good response to major tranquilizers

Schizophrenia

DSM–III schizophrenia

continues as the most severe and chronic of the disorders lasts more than 6 months

many psychotic persons with mood disorders join mood disorder due to lithium and antidepressants

Affective (Mood) Disorder

mood disorder emerges as greatly enlarged concept

"minor mood disorder" depressive neurosis changes to dysthymic disorder joins mood disorder

simple schizophrenia goes to "schizoid personality" and schizotypal personality

Neurotic Disorders "Middle Zone"

anxiety disorders

somatiform disorder

dissociative disorder

borderline schizophrenia goes to borderline personality and schizotypal personality

cyclothymic personality joins mood disorders as cyclothymic disorder

Personality Disorders Including Moral Insanity

axis II

avoidant and narcissistic personality joins axis II

brief sex therapy treats psychosexual dysfunction

crisis therapy treats adjustment disorder

DSM-III has defined eleven personality disorders that are clusters of some of the cardinal manifestations of mental disorders that we discussed in Part II. These personality disorders remain relatively stable over the years. DSM-III goes to considerable length to precisely define what it means by each personality disorder. Individuals who do not fully satisfy one of the particular descriptions would be said to have *"traits"* of that particular disorder.

Individuals who are essentially criminal and without conscience, who can use others for their own purposes and feel no guilt, and have a persistent pattern of violating the rights of others, never fit in the history of psychiatry into the classification of psychosis or of neurosis. These persons enter Axis II as *antisocial personality disorder.* Not only is it a life long and relatively stable disorder, but it has its roots early in childhood, and the DSM-III definition of the disorder requires a significant history of "violation of the rights of others" occurring before the age of fifteen.

A corresponding disorder in people under the age of eighteen is called *conduct disorder,* which is not an Axis II diagnosis, but would be diagnosed on Axis I in the case of a child. What we discussed as *aggressive violation of the rights of others* (page 40) and *non-aggressive violation of the rights of others* (page 40) together with what we discussed as the *attachment criterion* (page 35) form the basis of the definition.

In children there are four kinds of conduct disorder based on whether the violation of the rights of others is *aggressive* or *non-aggressive,* and based upon whether the child has the capacity to form a significant relationship with another person. If the child can form such a social relationship he is called socialized, if he can't he is called unsocialized.

Simple schizophrenia, mentioned when we were whittling down the definition of schizophrenia (page 185), was said to consist of a group of loners and drifters whose condition remained relatively stable throughout life. A good deal of research and study indicates that this is a stable condition that does not manifest the symptoms of schizophrenia as they have been defined by DSM-III.

It enters axis II as the *schizoid personality disorder,* a condition where there is little or no involvement with people, no interest in having such involvement, and an indifference to praise or criticism by others.

The *paranoid personality disorder* is characterized by suspiciousness and mistrust of others, together with a kind of hypersensitivity of being slighted, and a coldness and unemotionalness. It is distinguished from paranoid disorder, which is a psychosis, and is distinguished from paranoid schizophrenia which is schizophrenia with delusions of persecution, jealousy, grandiosity, or hallucinations with persecutory or jealous content.

Schizotypal personality disorder is a new phrase in the new language of psychiatry; it identifies a personality type characterized by certain kinds of odd thought, odd perception, odd behavior, together with distancing from others, and may also show features that are paranoid personality disorder features. Interestingly, the definition of schizotypal, which contains several criteria, actually does contain within it as one possible variety, all of the criteria of the paranoid personality disorder, so that there are several varieties of schizoptypal as defined by DSM-III.

The most important thing about schizotypal personality is that it consists of a set of traits that strongly resemble the characteristics of the prodrome of schizophrenia or the characteristics of the residual state of schizophrenia.

The *histrionic personality* is an overdramatic, vain, demanding, manipulative personality type that inherits what in older classifications were called "hysterical personality".

The *avoidant personality* is an effort by DSM-III to cope directly with individuals who are shy and remain shy as a life long trait. These are individuals who have minimal social relationships but who really want them, and are overly sensitive to rejection and criticism, and who will only involve themselves with other people when they are given unusually strong guarantees of uncritical acceptance.

The *dependent personality* wishes to set up a relationship with another person who takes care of him and is willing to put up with abuse from the person who takes care of him, allowing that person to make his major life decisions. It is a form of "never growing up".

The *passive-aggressive personality* was discussed under passive-aggressive manifestations of behavior (page 42).

The *compulsive personality* is overly perfectionistic, meticulous, placing emphasis on work and productivity to the exclusion of recreation and social relationships, and manifesting a kind of coldness, unemotionalness, and objectivity; he may appear unusually stiff, formal or stingy. They have a tendency to become preoccupied with small details and be unable to see "the big picture". Compulsive personality is a stable collection of personality traits and is not related to obsessive-compulsive personality disorder.

Two very interesting personality disorders that are new in DSM-III, and represent another door open to the future, are the *borderline* and the *narcissistic* personalities.

When we were discussing schizophrenia, we talked about a kind of person that the psychoanalysist didn't know what to do with, who was on the borderline between psychosis and neurosis (page 186).

The borderline personality disorder has unstable social relationships involving clinging, intense overvaluing and devaluing (or perhaps rapid shifts between the two), and a tendency at times to be manipulative of others, together with an inability to be alone and a craving to be with other people, together with distressing confusion about a variety of issues related to identity, and a lack of a stable sense of self.

Narcissistic personality is a relatively recent discovery. It also represents a door open to the future. Here an individual manipulates others, not for the purpose of gaining either goods or money, but for the purpose of obtaining a self-agrandizement and being admired. The individual displays a kind of immature quality. His social relating is characterized by this particular style of using others for his own purposes. The narcissistic personality is the one characterized by *entitlement* (page 44).

Our discussion of the evolution of the classification of mental disorders, and our discussion of what happened to the conditions in the middle zone, should not give the reader the impression that DSM-III has a disregard for psychoanalysis.

The disorders that have been taken in as narcissistic and borderline together with concepts behind the creation of Axis II as a necessary part of diagnosis, reflect important progress in psychoanalysis, which has moved on to look into the formation of deep and enduring traits in the personality, something that the psychoanalysts have called "character neurosis".

Some psychoanalysts have actually been able to treat these disorders through a modification of psychoanalytic technique that takes account of the unique characteristics of borderline and of narcissistic persons.

This is a breakthrough. It is now appreciated that a psychoanalysis that is properly conducted and directed specifically at the treatment of either the borderline or the narcissistic personality difficulty can often help such persons to achieve significant improvement.

While DSM-III purposely says little concerning the current theories about narcissistic and borderline personalities and about personality disorder in general, it is important to understand that all of these eleven kinds of personality problems are thought to represent difficulties in social relating that have their origin in very early childhood experiences. These are early experiences that are part of the process whereby children form their earliest attachments to people, develop their earliest sense of self in relation to others, and develop their first sense of whatever autonomy they have from their parents.

Certainly, most of the characteristics of these conditions make their first appearance in childhood, and some of them have corresponding Axis I diagnoses that can be made in children, such as schizoid disorder of childhood, conduct disorder, identity disorder (which corresponds to borderline personality disorder, but which is not quite as severe), avoidant disorder in childhood or adolescence, (which corresponds to the avoidant personality disorder), and oppositional behavior (page 41) that corresponds to passive-aggressive personality disorder in adulthood.

One of the important aspects of borderline personality disorder is that work with adolescents over the past decade has implicated problems of this kind in cases of a number of teenagers who were undergoing unusually tumultuous development during adolescence. While not representing neurosis, and falling short of being a psychotic disorder, these problems seemed to have been best understood and treated as an adolescent form of borderline personality disorder.

There is a spectrum here involving issues about sense of self and identity. *Identity disorder* is the softest and mildest version; borderline personality disorder is more serious; and finally a psychotic disorder like schizophrenia can represent the greatest degree of disorganization relating to sense of self and identity.

Traits Shared by Paranoid, Schizoid, Schizotypal Personality Disorders

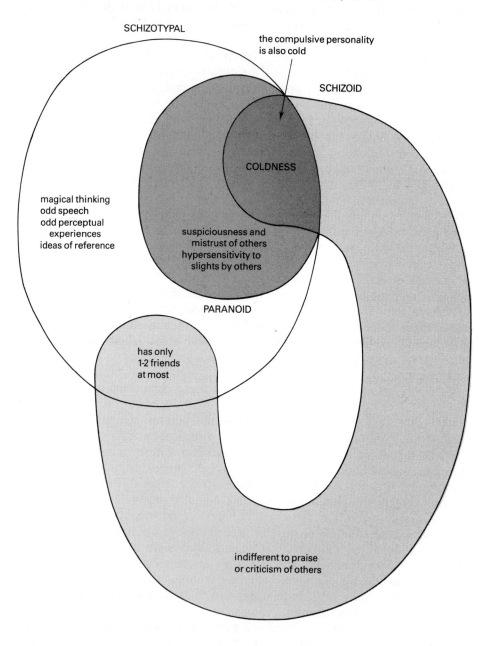

SCHIZOTYPAL

the compulsive personality
is also cold

SCHIZOID

COLDNESS

magical thinking
odd speech
odd perceptual
    experiences
ideas of reference

suspiciousness and
mistrust of others
hypersensitivity to
slights by others

PARANOID

has only
1-2 friends
at most

indifferent to praise
or criticism of others

notice that
1. schizotypal can contain all paranoid traits
2. coldness can occur in all 3
3. schizoid and schizotypal may have no friends

Traits Shared by Borderline, Narcissistic, Histrionic Personality Disorders

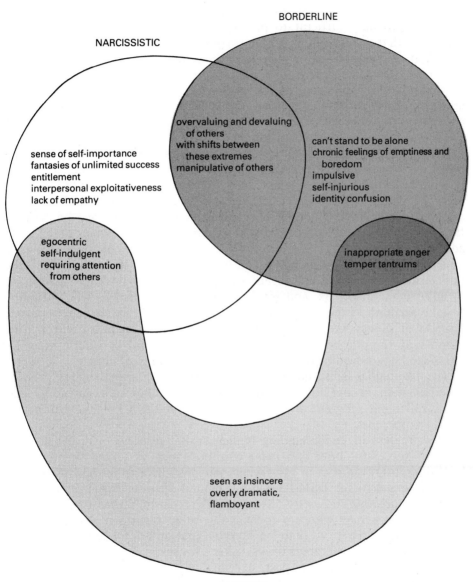

BORDERLINE

NARCISSISTIC

overvaluing and devaluing
of others
with shifts between
these extremes
manipulative of others

can't stand to be alone
chronic feelings of emptiness and
boredom
impulsive
self-injurious
identity confusion

sense of self-importance
fantasies of unlimited success
entitlement
interpersonal exploitativeness
lack of empathy

egocentric
self-indulgent
requiring attention
from others

inappropriate anger
temper tantrums

seen as insincere
overly dramatic,
flamboyant

HISTRIONIC

Interesting logical relationships exist between the categories in DSM-III of personality disorder that are illustrated in the two preceding figures. Notice individual criteria that are shared by some of the categories; these relationships between categories within the Axis II personality disorders make it extremely difficult to present any sort of flow chart or series of questions that would allow a user to quickly rule out all of the disorders. He might be taken around in a circle to the point where he started.

Finally, one of the disorders that was once thought to be a stable personality disorder—cyclothymic personality, where mood level goes up an down but is not usually severe—was recognized as a mild mood disorder and left to join its relatives in the family of mood disorders where it belongs. (Now it is called cyclothymic disorder).

Adjustment disorders are milder mental disorders that are distinctly linked to a recent life stress. DSM-III subdivides them according to the kind of symptom picture they present, such as depressed mood, conduct disorder features, social withdrawal, work or academic inhibitions, and so on, as opposed to DSM-II which divided adjustment disorders on the basis of the patient's age, having adjustment reactions of childhood, adolescence, adulthood, and so forth. Here too, the importance of psychotherapy, especially brief psychotherapy, and what has been learned about crisis intervention techniques has been incorporated both into the description of adjustment disorders, and into the concept of Axis IV, which attempts to take account of the life stress on the person in relationship to his current episode of illness. Adjustment disorders must have an onset within three months of the alleged life stress, and are understood to vanish when the stress can be removed or the patient finds a better way of coping.

The *paraphilias* and the *psychosexual dysfunctions* have been grouped together with gender identity disturbances [another new category (page 93)], reflecting progress that has been made in the whole field of gender identity problems.

The progress in understanding human sexual response, and the development of successful brief treatment methods, such as sexual therapy, have had an important impact in cases where persons suffer from these disorders.

Homosexuality for DSM-III is not a mental disorder. What DSM-III calls *"ego-dystonic homosexuality"* is a disorder that is rather rigidly defined as involving a person who has considerable subjective distress over a conflict between their strong wish to be heterosexual and a tendency to become sexually aroused by members of his or her own sex.

The experience of the past decades of use and abuse of so-called "recreational" drugs such as marijuana and LSD, cocaine, PCP, barbiturates, and amphetamines, as well as alcohol and narcotics, is reflected in DSM-III's extensive treatment of this subject.

There is firstly a description of drug specific syndromes of intoxication and withdrawal, and then of patterns of maladaptive behavior related to the use of these substances for purposes of becoming intoxicated.

DSM-III defines two *substance use problems: substance abuse* and *substance dependence,* where dependence is the more serious, involving the development of *tolerance* to a drug (needing more and more of it to produce the desired effect, or getting less and less of an effect from taking the same amount) together with a tendency to have physiologic disturbances upon cessation of use or reduction in the amount taken, indicating that the body has become used to receiving the drug and *dependent* on it.

DSM-III pays particular attention to problems resulting from alcohol and sets out criteria for alcohol abuse and alcohol dependence.

The category of *"pathological intoxication" to alcohol,* a condition where individuals taking relatively small amounts of alcohol behave in a highly uncharacteristic fashion, is included in DSM-III as *"alcohol idiosyncratic intoxication.* The old DSM-II category of alcoholic paranoia was dropped since it was felt that it was not a sufficiently distinctive condition from the specific DSM-III organic mental disorders that cover similar symptoms.

To use the term for an organic mental disorder when a drug is involved, the name of the drug is appended to the name of the disorder, so that delirium due to a drug like digitalis would be called *digitalis delirium* and an organic delusional syndrome which was due to digitalis would be called *digitalis delusional disorder,* where the word "organic" would be dropped to apply the name of the specific drug.

Drug specific intoxication or withdrawal would likewise append the name of the drug to the term "intoxication" or the term "withdrawal".

CHILDREN

One of the major changes in DSM-III was its treatment of childhood disorders. In the history we gave of the evolution of the classification of mental disorders, the reader will notice that we never mentioned children when we discussed the sane versus the insane, and when we discussed the psychotic group of patients versus the patients in the middle zone.

There is a reason for this.

Historically, child psychiatry had different roots than general psychiatry. Child psychiatry started in the child guidance clinics of the twenties and not in the offices of psychiatrists. Child psychiatry has been a separate stream that developed its own systems of classifying disorders of children, and identified a number of childhood disorders that were never a part of any official psychiatric language.

Conditions like early infantile autism, and attachment disorders and rumination disorders of babies, were psychiatric problems recognized by child psychiatrists that were part of their branch of knowledge and were not merged with the rest of psychiatry.

DSM-III has accomplished this fusion.

One of the ways it has done this is by allowing any diagnosis that can be made in an adult to also be made in a child. At the same time, DSM-III incorporates an extensive special section containing many disorders that child psychiatrists have studied, diagnosed, and treated in many children over the past several decades.

DSM-III describes the pervasive developmental disorders that includes infantile autism.

What used to be called "hyperkinetic reaction of childhood" in DSM-III (what the layman refers to as a hyperactive child) has been renamed and carefully defined as *attention deficit disorder,* where the problem is now seen as being largely one of difficulty in sustained attention, together with impulsiveness, and where the condition can be present both with and without hyperactivity.

DSM-III has also incorporated the knowledge that attention deficit disorder with hyperactivity is not usually a phase that children go through and then "grow out of", but often persists into adolescence and adulthood. This will now be diagnosed as *attention deficit disorder, residual state* in adults who have characteristics of the condition now, with a substantial history of having had the hyperactive variety attention deficit disorder as children.

The incorporation of Axis II for children, emphasizing learning disabilities as specific developmental delays in reading, arithmetic, receptive and expressive language, and articulation (pronunciation), is an important and major step in the careful diagnosis and treatment of children. Each examiner of children is now asked to look carefully for signs of such specific developmental delay which have been overlooked when children were being seen because of an acute episode or acute complaint such as lying, stealing, truancy, or a family argument.

Mental retardation has been very clearly defined as an IQ below seventy with corresponding impairment in adaptive functioning, where the condition must begin before age eighteen.

This represents a change because the group of persons previously diagnosed as having borderline mental retardation (IQ seventy-one to eighty-four), are not included as having a disorder in DSM-III. Their difficulties in adaptive functioning occur principally as a result of being in school, and after they leave the school system, for the most part, they blend rather well into the rest of society.

It is important to note that low IQ alone does not mean a diagnosis of mental retardation; there must be a corresponding impairment in adaptive functioning.

Disorders such as anorexia nervosa, bulimia, pica, sleep terror disorder, sleepwalking disorder have all been incorporated into the new language of psychiatry as part of DSM-III's effort to embrace all of these other areas where important work has been done.

The inclusion of infant psychiatric disorders is noteworthy because the new field of infant psychiatry has been firmly established by the first International Congress on Infant Psychiatry that was held recently in Portugal.

This too is a door open to the future. We are looking to infants in an effort to learn more about social relatedness, to understand what it is that a person learns and develops in his or her first social relationship with his or her mother or other caretaker, and to try to understand what difficulties her disturbances may arise when that first social relationship is interfered with.

Another point on the application of DSM-III to children: Now that all of DSM-III, including the childhood section of DSM-III, applies to children, there are roughly four times as many diagnoses that can be given to a child. Some of the criteria in DSM-III for certain disorders are specially constructed to allow them to apply to children (such as the definition in DSM-III of a major depressive episode, which contains special instructions for how to use it in the case of children).

It is an important step forward that mental disorder in children, a concept which was always difficult for the layman, for the health professional, and even for the adult psychiatrist to recognize and to appreciate, has now, with DSM-III, been accorded that important recognition.

Child psychiatry, as we mentioned, came from a different source and was not officially recognized by the rest of psychiatry as a distinct subspecialty until 1957; it now flows in the mainstream.

The reader needs to appreciate that a problem arises in attempting to apply the DSM-III categories to children. First of all, there is a lot of controversy in child psychiatry over what some diseases like affective disorder really look like when they occur in childhood—and there is considerable controversy among several different schools of thought just on that point alone. Some individuals maintain that there doesn't even exist such a condition as depression in childhood; other schools of thought feel that there is some condition that could be called depression in childhood but that it looks different from depression in adulthood.

And there is yet another school that feels that if we try to look for certain "core symptoms" of depression in children that correspond to adult symptoms, we can find children whose difficulties bear a strong resemblance to adult depression.

Just as we saw certain adult diseases as being major when we looked at the classification of the sane versus the insane, with the creation of the middle zone, so are there certain conditions in children that are major and very serious; these include organic disorders, psychotic disorders such as schizophrenia (which can be seen rarely in children), the pervasive developmental disorders (that include infantile autism and other "psychoses of childhood") and major affective disorder (for which there is increasing evidence today that it does occur and when it occurs, it is serious).

Conduct disorder disturbances in children are Axis I conditions and are relatively serious, not only because they could lead to the adult problems of antisocial personality, but because studies have shown that in children, a sizable number of those children who do commit suicide suffer from conduct disorder disturbances (this is in sharp contrast to adults where antisocial personality disorder makes relatively little contribution to completed suicides.)

Psychosis in children can mean something different. The term psychosis, as we defined it in Chapter II, involving reality testing or involving delusions, has to undergo some modification for use in children.

Most children normally have thoughts that would be signs of psychosis in adults. For example, at least one third of all children have had an imaginary playmate. If an adult had an imaginary person whom they talked to all the time, and bought presents for, and left food on the table for, they would be psychotic. Children have license with fantasy.

There are similar problems in applying concepts of adult anxiety. Children can *normally* have incredible fears, such as fears of being "eaten up by something that lurks in the dark".

This is what makes them children and this is where correct use of DSM-III relies on the examiner's knowledge of what constitutes normal behavior for children of a particular age.

What constitutes normal behavior changes during childhood as children grow older and develop, and what is age appropriate behavior at four will not be age appropriate behavior at eight.

There is a big difference between a well-functioning child of four who might nevertheless have no idea of how to share, and a healthy well-functioning child of eight who can be so strict about fair play that it borders on compulsiveness. What is normal in children is beyond what DSM-III or what any book can teach, and sometimes even years of experience with children will not provide this answer.

CONCLUSION

It is important to remember that DSM-III, the New Language of Psychiatry, except for the optional Axis V, does not emphasize the strengths of people, but rather points out the things that can be "wrong" with them. This is a feeling the reader may have gotten in going through Chapter II.

DSM-III is not a language that describes a person's strong points, and this is another area where the users of DSM-III must go further than a blind application of criteria and definitions.

We need to know, with every human being, child, adolescent, or adult, not only what their complaint is, and what their disorders are, but what are their strengths, what are the capacities that they can use to go beyond the difficulty in which they find themselves.

DSM-III embodies much of what has been learned in the passing decades from the time when all mental disorder was hopeless to the situation in 1980, where major progress has been made in almost every area of serious mental disorder, and where doors are open to the future. The New Language of Psychiatry has been designed so that if it is correctly used, and if diagnoses can be correctly made and carefully applied, then years from now, when psychiatrists perform that truly important kind of diagnosis that is done in retrospect, they will have the information that will allow for continuing progress. Someday this will be reflected in a language they will write, that will be called DSM-IV.

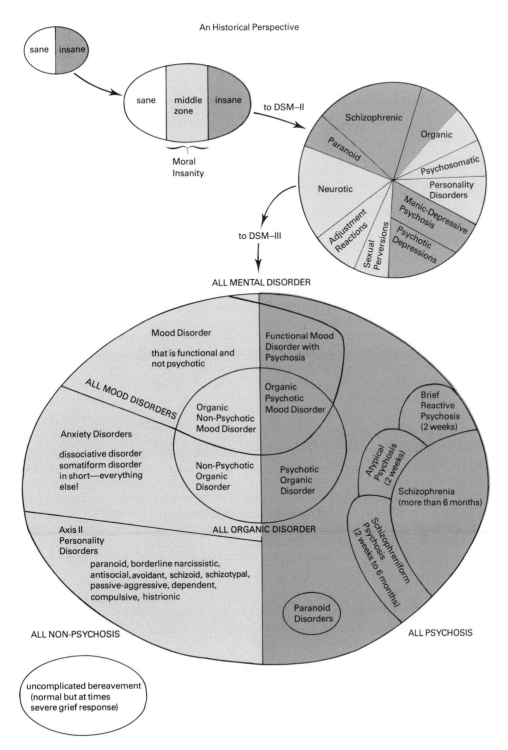

An Historical Perspective

sane | insane

sane | middle zone | insane

Moral Insanity

to DSM–II

Schizophrenic

Paranoid

Organic

Psychosomatic

Neurotic

Personality Disorders

Manic-Depressive Psychosis

Adjustment Reactions

Sexual Perversions

Psychotic Depressions

to DSM–III

ALL MENTAL DISORDER

Mood Disorder

that is functional and not psychotic

Functional Mood Disorder with Psychosis

ALL MOOD DISORDERS

Organic Psychotic Mood Disorder

Organic Non-Psychotic Mood Disorder

Brief Reactive Psychosis (2 weeks)

Anxiety Disorders

dissociative disorder somatiform disorder in short—everything else!

Non-Psychotic Organic Disorder

Psychotic Organic Disorder

Atypical Psychosis (2 weeks)

Schizophrenia (more than 6 months)

Axis II Personality Disorders

ALL ORGANIC DISORDER

Schizophreniform Psychosis (2 weeks to 6 months)

paranoid, borderline narcissistic, antisocial, avoidant, schizoid, schizotypal, passive-aggressive, dependent, compulsive, histrionic

Paranoid Disorders

ALL NON-PSYCHOSIS

ALL PSYCHOSIS

uncomplicated bereavement (normal but at times severe grief response)

SELF-STUDY QUESTIONS, PART III

1. Discuss the important changes that have taken place in DSM-III's concept of schizophrenia.

2. Discuss the role of affective disorder as an organizing principle in DSM-III.

3. In a patient who had a full picture of severe manic mood together with psychosis, which way do you think DSM-III is fundamentally biased in regard to the two following diagnoses?
   1. Acute schizophrenia with features of manic mood
   2. Bipolar disorder—manic type with psychosis

4. What has become of the category of schizoaffective disorder?

5. Discuss the two principal kinds of organic mental disorders. What are their essential features?
   What are the other seven varieties of organic mental disorders and how would you characterize them?

   Answer: The two fundamental pictures are delirium and dementia. Delirium is characterized primarily by clouding of consciousness together with disorientation and disturbances of memory. It comes on acutely and has a fluctuating course.
   Dementia is not characterized by clouding of consciousness but rather by a decline in intellectual ability or memory disturbance, disturbances of judgment, and one of a number of various neurological complaints that indicate damage to the nervous system.
   The other seven kinds of organic mental disorder are *amnestic syndrome* that occurs in a clear consciousness (distinguishing it from delirium) and is character- ized by impairment of both short- and long-term memory without general loss of intellectual ability as in dementia, *organic delusional syndrome* that occurs in a clear consciousness but where there are delusions, *organic hallucinosis* that occurs in a clear consciousness but where there are hallucinations, *organic affective syndrome* that occurs in a clear consciousness but where there is affective disorder such as depression, *organic personality disorder* that occurs in a clear consciousness and where there is a specific kind of personality change involving lability of affect, suspiciousness, poor social judgment, and other features. *Intoxication* refers to a drug specific syndrome that results when a person is given too much of a drug—you would have to know what the specific syndrome of the drug is—and *withdrawal* which is similiarly a drug specific problem resulting from withdrawal (intoxication and withdrawal can only be diagnosed in a case of a particular drug when the picture produced is not that of any of the other mental disorders such as delirium or organic delusional syndrome and so on).

6. How old do you have to be before you can be sure that you will never contract schizophrenia?

   Answer: You cannot get schizophrenia when you are older than forty-five. Remember that the prodrome is part of the illness and the illness starts when the prodrome starts. Therefore the prodrome of the schizophrenic-like illness, if it occurs before the age of forty-five means schizophrenia. If it occurs afterwards, it is atypical psychosis.

7. Describe the two kinds of psychoses that are used to discuss psychotic disorders without a predominant mood disturbance that have lasted less than two weeks. What is the basis of distinguishing between the two?

   Answer: The two conditions are brief reactive psychosis and atypical psychosis. Brief reactive psychosis is used when there is a definite psychosocial stressor that occurs in relationship to the disorder.

8. What are the two kinds of major affective disorder?

   Answer: The two kinds of major affective disorders are major depression and bipolar disorder.

9. What's the difference?

   Answer: Bipolar disorder has had at least one attack of full mania. Major depression is a condition characterized by severe depression but where mania has never occurred.

10. In bipolar disorder after a patient has had one episode of mania, what do we say when he or she develops hypomania?

    Answer: He doesn't need the full picture of mania after a first episode in order for it to count as a recurrence of the disease.

11. In bipolar disorder, when a person has had at least one major depression, what do we say when he or she becomes mildly depressed?

    Answer: We call it bipolar disorder depressed because the patient doesn't need the full picture of major depression again in order for it to count as a recurrence of the disorder.

12. In major depression, recurrent, what do we say when the person develops a mild depression?

    Answer: We do not call it major depression, recurrent. In major depression each episode has to be a full picture of major depressive episode as defined in DSM-III. However, it is possible for individuals who have had major depression to develop a dysthymic disorder or for individuals with dysthymic disorder to have major depression superimposed upon it.

13. In what appeared to be a severe depression, what two cardinal manifestations of mental disorder would raise immediately the question that the patient might have schizophrenia?

    Answer: 1. Mood-incongruent delusions or hallucinations
            2. Bizarre behavior

14. What is the specific treatment for mania?

    Answer: Lithium

15. What happened to neurosis? Explain it in your own words.

16. What specific drug treatment was discovered for agoraphobia with panic attacks?

    Answer: Imipramine was used to treat panic attacks, mild tranquilizers were found to be helpful with the anticipatory anxiety concerning future panic attacks and a combination of these treatments was found to be of significant benefit to even severe agoraphobics.

17. What condition related to agoraphobia in a number of ways was found also to benefit from treatment with imipramine?

    Answer: Separation anxiety disorder in children.

18. The old category, used many many years ago, of moral insanity found its way into DSM-III in a special form. What is it?

    Answer: It found its way into Axis II and is largely covered by what is now described as antisocial personality disorder.

19. Of what use is Axis II in children?

    Answer: To list specific learning disabilities involving specific developmental delays in arithmetic, reading, language skills, both receptive and expressive language, and articulation.

20. What are the severe disorders in children that must always be thought of first when attempting to apply DSM-III to a child?

    Answer: Organic mental disorders do occur in children—they are serious. Psychotic disorders do occur in children—they must definitely be ruled out. Depressions and affective disorders do occur in children—they must be ruled out. Conduct disorder is serious for several reasons. Attention deficit disorders can cause a variety of difficulties if not properly diagnosed and handled, and other disorders in children such as the separation anxiety disorder, avoidant disorder of children, schizoid disorder of childhood and adolescence can severely impair social relatedness and are Axis I conditions in childhood. Some child psychiatrists believe that some of these conditions can improve with proper treatment that may, however, be lengthy and require a considerable dedication on the part of the therapist.

Afterword

Terms that are often used by the general public such as "emotionally disturbed", "emotionally ill", "emotionally handicapped", "nervous breakdown" and so on do not appear in DSM-III, and should never be used because these terms are too vague.

There are also some less fancy terms used by the general public such as "crazy", "nuts", "unbalanced", "screwy", and so on. These are not kind words and are often applied to people in a hostile and fearful way.

The fancier words, like "emotionally disturbed", are just as stigmatizing because they are merely euphemisms for "crazy". These terms—all of them—are applied to people out of ignorance. That is, they are used by persons who don't know one psychiatric diagnosis from another, and who lack understanding about how to help or what to do.

The vagueness of these words makes them useless—they cover everything from mild adjustment disorders that will get better in a short time to the most serious mental disorders where the patient can be a danger to others.

These terms are unworkable. They do not work because they cover such a hodgepodge of different problems, from the mildest to the most serious, that they are useless to the psychiatrists in the same way that a word like "sick" or a word like "cripple" is useless to the doctor who treats physical disorder.

A word like "cripple" covers everything from persons who have a slight impairment using one of their thumbs to persons who can never walk.

A doctor doesn't know how to help a "cripple" but he knows ways to help a person who has trouble with his thumb and he knows ways today to help even persons who can never walk.

Similarly a doctor (or anyone else) doesn't know what to do for a "sick" person but doctors know how to operate a vast technology to help most persons who suffer from most diseases.

In the same way, generic euphemisms for insanity like "emotionally disturbed" are unworkable concepts. No one knows what to do about a person who is "emotionally disturbed", but the reader already understands that there are today ways to deal even with schizophrenia. Therefore, these words, like "emotionally disturbed", should be eliminated from our vocabularly and sent to the same museum where we have put the concept of the flat earth.

These words, like "emotionally disturbed", serve to stigmatize people when they are written down in permanent records handled by schools, personnel offices, motor vehicle bureaus, and so on. By their vagueness, such terms leave to the imagination of untrained persons the decision about what they mean. A term like "emotional problems" could mean anything from "has trouble falling asleep at night" to "has delusions" and it would be better to be specific about people's problems because it is only when we know precisely what his individual unique problems are that we can also start to know what a person's individual unique strengths and resources are. The individual strengths and resources of persons is what every form of therapy relies on, and the strengths and resources of persons are as important to the overcoming of a mental disorder as they are to the overcoming of a physical disorder.

It is only by taking stock of each person's individual strengths and individual resources that any person with any kind of problem can receive any genuine help. It is by attending to people's individual differences that we can do them a service and it is when we start closing our eyes to these individual differences and lumping a person together with thousands of other people under the same label that we take a step in the other direction. In fact, we take a chance that treating such an individual as though he is like thousands of other people with a similar problem could be the very thing that does him harm.

When psychiatrists learn in a permanent record only that a person is "emotionally ill", they do not know what problem is meant by such a term anymore than medical doctors would know what was troubling someone described in a permanent school record only as "sick" or as "crippled".

If medical doctors know that a so-called crippled or handicapped person cannot walk, they know something about the person's capacity to deal with the problem—because they know that the patient can use his or her arms and they can wonder whether the person has developed skills with a wheelchair.

If they know that a person described as crippled has trouble using one thumb, then they know that the person can see, hear, and walk; they know something about what could be done to help, and they can wonder if these things have been done.

In the same way, the psychiatrists have many ways today to help in most mental disorders, and much is known about how each mental disorder responds to various interventions.

We do need to be afraid of some persons with mental disorder, and only by specifying each person's unique problem can we know whether or not we need to be afraid. Only by specifying each person's problem when we do need to be afraid can we know what to be afraid of, what precautions to take, and how to change the situation when change is possible. But we cannot know these things from vague words like "emotionally disturbed".

By lumping all persons together, the harmless and the dangerous, under terms like emotionally disturbed, we do both a disservice—we do not know whom to treat with caution, and are therefore cautious and wary of all persons called "emotionally disturbed". We remain ignorant about what to do to help any patient, and ignorant about how to deal effectively with a dangerous patient.

The situation is similar with physical diseases. There are physical diseases that we need to be afraid of, such as certain contagious diseases, but only by specifying each patient's problem with their particular disease can we know which patients will put others in danger and which ones will not. Labels like "sick", or "ill", or even "contagious" are too vague, and only by knowing exactly what contagious disease a patient has can we know what to do to safeguard others from danger.

It would be better to describe one person as having trouble going to sleep at night and another as having schizophrenia than to lump both persons together in an unworkable classification such as "emotionally disturbed" and stigmatize both of them.

By being specific and using the terms that DSM-III provides, we have a workable system that can also be used to eliminate the stigma in all of the generic euphemisms for "crazy". But emotionally ill, mentally ill, and so on, do not appear in DSM-III; they do not describe what DSM-III describes and they harken back to the dark ages of psychiatry, which is where such terms are from, and which is where they belong.

Worse than the stigmatizing words used by the general public are the words used by the law that come out of the same unworkable ideas, except that such words have been given a dangerous official status as a key that can unlock public funds.

Using such terms as "emotionally handicapped", children can be labeled and sorted and stigmatized for a lifetime through their school records. And similar words that unlock social security money, Medicare money, or other public health or public job programs can stigmatize adults and allow bureaucrats to label them and to harm them at the same time.

The terms used by the government are useless to the psychiatrist and are just as unworkable as the words used by the general public, except that now the word is more stigmatizing because it has a legal sanction and is not merely a piece of gossip.

The author believes that it is time to close the gap between the law and our current knowledge about mental disorder, and to strike out from the law these vague, damaging, and totally unworkable classifications.

In this book I have tried to explain what mental disorder is, and in these last few pages I have attempted to explain what mental disorder is not.

Our laws and our permanent records about people should at least reflect our knowledge, and not serve to damage people by being the vehicle for the ignorance of an earlier era.

The government, like the general public, stigmatizes by being too vague. All persons with mental disorders should be described by the new language of psychiatry. The argument that such an approach is too complex fails to deal with the fact that it is people themselves who are complex, and people's problems require a complex language. The general public, as well as the law, understand that automobiles are complex objects, an it is clear that not much is communicated by a term like "car trouble" about what needs to be done for an automobile: the public understands and is willing to talk today about such complex parts as carburetors, transmissions, fuel lines, air pollution control devices, specific safety design features, and the like.

In the same way it is time to recognize that people are at least as complicated as automobiles, and that only a workable language like DSM-III can describe their difficulties and only such a workable language should be sanctioned by law.

The term *"Mental Disorder"* used by DSM-III is not merely a substitute for vague euphemisms. *Mental Disorder* as defined by DSM-III (see page 3) is the general term that was chosen to designate all of those things covered by DSM-III".

DSM-III concerns itself with a number of conditions that were never linked to concepts of insanity in the past such as Axis II "specific developmental delays of children" (that include disorders that have gone previously by other names, such as dyslexia and learning disability) and "stuttering".

This is one reason why the term "mental disorder" cannot be used as a replacement for the terms used by the general public that we have condemned such as "emotionally ill". The disorders that we have discussed in DSM-III are *simply that: they are the disorders that are discussed in the new system,* and no implication is to be drawn from that discussion about whether the disorder should be linked in someone's mind with other concepts, or with earlier ideas about insanity.

DSM-III is a book and "Mental Disorder" is the general term used to denote *every condition found in that system.*

The places in part III of this book where some of the generic euphemisms now condemned have been used were occasions where they served as a bridge to carry the reader's understanding from the simpler, older concepts to the concepts of DSM-III; having made the crossing from the past to the present, the reader is urged to abandon all of the older words.

appendix A

Fifth-Digit Code Numbers

Ten disorders have special coding numbers in the fifth-digit position of the number.

1. *Mental Redardation,* where 1 or 0 in fifth digit codes whether or not there are *"other behavioral symptoms"* respectively.

2. *Pervasive Developmental Disorders* where 1 or 0 in 5th digit indicates either *"residual state"* or *"full syndrome present".*

3. *Attention Deficit Disorder* where 1 or 0 in 5th digit means *"with hyperactivity"* or *"without hyperactivity".*

4. *Dementias that use ICD-9-CM* code numbers and where 5th digit codes *symptom picture.* Primary degenerative dementia and multi-infarct dementia have 0, 1, 2, or 3 in 5th digit and that means 0 - umcomplicated, 1 - with delirium, 2 - with delusions, 3 - with depression.

5. *Alcohol induced Organic mental Disorders* that use ICD-9-CM code numbers where the *degree of severity of any dementia* present is coded in 5th digit as 0 - unspecified, 1 - mild, 2 - moderate, 3 - severe. These include alcohol intoxication, alcohol idiosyncratic intoxication, alcohol withdrawal, alcohol withdrawal delirium, alcohol hallucinosis, alcohol amnestic disorder.

6. *Substance Use disorders*
   Where 5th digit shows the course
   0 - unspecified, 1 - continuous, 2 - episodic, 3 - in remission
   Thus Alcoholism, now in DSM-III called "Alcohol Dependence," has code No. 303.9x;

to indicate alcohol dependence in remission you write 303.93. Narcotic addiction is now called opiod dependence and has code No. 304.0x. To indicate continuous use write 304.01.

7. *Schizophrenia* is coded for course in 5th digit and the numbers are
   0 - unspecified,
   1 - sub-chronic, (continuous illness for more than 6 months but less than 2 years)
   2 - chronic (continuous illness for more than 2 years)
   3 - sub-chronic with re-exacerbation
   4 - chronic with re-exacerbation
   5 - in remission *(totally* symptom free, not just in residual state)

8. & 9. *Affective Disorders* of Bipolar Disorder & Major Depression
   5th digit codes *Symptom Pictures*
   0 - unspecified
   2 - without melancholia
   3 - with melancholia
   4 - with psychosis
   6 - in remission
   7 - unofficial ICD-9-CM number to indicate psychosis present with mood incongruent features

10. The Gender Identity Disorder of Transsexualism coded in 5th digit to indicate *pattern of sexual activity* as 0 - unspecified, 1 - asexual, 2 - homosexual, 3 - heterosexual.

appendix B

Alphabetical List
of Disorders

Abuse, barbiturate or similarly acting sedative or hypnotic, in remission (305.43).

Abuse, substance, mixed or unspecified (305.9x).

Abuse, substance, mixed or unspecified, continuous (305.91).

Abuse, substance, mixed or unspecified, episodic (305.92).

Abuse, substance, mixed or unspecified, in remission (305.93).

Abuse, opioid (305.5x).

Abuse, (PCP,) phencyclidine or similar (305.9x). See other PCP disorders.

Academic problem (V62.30). This is not a mental disorder.

Acute paranoid disorder (298.30).

Adjustment disorder with anxious mood. (309.24).

Adjustment disorder with atypical features (309.90).

Adjustment disorder, with depressed mood (309.00).

Adjustment disorder with disturbance of conduct (309.30).

Adjustment disorder with mixed disturbance of emotions and conduct (309.40).

Adjustment disorder with mixed emotional features (309.28).

Adjustment disorder with withdrawal (309.83).

Adjustment disorder with work (or academic) inhibition (309.23).

225

Adult, antisocial behavior (V71.01). This is not a mental disorder.

Affective disorder, hallucinogen (292.84).

Affective disorder, other or unspecified substance (292.84).

Agoraphobia, with panic attacks (300.21).

Agoraphobia, without panic attacks (300.22).

Alcohol abuse (305.0x).

Alcohol abuse, continuous (305.01).

Alcohol abuse, episodic (305.02).

Alcohol abuse, in remission (305.03).

Alcohol abuse, unspecified (305.00).

Alcohol dependence (alcoholism) (303.9x).

Alcohol dependence (alcoholism), continuous (303.91).

Alcohol dependence (alcoholism), episodic (303.92).

Alcohol dependence, (alcoholism), in remission (303.93).

Alcohol dependence, (alcoholism), unspecified (303.90).

Amnesia, psychogenic (300.12).

Amnestic disorder, alcohol (291.10).

Amnestic disorder, barbiturate, similar acting sedative or hypnotic (292.83).

Amnestic disorder, other or unspecified substance (292.83).

Amnestic, syndrome (294.00).

Amphetamine (or similar) abuse (305.7x).

Amphetamine (or similar) abuse, continuous (305.71).

Amphetamine (or similar) abuse, episodic (305.72).

Amphetamine (or similar) abuse, in remission (305.73).

Amphetamine (or similar) abuse, unspecified (305.70).

Amphetamine (or similar) dependence, (304.4x).

Amphetamine (or similar) dependence, continuous (304.41).

Amphetamine (or similar) dependence, episodic (304.42).

Amphetamine (or similar) dependence, in remission (304.43).

Amphetamine (or similar) dependence, unspecified (304.40).

Anorexia nervosa (eating disorder) (307.10).

Antisocial behavior, adult (V71.01). This is not a mental problem.

Antisocial behavior, childhood or adolescent (V71.02). This is not a mental problem.

Antisocial personality disorder (301.70). Coded on Axis II.

Anxiety disorder, atypical, post-traumatic, stress (300.00).

Anxiety disorder, generalized (200.02).

Arithmetic disorder, developmental (315.10). Coded on Axis II.

Articulation disorder, developmental (315.39). Coded on Axis II.

Attention deficit disorder, with hyperactivity (314.01).

Attention deficit disorder, without hyperactivity (314.00).

Attention deficit disorder, residual type (314.80).

Atypical bipolar disorder (296.70).

Atypical depression (296.82).

Atypical dissociative disorder (300.15).

Atypical impulse control disorder (312.39).

Atypical gender identity disorder (302.85).

Atypical paranoid disorder (297.90).

Atypical paraphilia (302.90).

Atypical, personality disorder, mixed or other (301.89). Coded on Axis II.

Atypical psychosexual dysfunction (302.70).

Atypical psychosis (298.90).

Atypical somatoform disorder (300.70).

Autism, infantile (299.0x).

Autism, infantile, full syndrome present (299.00).

Autism, infantile, residual state (299.01).

Avoidant personality disorder (301.82). Coded on Axis II.

Avoidant disorder or childhood or adolescence, anxiety disorder of childhood or adolescence (313.21).

Barbiturate, or similarly acting sedative or hypnotic abuse (305.4x).

Barbiturate or similarly acting sedative or hypnotic abuse, continuous (305.41).

Barbiturate or similarly acting sedative or hypnotic abuse, episodic (305.42).

Barbiturate or similarly acting sedative or hypnotic abuse, unspecified (305.40).

Barbiturate or similarly acting sedative or hypnotic dependence (304.1x).

Barbiturate or similarly acting sedative or hypnotic dependence, continuous (304.11).

Barbiturate or similarly acting sedative or hypnotic dependence, episodic (304.12).

Barbiturate or similarly acting sedative or hypnotic dependence, in remission (304.13).

Barbiturate or similarly acting sedative or hypnotic dependence. unspecified (304.10).

Bereavement, uncomplicated (V62.82). This is not a mental problem.

Bipolar disorder, atypical (296.70).

Bipolar disorder, depression (296.5x).

Bipolar disorder, depression, major depressive episode with melancholia (296.53).

Bipolar disorder, depression, major depressive episode without melancholia (296.53).

Bipolar disorder, depression, major depressive episode without melancholia (296.52).

Bipolar disorder, depression, major depressive episode with psychotic features (296.54), (296.57) (psychotic features are mood-incongruent).

Bipolar disorder, depression, major depressive episode in remission (296.56).

Bipolar disorder, depression, major depressive episode unspecified (296.50).

Bipolar disorder, depression, manic episode with psychotic features (296.54), (296.57) (psychotic features are mood-incongruent).

Bipolar disorder, depression, manic episode without psychotic features.

Bipolar disorder, depression, manic episode in remission (296.56).

Bipolar disorder, depression, manic episode, unspecified (296.50).

Bipolar disorder, manic (296.4x).

Bipolar disorder, manic, major depressive episode with melancholia (296.43).

Bipolar disorder, manic, major depressive episode without melancholia (296.42).

Bipolar disorder, manic, major depressive episode with psychotic features (296.44), (296.47) (psychotic features are mood incongruent).

Bipolar disorder, manic, major depressive episode in remission (296.46).

Bipolar disorder, manic, major depressive episode, unspecified (296.40).

Bipolar disorder, manic, manic episode with psychotic features (296.44), (296.47) (Psychotic features are mood incongruent).

Bipolar disorder, manic, manic episode without psychotic features (296.42).

Bipolar disorder, manic, manic episode in remission (296.46).

Bipolar disorder, manic, manic episode, unspecified (296.40).

Bipolar disorder, mixed (296.6x).

Bipolar disorder, mixed, major depressive episode with melancholia (296.63).

Bipolar disorder, mixed, major depressive episode without melancholia (296.62).

Bipolar disorder, mixed, major depressive episode with psychotic features (296.64), (296.67) (psychotic features are mood-incongruent).

Bipolar disorder, mixed, major depressive episode in remission (296.66).

Bipolar disorder, mixed, major depressive episode, unspecified (296.60).

Bipolar disorder, mixed, manic episode with psychotic features (296.64), (296.67) (psychotic features are mood-incongruent)

Bipolar disorder, mixed, manic episode without psychotic features (296.62).

Bipolar disorder, mixed, manic episode in remission (296.66).

Bipolar disorder, mixed, manic episode unspecified (296.60).

Borderline intellectual functioning (V62.89). This is not a mental problem.

Borderline personality disorder, Coded on Axis II (301.83).

Brief reactive psychosis (298.80).

Bulima (eating disorder) (307.51).

Cannabis abuse (305.2x).

Cannabis abuse, continuous (305.21).

Cannabis abuse, episodic (305.22)

Cannabis abuse, in remission (305.23).

Cannabis abuse, unspecified (305.20).

Cannabis dependence (304.3x).

Cannabis dependence, continuous (304.31).

Cannabis dependence, episodic (304.32).

Cannabis dependence, in remission (304.33).

Cannabis dependence, unspecified (304.30).

Cannabis intoxication (305.20).

Child-parent problem (V61.20). This is not a mental problem.

Childhood or adolescent antisocial behavior (V71.02). This is not a mental problem.

Circumstances, family, other specified (V61.80). This is not a mental problem.

Cocaine abuse (305.6x).

Cocaine abuse (305.61) continuous.

Cocaine abuse, episodic (305.62).

Cocaine abuse, in remission (305.63).

Cocaine abuse, unspecified (305.60).

Compulsive disorder, obsessive (or compulsive neurosis, obsessive) (300.30).

Compulsive personality disorder. Coded on Axis II (301.40).

Conduct disorder, atypical (312.90).

Conduct disorder, socialized, aggressive (312.23).

Conduct disorder, socialized, nonaggressive (312.21).

Conduct disorder, undersocialized, aggressive (312.00).

Conduct disorder, undersocialized, nonaggressive (312.10).

Conversion disorder (300.11).

Cyclothymic disorder (301.13).

Deferred on Axis II, diagnosis (799.90).

Deferred on Axis I, diagnosis (799.90).

Delirium (293.00).

Delirium, amphetamine, etc. (292.81).

Delirium, phencyclidine (PCP) etc. (292.81). See specific other PCP disorders.

Delirium, other or unspecified substance (292.81).

Delusional disorder, amphetamine, etc. (292.11).

Delusional disorder, cannabis (292.11).

Delusional disorder, hallucinogen (292.11).

Delusional disorder, other or unspecified substance (292.11). See general discussion.

Dementia (294.10).

Dementia associated with alcohol (291.2x).

Dementia associated with alcohol, mild (291.21).

Dementia associated with alcohol, moderate (291.22).

Dementia associated with alcohol, severe (291.23).

Dementia associated with alcohol, unspecified (291.20).

Dementia, multi-infarct (290.4x).

Dementia, multi-infarct, with delirium (290.41).

Dementia, multi-infarct, with delusions (290.42).

Dementia, multi-infarct, with depression (290.43).

Dementia, multi-infarct, uncomplicated (290.40).

Dementia, other or unspecified substance (292.82).

Dementia, primary degenerative, presenile onset (290.1x).

Dementia, primary degenerative, presenile onset, with delirium (290.11).

Dementia, primary degenerative, presenile onset, with delusions (290.12).

Dementia, primary degenerative, presenile onset, with depression (290.13).

Dementia, primary degenerative, presenile onset, uncomplicated (290.10).

Dementia, primary degenerative, senile onset, with delirium (290.30).

Dementia, primary degenerative, senile onset, with delusions (290.20).

Dementia, primary degenerative, senile onset, with depression, (290.21).

Dementia, primary degenerative, senile onset, uncomplicated (209.00).

Dependence, combination of opioid and other nonalcoholic substance, (304.7x).

Dependence, combination of opioid and other nonalcoholic substance, continuous, (304.71).

Dependence, combination of opioid and other nonalcoholic substance, episodic, (304.72).

Dependence, combination of opioid and other nonalcoholic substance, in remission (304.73).

Dependence, combination of opioid and other nonalcoholic substance, unspecified (304.70).

Dependence, combination of substances excluding opioids and alcohol (304.8x).

Dependence, combination of substances excluding opioids and alcohol, continuous (304.81).

Dependence, combination of substances excluding opioids and alcohol, episodic (304.82).

Dependence, combination of substances excluding opioids and alcohol, in remission (304.83).

Dependence, combination of substances excluding opioids and alcohol, unspecified (304.80).

Dependent personality disorder, coded on Axis II (301.60).

Depersonalization disorder (or neurosis) (300.60).

Depression - see bipolar disorder depression.

Depression, atypical (296.82).

Depression, major, recurrent, (296.3x).

Depression, major, recurrent, major depressive episode with melancholia (296.33).

Depression, major, recurrent, major depressive episode without melancholia (296.33).

Depression, major, recurrent, major depressive episode with psychotic features (296.34), (296.37) (psychotic features are mood-incongruent).

Depression, major, recurrent, major depressive episode, in remission (296.36).

Depression, major, recurrent, major depressive episode, unspecified (296.30).

Depression, major, recurrent, manic episode with psychotic features (296.34), (296.37) (psychotic features are mood-incongruent).

Depression, major, recurrent, manic episode without psychotic features (296.32).

Depression, major, recurrent, manic episode, in remission (296.36).

Depression, major, recurrent, manic episode, unspecified (396.30).

Depression, major, single episode (296.2x).

Depression, major, single episode, major depressive episode with melancholia (296.23).

Depression, major, single episode, major depressive episode without melancholia (296.22).

Depression, major, single episode, major depressive episode with psychotic features (296.24), (296.27) (psychotic features are mood-incongruent).

Depression, major, single episode, major depressive episode in remission (296.26).

Depression, major, single episode, major depressive episode, unspecified (296.20).

Depression, major, single episode, manic episode with psychotic features (296.24), (296.27) (psychotic features are mood-incongruent).

Depression, major, single episode, manic episode, without psychotic features (296.22).

Depression, major, single episode, manic episode in remission (296.26).

Depression, major, single episode, manic episode unspecified (296.20).

Depressive neurosis (dysthymic disorder) (300.40).

Developmental disorder, atypical, specific, Coded on Axis II (315.90).

Developmental disorder, mixed, specific, Coded on Axis II (315.50).

Diagnosis, or condition, deferred on Axis I (799.90).

Diagnosis, or condition, deferred on Axis II (799.90).

Diagnosis, or condition, no, on Axis I (V71.09). This is not a mental problem.

Diagnosis, or condition, no on Axis II (V71.09). This is not a mental problem.

Dissociative disorder, atypical (300.15) P.

Dyspareunia, functional (302.76).

Dysthymic disorder (or depressive neurosis) (300.40).

Eating disorder, atypical (307.50).

Ego-dystonic homosexuality (302.00).

Exhibitionism (302.40).

Explosive disorder, intermittent (312.34).

Explosive disorder, isolated (312.35).

Factitious disorder, atypical, with physical symptoms (300.19).

Factitious disorder, chronic, with physical symptoms (301.51).

Factitious disorder with psychological symptoms (300.16).

Family circumstances, other specified (V61.80). This is not a mental disorder.

Fetishism (302.81).

Fugue, psychogenic (300.13).

Functional dyspareunia (302.76).

Functional encopresis (307.70).

Functional enuresis (307.60).

Functional vaginismus (306.51).

Gambling, pathological (312.31).

Gender identity disorder, atypical (302.85).

Gender identity disorder, of childhood (302.60).

Hallucinogen, abuse (305.3x).

Hallucinogen, abuse, unspecified (305.30).

Hallucinogen abuse, continuous (305.31).

Hallucinogen abuse, episodic (305.32).

Hallucinogen, hallucinosis (305.30).

Hallucinosis, alcohol (291.30).

Hallucinosis, other or unspecified substance (292.12).

Hallucinogen abuse, in remission (305.33).

Histrionic personality disorder, Coded on Axis II (301.50).

Homosexuality, ego-dystonic (302.00)

Hypochondriasis (300.70).

Hypochondrical neurosis (300.70).

Hysterical neurosis, conversion type (300.11).

Identity disorder, (313.82).

Idiosyncratic intoxication, alcohol (291.40).

Impulse control disorder, atypical (312.39).

Intermittent explosive disorder (312.34).

Interpersonal problem, other (V62.81). This is not a mental problem.

Intoxication, alcohol (303.00).

Intoxication, amphetamine or similar acting sympathomimetic (305.70).

Intoxication, barbiturate or similar acting sedative or hypnotic (305.40).

Intoxication, caffeine (305.90).

Intoxication, cocaine (305.60).

Intoxication, opioid (305.50).

Intoxication, phencyclidine (PCP) or similarly acting arylcyclohexylamine (305.90). See specific other PCP disorders.

Intoxication, other or unspecified substance (305.90).

Isolated explosive disorder (312.35).

Kleptomania (312.32).

Language disorder, developmental, coded on Axis II (315.31).

Life problem, phase of, or other life circumstance problem (V62.89). This is not a mental problem.

Malingering (V65.20). This is not a mental problem.

Manic (*see* Bipolar disorder, manic).

Marital Problem (V61.10). This is not a mental problem.

Masochism, sexual (302.83).

Mental retardation, mild (317.0x).

Mental retardation, mild, with other behavioral symptoms (requiring attention or treatment and that are not part of another disorder) (317.01).

Mental retardation, mild, without other behavioral symptoms (requiring attention or treatment and that are not part of another disorder) (317.00).

Mental retardation, moderate (318.0x).

Mental retardation, moderate, with other behavioral symptoms (requiring attention or treatment and that are not part of another disorder) (318.01).

Mental retardation, moderate, without other behavioral symptoms (requiring attention or treatment and that are not part of another disorder) (318.00).

Mental retardation, profound (318.2x).

Mental retardation, profound, with other behavioral symptoms (requiring attention or treatment and that are not part of another disorder) (318.21).

Mental retardation, profound, without other behavioral symptoms (requiring attention or treatment and that are not part of another disorder) (318.20).

Mental retardation, severe (318.1x).

Mental retardation, severe, with other behavioral symptoms (requiring attention or treatment and that are not part of another disorder) (318.11).

Mental retardation, severe, without other behavioral symptoms (requiring attention or treatment and that are not part of another disorder) (318.10).

Mental retardation, unspecified (319.0x).

Mental retardation, unspecified, with other behavioral symptoms (requiring attention or treatment and that are not part of another disorder) (319.01).

Mental retardation, unspecified, without other behavioral symptoms (requiring attention or treatment and that are not part of another disorder) (319.00).

Motor tic disorder, chronic (movement disorder – stereotyped) (307.22).

Multiple personality (300.14).

Mutism, elective (313.23).

Narcissistic personality disorder, coded on Axis II (301.81).

Noncompliance with medical treatment (V15.81). This is not a mental problem.

Obsessive compulsive disorder (or obsessive compulsive neurosis) (300.30).

Occupational problem (V62.20). This is not a mental problem.

Opioid abuse, continuous (305.51).

Opioid abuse, episodic (305.52).

Opioid abuse, in remission (305.53).

Opioid abuse, unspecified (305.50).

Opioid dependence (304.0x).

Opioid dependence, continuous (304.01).

Opioid dependence, episodic (304.02).

Opioid dependence, in remission (304.03).

Opioid dependence, unspecified (304.00).

Oppositional disorder (313.81).

Organic affective syndrome (293.83)

Organic brain syndrome, atypical or mixed (294.80).

Organic delusional syndrome (293.81).

Organic hallucinosis (293.82).

Organic mental disorder, atypical or mixed, other or unspecified substance (292.90).

Organic mental disorder, mixed, Phencyclidine (PCP) (292.90).

Organic personality syndrome (310.10).

Orgasm, female inhibited (302.73).

Orgasm, male, inhibited (302.74).

Other personality disorder, mixed or atypical, coded on Axis II (301.89).

Overanxious disorder, anxiety disorder of childhood or adolescence (313.00).

Panic disorder (300.01).

Paranoia (297.10).

Paranoid disorder, acute (298.30).

Paranoid disorder, atypical (297.90).

Paranoid disorder, shared (297.30).

Paranoid personality disorder, coded on Axis II (301.00).

Paraphilia, atypical (302.90).

Parent-child problem (V61.20). This is not a mental problem.

Passive-aggressive personality disorder, coded on Axis II (301.84).

Pathological gambling (312.31).

Personality disorder, other or unspecified substance (292.89).

Pervasive developmental disorder, atypical (299.8x).

Pervasive developmental disorder, atypical, full syndrome present (299.80).

Pervasive developmental disorder, atypical, residual state (299.81).

Pervasive developmental disorder, childhood onset (299.9x).

Pervasive developmental disorder, childhood onset, full syndrome present (299.90).

Pervasive developmental disorder, childhood onset, residual state (299.91).

Phobia, simple (300.29).

Phobia, social (300.23).

Pedophilia (302.20).

Phase of life problem, or other life circumstance problem. This is not a mental problem (V62.89).

Phencyclidine (PCP) or similar abuse, continuous (305.91). See other PCP disorders.

Phencyclidine (PCP) or similar abuse, episodic (305.92). See other PCP disorders.

Phencyclidine (PCP) or similar abuse, in remission (305.93). See other PCP disorders.

Phencyclidine (PCP) or similar abuse, unspecified (305.90). See other PCP disorders.

Pica (eating disorder) (307.52).

Post-traumatic stress disorder, acute (308.30).

Post-traumatic stress disorder, atypical anxiety disorder (300.00).

Post-traumatic stress disorder, chronic or delayed (309.81).

Premature ejaculation (302.75).

Psychogenic amnesia (300.12).

Psychological factors affecting physical condition (specify physical condition on Axis III) (316.00).

Psychosexual disorder not elsewhere classified (302.89).

Psychogenic fugue (300.13).

Psychogenic pain disorder (307.80).

Psychosexual dysfunction, atypical (302.70).

Psychosis, atypical (298.90).

Psychosis, brief reactive (298.80).

Pyromania (312.33).

Reactive attachment disorder of infancy (313.89).

Reading disorder, developmental, coded on Axis II (315.00).

Rumination disorder of infancy (eating disorder) (307.53).

Sadism, sexual (302.84).

Schizoaffective disorder (295.70).

Schizoid disorder of childhood or adolescence (313.22).

Schizoid personality disorder, coded on Axis II (301.20).

Schizophrenia, catatonic (295.2x).

Schizophrenia, catatonic, chronic (295.22).

Schizophrenia, catatonic, chronic with acute exacerbation (295.24).

Schizophrenia, catatonic, in remission (295.25).

Schizophrenia, catatonic, subchronic (295.21).

Schizophrenia, catatonic, subchronic with acute exacerbation (295.23).

Schizophrenia, catatonic, unspecified (295.20).

Schizophrenia, disorganized (295.1x).

Schizophrenia, disorganized, chronic (295.12).

Schizophrenia, disorganized, chronic with acute exacerbation (295.14).

Schizophrenia, disorganized, in remission (295.15).

Schizophrenia, disorganized, subchronic (295.11).

Schizophrenia, disorganized, subchronic with acute exacerbation (295.13).

Schizophrenia, disorganized, unspecified (295.10).

Schizophrenia, residual (295.6x).

Schizophrenia, residual, chronic (295.62).

Schizophrenia, residual, chronic with acute exacerbation (295.64).

Schizophrenia, residual, in remission (295.65).

Schizophrenia, residual, subchronic (295.61).

Schizophrenia, residual, subchronic with acute exacerbation (295.63).

Schizophrenia, residual, unspecified (295.60).

Schizophrenia, undifferentiated (295.9x).

Schizophrenia, undifferentiated, chronic (295.92).

Schizophrenia, undifferentiated, chronic with acute exacerbation (295.94).

Schizophrenia, undifferentiated, in remission (295.95).

Schizophrenia, undifferentiated, subchronic (295.91).

Schizophrenia, undifferentiated, subchronic with acute exacerbation (295.93).

Schizophrenia, undifferentiated, unspecified (295.90).

Schizophrenia, paranoid (295.3x).

Schizophrenia, paranoid, chronic (295.32).

Schizophrenia, paranoid, chronic with acute exacerbation (295.34).

Schizophrenia, paranoid, in remission (295.35).

Schizophrenia, paranoid, subchronic (295.31).

Schizophrenia, paranoid, subchronic with acute exacerbation (295.33).

Schizophrenia, paranoid, unspecified (295.30).

Schizophrenic (*see* Schizophrenia).

Schizophreniform disorder (295.40).

Schizotypal personality disorder, coded on Axis II (301.22).

Sexual desire, inhibited (302.71).

Sexual excitement, inhibited (302.72).

Sexual masochism (302.83).

Sexual sadism (302.84).

Separation anxiety disorder, anxiety disorders of childhood or adolescence (309.21).

Shared paranoid disorder (297.30).

Simple phobia (300.29).

Sleep terror disorder (307.46).

Sleepwalking disorder (307.46).

Social phobia (300.23).

Somatization disorder (300.81).

Somatoform disorder, atypical (300.70).

Stereotyped movement, disorder, atypical (307.30).

Stuttering (307.00).

Substance abuse, mixed or unspecified, unspecified (305.90).

Substance dependence, other, specified (304.6x).

Substance dependence, other, specified, continuous (304.61).

Substance dependence, other specified, episodic (304.62).

Substance dependence, other specified, in remission (304.63).

Substance dependence, other specified, unspecified (304.60).

Substance dependence, unspecified (304.9x).

Substance dependence, unspecified, continuous (304.91).

Substance dependence, unspecified, episodic (304.92).

Substance dependence, unspecified, in remission (304.93).

Substance dependence, unspecified, unspecified (304.90).

Tic disorder, atypical (movement disorder - stereotyped) (307.20).

Tic disorder, transient (movement disorder - stereotyped) (307.21).

Tobacco dependence (305.1x).

Tabacco dependence, continuous (305.11).

Tobacco dependence, episodic (305.12).

Tobacco dependence, in remission (305.13).

Tobacco dependence, unspecified (305.10).

Tourette's disorder, (movement disorder - stereotyped) (307.23).

Transsexualism (302.5x).

Transsexualism, asexual (302.51).

Transsexualism, heterosexual (302.53).

Transsexualism, homosexual (302.52).

Transsexualism, unspecified (302.50).

Transvestism (302.30).

Unspecified mental disorder (nonpsychotic) (300.90).

Vaginismus, functional (306.51).

Voyeurism (302.82).

Withdrawal, alcohol (291.80).

Withdrawal, amphetamine etc. (292.00).

Withdrawal, barbiturate, similar acting sedative or hypnotic (292.00).

Withdrawal delirium, alcohol (291.00).

Withdrawal delirium, barbiturate or similar acting sedative or hypnotic (292.00).

Withdrawal, opioid (292.00).

Withdrawal, other or unspecified substance (292.00).

Withdrawal, tobacco (292.00).

Zoophilia (302.10).

appendix C

Numerical List
of Disorders

200.02	Anxiety disorder, generalized
209.00	Dementia, primary degenerative, senile onset, uncomplicated
290.1x	Dementia, primary degenerative, presenile, onset
290.10	Dementia, primary degenerative, presenile onset, uncomplicated
290.11	Dementia, primary degenerative, presenile onset, with delirium
290.12	Dementia, primary degenerative, presenile onset, with delusions
290.13	Dementia, primary degenerative, presenile onset, with depression
290.20	Dementia, primary degenerative, senile onset, with delusions
290.21	Dementia, primary degenerative, senile onset, with depression
290.30	Dementia, primary degenerative, senile onset, with delirium
290.4x	Dementia, multi-infarct
290.40	Dementia, multi-infarct, uncomplicated
290.41	Dementia, multi-infarct, with delirium
290.42	Dementia, multi-infarct, with delusions
290.43	Dementia, multi-infarct, with depression
291.00	Withdrawal delirium, alcohol
291.10	Amnestic disorder, alcohol

291.2x	Dementia associated with alcohol
292.21	Dementia associated with alcohol, mild
291.22	Dementia associated with alcohol, moderate
291.20	Dementia associated with alcohol, unspecified
291.30	Hallucinosis, alcohol
291.40	Idiosyncratic intoxication, alcohol
291.23	Dementia associated with alcohol, severe
291.80	Withdrawal, alcohol
*292.00	Withdrawal, opioid Withdrawal, barbiturate, similiar acting dedative or hypnotic Withdrawal, tobacco Withdrawal, other or unspecified substance Withdrawal, amphetamine, etc. Withdrawal, delirium, barbiturate or similar acting sedative or hypnotic
*292.11	Delusional disorder, other or unspecified substance Delusional disorder, cannabis Delusional disorder, hallucinogen Delusional disorder, amphetamine, etc.
292.12	Hallucinosis, other or unspecified substance
*292.81	Delirium, other or unspecified substance Delirium, phencyclidine (PCP), etc. Delirium, amphetamine, etc.
*292.82	Dementia, other or unspecified substance
*292.83	Amnestic disorder, other or unspecified substance Amnestic disorder, barbiturate, similiar acting sedative or hypnotic
*292.84	Affective disorder, other or unspecified substance Affective disorder, hallucinogen
292.89	Personality disorder, other or unspecified substance
292.90	Organic mental disorder, atypical or mixed, other or unspecified substance Organic mental disorder, mixed, Phencyclidine (PCP)
293.00	Delirium
293.81	Organic delusional syndrome
293.82	Organic hallucinosis
293.83	Organic affective syndrome

* = Not Specifically Discussed. See General Discussion.

294.00   Amnestic, syndrome

294.10   Dementia

294.80   Atypical or mixed organic brain syndrome

295.1x   Schizophrenia, disorganized

295.10   Schizophrenia, disorganized, unspecified

295.11   Schizophrenia, disorganized, subchronic

295.12   Schizophrenia, disorganized, chronic

295.13   Schizophrenia, disorganized, subchronic with acute exacerbation

295.14   Schizophrenia, disorganized, chronic with acute exacerbation

295.15   Schizophrenia, disorganized, in remission

295.2x   Schizophrenia, catatonic

295.20   Schizophrenia, catatonic, unspecified

295.21   Schizophrenia, catatonic, subchronic

295.22   Schizophrenia, catatonic, chronic

295.23   Schizophrenia, catatonic, subchronic with acute exacerbation

295.24   Schizophrenia, catatonic, chronic with acute exacerbation

295.25   Schizophrenia, catatonic, in remission

295.3x   Schizophrenia, paranoid

295.30   Schizophrenia, paranoid, unspecified

295.31   Schizophrenia, paranoid, subchronic

295.32   Schizophrenia, paranoid, chronic

295.33   Schizophrenia, paranoid, subchronic with acute exacerbation

295.34   Schizophrenia, paranoid, chronic with acute exacerbation

295.35   Schizophrenia, paranoid, in remission

295.40   Schizophreniform disorder

295.6x   Schizophrenia, residual

295.60   Schizophrenia, residual, unspecified

295.61   Schizophrenia, residual, subchronic

295.62   Schizophrenia, residual, chronic

295.63   Schizophrenia, residual, subchronic with acute exacerbation

295.64   Schizophrenia, residual, chronic with acute exacerbation

295.65   Schizophrenia, residual, in remission

295.70   Schizoaffective disorder

295.9x   Schizophrenia, undifferentiated

295.90   Schizophrenia, undifferentiated, unspecified

295.91   Schizophrenia, undifferentiated, subchronic

295.92   Schizophrenia, undifferentiated, chronic

295.93   Schizophrenia, undifferentiated, subchronic with acute exacerbation

295.94   Schizophrenia, undifferentiated, chronic with acute exacerbation

295.95   Schizophrenia, undifferentiated, in remission

296.2x   Depression, major, single episode

296.20   Depression, major, single episode, manic episode unspecified
Depression, major, single episode, major depressive episode unspecified

296.22   Depression, major, single episode, manic episode without psychotic features
Depression, major, single episode, major depressive episode without melancholia

296.23   Depression, major, single episode, major depressive episode with melancholia

296.24   Depression, major, single episode, manic episode with psychotic features
Depression, major, single episode, major depressive episode with psychotic features

296.26   Depression, major, single episode, major depressive episode in remission
Depression, major, single episode manic episode in remission

296.3x   Depression, major, recurrent

296.30   Depression, major, recurrent, manic episode unspecified
Depression, major, recurrent, major depressive episodic unspecified

296.32   Depression, major, recurrent, manic episode without psychotic features
Depression, major, recurrent, major depressive episode, without melancholia

296.33   Depression, major, recurrent, major depressive episode with melancholia

296.34   Depression, major, recurrent, manic episode with psychotic features

296.34   Depression, major, recurrent, major depressive episode with psychotic features

296.36   Depression, major, recurrent, major depressive episode in remission
Depression, major, recurrent, manic episode in remission

296.4x   Bipolar disorder, manic

296.40   Bipolar disorder, manic, manic episode unspecified

296.40	Bipolar disorder, manic, major depression episode unspecified
296.42	Bipolar disorder, manic, major depressive episode without melancholia Bipolar disorder, manic, manic episode without psychotic features
296.43	Bipolar disorder, manic, major depressive episode with melancholia
296.44	Bipolar disorder, manic, manic episode with psychotic features Bipolar disorder, manic, major depressive episode with psychotic features
296.46	Bipolar disorder, manic, major depressive episode in remission Bipolar disorder, manic, manic episode in remission
296.5x	Bipolar disorder, depression
296.50	Bipolar disorder, depression, manic episode unspecified Bipolar disorder, depression, major depressive episode in unspecified
296.52	Bipolar disorder, depression, major depressive episode without melancholia Bipolar disorder, depression, manic episode without psychotic features
296.53	Bipolar disorder, depression, major depressive episode with melancholia
296.54	Bipolar disorder, depression, manic episode with psychotic features Bipolar disorder, depression, major depressive episode with psychotic features
296.56	Bipolar disorder, depression, major depressive episode in remission Bipolar disorder, depression, manic episode in remission
296.6x	Bipolar disorder, mixed
296.60	Bipolar disorder, mixed, manic episode unspecified Bipolar disorder, mixed, major depressive episode unspecified
296.62	Bipolar disorder, mixed, manic episode without psychotic features Bipolar disorder, mixed, major depressive episode without melancholia
296.63	Bipolar disorder, mixed, major depressive episode with melancholia
296.64	Bipolar disorder, mixed, manic episode with psychotic features Bipolar disorder, mixed, major depressive episode with psychotic features
296.66	Bipolar disorder, mixed, major depressive episode in remission Bipolar disorder, mixed, manic episode in remission
296.70	Bipolar disorder, atypical
296.82	Depression, atypical
297.10	Paranoia
297.30	Paranoid disorder, shared
297.90	Atypical paranoid disorder
298.30	Paranoid disorder, acute
298.80	Brief reactive psychosis

298.90	Atypical psychosis
299.0x	Autism, infantile
299.00	Autism, infantile, full syndrome present
299.01	Autism, infantile, residual state
299.8x	Pervasive developmental disorder, atypical
299.80	Pervasive developmental disorder, atypical, full syndrome present
299.81	Pervasive developmental disorder, atypical, residual state
299.9x	Pervasive developmental disorder, childhood onset
299.90	Pervasive developmental disorder, childhood onset, full syndrome present
299.91	Pervasive developmental disorder, childhood onset, residual state
300.00	Post-traumatic stress disorder, atypical anxiety disorder
300.01	Panic disorder
300.11	Conversion disorder Hysterical neurosis, conversion type
300.12	Psychogenic amnesia
300.13	Fugue, psychogenic
300.14	Multiple personality
300.15	Atypical dissociative disorder
300.16	Factitious disorder with psychological symptoms
300.19	Factitious disorder, atypical, with physical symptoms
300.21	Agoraphobia with panic attacks
300.22	Agoraphobia without panic attacks
300.23	Social phobia
300.29	Simple phobia
300.30	Obsessive compulsive disorder
300.40	Dysthymic disorder (or depressive neurosis)
300.60	Depersonalization disorder (or neurosis)
300.70	Hypochondriasis Hypochondrical neurosis Atypical somatoform disorder
300.81	Somatization disorder
300.90	Unspecified mental disorder (non-psychotic)

301.00	Paranoid personality disorder, coded on Axis II
301.13	Cyclothymic disorder
301.20	Schizoid personality disorder, coded on Axis II
301.22	Schizotypal personality disorder, coded on Axis II
301.40	Compulsive personality disorder, coded on Axis II
301.50	Histrionic personality disorder, coded on Axis II
301.51	Factitious disorder, chronic, with physical symptoms
301.60	Dependent personality disorder, coded on Axis II
301.70	Antisocial personality disorder, coded on Axis II
301.81	Narcissistic personality disorder, coded on Axis II
301.82	Avoidant personality disorder, coded on Axis II
301.83	Borderline personality disorder, coded on Axis II
301.84	Passive-aggressive personality disorder, coded on Axis II
301.89	Atypical, mixed or other personality disorder, coded on Axis II
302.00	Homosexuality, ego-dystonic
302.10	Zoophilia
302.20	Pedophilia
302.30	Transvestism
302.40	Exhibitionism
302.5x	Transsexualism
302.50	Transsexualism, unspecified
302.51	Transsexualism, asexual
302.52	Transsexualism, homosexual
302.53	Transsexualism, heterosexual
302.60	Gender identity disorder of childhood
302.70	Psychosexual dysfunction, atypical
302.71	Inhibited sexual desire
302.72	Inhibited sexual excitement
302.73	Inhibited female orgasm
302.74	Inhibited male orgasm
302.75	Premature ejaculation

302.76	Functional dyspareunia
302.81	Fetishism
302.82	Voyeurism
302.83	Masochism, sexual
302.84	Sadism, sexual
302.85	Atypical gender identity disorder
302.89	Psychosexual disorder not elsewhere classified
302.90	Atypical paraphilia
303.00	Intoxication, alcohol
303.9x	Alcohol dependence (alcoholism)
303.90	Alcohol dependence, unspecified
303.91	Alcohol dependence (alcoholism), continuous
303.92	Alcohol dependence (alcoholism), episodic
303.93	Alcohol dependence (alcoholism), in remission
304.0x	Opioid dependence
304.00	Opioid dependence, unspecified
304.01	Opioid dependence, continuous
304.02	Opioid dependence, episodic
304.03	Opioid dependence, in remission
304.1x	Barbiturate or similarly acting sedative or hypnotic dependence
304.10	Barbiturate or similarly acting sedative or hypnotic dependence, unspecified
304.11	Barbiturate or similarly acting sedative or hypnotic dependence, continuous
304.12	Barbiturate or similarly acting sedative or hypnotic dependence, episodic
304.13	Barbiturate or similarly acting sedative or hypnotic dependence, in remission
304.3x	Cannabis dependence
304.30	Cannabis dependence, unspecified
304.31	Cannabis dependence, continuous
304.32	Cannabis dependence, episodic
304.33	Cannabis dependence, in remission
304.4x	Amphetamine (or similar) dependence
304.40	Amphetamine (or similar) dependence, unspecified

304.41	Amphetamine (or similar) dependence, continuous
304.42	Amphetamine (or similar) dependence, episodic
304.43	Amphetamine (or similar) dependence, in remission
304.6x	Substance dependence, other specified
304.60	Substance dependence, other specified, unspecified
304.61	Substance dependence, other specified, continuous
304.62	Substance dependence, other specified, episodic
304.63	Substance dependence, other specified, in remission
304.7x	Combination dependence of opioid and other nonalcoholic substance
304.70	Combination dependence of opioid and other nonalcoholic substance, unspecified
304.71	Combination dependence of opioid and other nonalcoholic substance, continuous
304.72	Combination dependence of opioid and other nonalcoholic substance, episodic
304.73	Combination dependence of opioid and other nonalcoholic substance, in remission
304.8x	Combination dependence of substances, excluding opioids and alcohol
304.80	Combination dependence of substances excluding opioids and alcohol, unspecified
304.81	Combination dependence of substances, excluding opioids and alcohol, continuous
304.82	Combination dependence of substances, excluding opioids and alcohol, episodic
304.83	Combination dependence of substances excluding opioids and alcohol, in remission
304.9x	Substance dependence, unspecified
304.90	Substance dependence, unspecified, unspecified
304.91	Substance dependence, unspecified, continuous
304.92	Substance dependence, unspecified, episodic
304.93	Substance dependence, unspecified, in remission
305.0x	Alcohol abuse
305.00	Alcohol abuse, unspecified
305.01	Alcohol abuse, continuous

305.02	Alcohol abuse, episodic
305.03	Alcohol abuse, in remission
305.1x	Tobacco dependence
305.10	Tobacco dependence, unspecified
305.11	Tobacco dependence, continuous
305.12	Tobacco dependence, episodic
305.13	Tobacco dependence, in remission
305.2x	Cannabis abuse
*305.20	Cannabis intoxication
305.21	Cannabis abuse, continuous
305.22	Cannabis abuse, episodic
305.23	Cannabis abuse, in remission
305.3x	Hallucinogen abuse
*305.30	Hallucinogen, Hallucinosis
305.31	Hallucinogen abuse, continuous
305.32	Hallucinogen abuse episodic
305.33	Hallucinogen abuse, in remission
*305.4x	Barbiturate or similarly acting sedative or hypnotic abuse
*305.40	Barbiturate or similarly acting sedative or hypnotic abuse, unspecified
305.41	Barbiturate or similarly acting sedative or hypnotic abuse, continuous
305.42	Barbiturate or similarly acting sedative or hypnotic abuse, episodic
305.43	Barbiturate of similarly acting sedative or hypnotic abuse, in remission
305.5x	Opioid abuse
*305.50	Opioid abuse, unspecified Opioid intoxication
305.51	Opioid abuse, continuous
305.52	Opioid abuse, episodic
305.53	Opioid abuse, in remission
305.6x	Cocaine abuse
*305.60	Cocaine abuse, unspecified Cocaine intoxication
305.61	Cocaine abuse, continuous

305.62   Cocaine abuse, episodic

305.63   Cocaine abuse, in remission

305.7x   Amphetamine (or similar) abuse

305.70   Amphetamine (or similar) abuse, unspecified

305.71   Amphetamine (or similar) abuse, continuous

305.72   Amphetamine (or similar) abuse, episodic

305.73   Amphetamine (or similar) abuse, in remission

305.9x   Substance abuse, mixed or unspecified
          Phencyclidine (PCP) (or similar) abuse (*see* other PCP disorders)

*305.90   Phencyclidine (PCP) or similarly acting arylcyclohexylamine intoxication
          See specific other PCP disorders
          Caffeine intoxication
          Other or unspecified substance intoxication
          Substance abuse, mixed or unspecified, unspecified
          Phencyclidine (PCP) (or similar) abuse, unspecified (*see* other specific PCP
          disorders

305.91   Substance abuse, mixed or unspecified, continuous
          Phencyclidine (PCP) (or similar) abuse, continuous (*see* other PCP disorders)

305.92   Substance abuse, mixed or unspecified, episodic

305.93   Substance abuse, mixed or unspecified, in remission
          Phencyclidine (PCP) (or similar) abuse, in remission (*see* other PCP disorders)

306.51   Functional vaginismus

307.00   Stuttering

307.10   Anorexia nervosa (eating disorder)

307.20   Atypical tic disorder (movement disorder) (stereotyped)

307.21   Transient tic disorder (movement disorder) (stereotyped)

307.22   Chronic motor tic disorder (movement disorder) (stereotyped)

307.23   Tourette's disorder (movement disorder) (stereotyped)

307.30   Atypical stereotyped movement disorder

307.46   Sleep terror disorder

307.46   Sleepwalking disorder

307.50   Atypical eating disorder

---

* Amphetamine or similar acting sympathomimetic intoxication.

307.51	Bulimia (eating disorder)
307.52	Pica (eating disorder)
307.53	Rumination disorder of infancy (eating disorder)
307.60	Functional enuresis
307.70	Functional encopresis
307.80	Psychogenic pain disorder
308.30	Post-traumatic stress disorder, acute
309.00	Adjustment disorder, with depressed mood
309.21	Anxiety disorders of childhood or adolescence. Separation Anxiety disorder
309.23	Adjustment disorder with work (or academic) inhibition
309.24	Adjustment disorder with anxious mood
309.28	Adjustment disorder with mixed emotional features
309.30	Adjustment disorder with disturbance of conduct
309.40	Adjustment disorder with mixed disturbance of emotions and conduct
309.81	Post-traumatic stress disorder, chronic or delayed
309.83	Adjustment disorder with withdrawal
309.90	Adjustment disorder with atypical features
310.10	Organic personality syndrome
312.00	Conduct disorder, undersocialized, aggressive
312.10	Conduct disorder, undersocialized, nonaggressive
312.31	Pathological gambling
312.32	Kleptomania
312.33	Pyromania
312.34	Explosive disorder, intermittent
312.35	Explosive disorder, isolated
312.39	Impulse control disorder, atypical
312.21	Conduct disorder, socialized, nonaggressive
312.23	Conduct disorder, socialized, aggressive
312.90	Conduct disorder, atypical
313.00	Anxiety disorders of childhood or adolescence; Overanxious disorder
313.21	Anxiety disorders of childhood or adolescence. Avoidant disorder of childhood or adolescence

312.22   Schizoid disorder of childhood or adolescence

313.23   Elective mutism

313.81   Oppositional disorder

313.82   Identity disorder

313.89   Reactive attachment disorder of infancy

314.00   Attention deficit disorder, without hyperactivity

314.01   Attention deficit disorder, with hyperactivity

314.80   Attention deficit disorder, residual type

315.00   Reading disorder, developmental, coded on Axis II

315.10   Arithmetic disorder, developmental, coded on Axis II

315.31   Language disorder, developmental, coded on Axis II

315.39   Articulation disorder, developmental, coded on Axis II

315.50   Mixed specific developmental disorder, coded on Axis II

315.90   Mixed specific developmental disorder, atypical, coded on Axis II

316.00   Psychological factors affecting physical condition (specify physical condition on Axis III)

317.0x   Mental retardation, mild

317.00   Mental retardation, mild without other behavioral symptoms

317.01   Mental retardation, mild with other behavioral symptoms (requiring attention or treatment and that are not part of another disorder)

318.0x   Mental retardation, moderate

318.00   Mental retardation, moderate without other behavioral symptoms

318.01   Mental retardation, moderate with other behavioral symptoms (requiring attention or treatment and that are not part of another disorder)

318.1x   Mental retardation, severe

318.10   Mental retardation, severe without other behavioral symptoms

318.11   Mental retardation, severe with other behavioral symptoms (requiring attention or treatment and that are not part of another disorder)

318.2x   Mental retardation, profound

318.20   Mental retardation, profound without other behavioral symptoms

318.21   Mental retardation, profound with other behavioral symptoms (requiring attention or treatment and that are not part of another disorder)

319.0x   Mental retardation, unspecified

319.00	Mental retardation, unspecified without other behavioral symptoms
319.01	Mental retardation, unspecified, with other behavioral symptoms (requiring attention or treatment and that are not part of another disorder)
799.90	Diagnosis or condition deferred on Axis I
799.90	Deferred on Axis II, diagnosis or condition

V CODES

V15.81	Noncompliance with medical treatment. This is not a mental disorder
V61.10	Marital problem. This is not a mental disorder
V61.20	Child-parent problem. This is not a mental problem
V61.80	Family circumstances, other specified. This is not a mental disorder
*V62.20	Occupational problem. This is not a mental disorder
*V62.30	Academic problem. This is not a mental disorder
V62.81	Interpersonal problem (other). This is not a mental problem
*V62.82	Uncomplicated bereavement. This is not a mental disorder
V62.89	Borderline intellectual functioning. This is not a mental problem
*V62.89	Phase of life problem or other life circumstance problem. This is not a mental problem
V65.20	Malingering. This is not a mental problem
*V71.01	Adult antisocial behavior. This is not a mental problem
*V71.02	Childhood or adolescent antisocial behavior. This is not a mental problem
V71.09	No diagnosis or condition on Axis I
V71.09	No diagnosis on Axis II

appendix D

DSM-III Disorders and Their Cardinal Manifestations

The aim in these tables is to present a description of the DSM-III definition of each mental disorder in a way that accurately summarizes each item as it appears in the DSM-III manual.

The complexities of these tables are necessary to reproduce the DSM-III definitions. As you begin to use these tables you should acquaint yourselves with the symbols or elements that represent the sometimes complex logic of a DSM-III definition. Once the elements are familiar you can use the tables as a quick reference to compare the description of one disorder against another.

These tables list all of the DSM-III disorders that are defined by a list of specific criteria. The tables list the mental disorders going down the page in the left margin; specific symptoms are across the top of the table reading from left to right.

Thus each *disorder* has a separate row or line horizontally across the table, and each specific *symptom* has a list that can be followed down the page in that specific column. When a mental disorder on a given line intersects with a column representing a specific symptom, often a symbol will appear indicating how that symptom is involved in the description of the disorder.

By looking down a column, for example, all of the disorders that *require* a particular symptom can be instantly picked out. Such information as the comparative length of time that symptoms have to be present, or a comparison of the kinds of disorders that must be excluded before a given diagnosis can be applied to a patient can be easily appreciated. If a box has no element or symbol, the DSM-III description of the disorder does not mention that particular symptom, so it is not related to the description of the disorder.

If you have a diagnosis and wish to read about its symptoms, find the diagnosed disorder in the left-hand column of the appropriate table. Read that line across the width of the table to identify the symptoms. If you wish to project a possible diagnosis from symptoms you observe, find those symptoms across the top of the tables, then read down to find disorders which may be indicated by the symptom. (You may have to scan all the tables, but a given symptom appears only once in a given table, and you will only have to read down one page.)

The following symbols are used to identify the relationship of the symptom to the disorder.

● Means that this cardinal manifestation of a mental disorder is always required to accord with a diagnosis.

No Means that this symptom is always excluded.

1, 2, 3, etc. Whenever a number appears, it means that the symptom is part of a group of symptoms of which one or more is required. *How many* symptoms are required is identified by the number; how many are in the group from which that number is drawn is identified by the items marked with the number. (A "2" noted under five symptoms means any 2 of those 5 make up a required diagnostic criterion).

○ □ ◇ These geometric symbols are used to separate different groups involved in the diagnosis of a disorder (if you need two of one group of four, and two of another group of five, you may find four 2s enclosed in squares and five 2s in circles).

*, 1 and * The symptom marked with "1 and *" only counts when any one of the symptoms marked "*" occurs with it; it is then considered, along with any other "1" in its group, as above.

● M, N
● P, R
● S, T A solid dot with any of the superscripts ^{M}, ^{P}, or ^{S} identifies a required symptom, as with any solid dot. The related superscripts identify related symptoms which must also occur as expansions or additional features. The related superscripts will be applied to numbers which, as above, refer to groupings of symptoms that are required for a certain diagnosis.

Could Not required by DSM-III, but often occurs with the given disorder.

✪, *italics* Words in italics, and the symbol ✪ identify information not in DSM-III which the author considers to have a bearing on the disorder in question. Not required for a DSM-III diagnosis.

KEY TO SUPERSCRIPT LETTERS

A Other disturbances of higher cortical function (aphasia, apraxia, agnosia, constructional difficulty).

B Significant cerebrovascular disease is the organic factor.

C May have to be inferred in a child under 6 from behavior, facial expression, etc.

D Depressed mood can alternate or intermingle with manic mood in a manic episode.

E Less severe than in major mood disorders.

F Only 3 symptoms are needed when child under 6 has the disorder; 4 are needed when patient is older than 6.

G Or apathy.

H Either of these.[†]

I Patient only needs hypomania now if he has had mania before to get diagnosis now of *bipolar disorder, manic,* and only needs mild depression (not full major depressive episode) if he has had major depressive episode before to get diagnosis now of *bipolar disorder, depressed.*

J While these appear to be similar categories, DSM-III uses them without attempting to merge them; therefore, they are presented literally and the user of DSM-III must decide in the case of an individual patient whether they represent the same or different ways of categorizing information.

K 3 or 4, depending on whether the mood is predominantly euphoric or irritable, respectively.

L Not prominent.

M and N See above.
P and R
S and T

O When an organic factor does exist, it is not enough to account for the patient's complaint or disability; here, "organic" doesn't refer to organic mental disorders but means "physical illness."

Q Panic attack can occur when in contact with the feared object or situation; when an obsession occurs; or when a compulsion is resisted.

U Both or "all of these." [†]

V Both or "all of these." [†]

W When psychosis looks just like schizophrenia but the patient is older than 45 (late paraphrenia).

X When psychosis looks just like schizophrenia and lasts or has lasted less than 2 weeks.

Y This is largely a disorder of women, only rarely seen in men; about 1 percent of women have it; the onset is before 30 years of age, usually in *adolescence* (otherwise it is diagnosed as *Atypical Somatiform Disorder).* The female patient must have a history, as described, of 12 of these 37 symptoms; 14 of the 37 symptoms must be present in male. While onset can be in the teens, the disorder is usually lifelong, with rarely a year going by without the patient needing attention. It is also diagnosed as *Atypical Somatiform Disorder* when the required number of symptoms have not been met, but the condition is strongly suspected.

Z Either of these (when H is already used). [†]

% Could precede another mental disorder and in that case only should be noted. By definition this illness cannot be said to coexist with other mental disorders capable of causing the same symptoms when the rest of the criteria for the other disorder are met.

a As the single primary symptom of the disorder.

b In a person who apparently has alcohol dependence.

[†] The superscript letters meaning "either of these" and "both or all of these" are applied to numbers which identify a group in which these symptoms must be present, as discussed above. Those in the group with the superscript must be considered as a single one of that number (for instance, in the grouping 2 2 2^U 2^U, *both* of the symptoms marked 2^U must be present along with one of the other 2s; otherwise both of the 2s will suffice, but *not* a 2 and only one 2^U).

d Or where there are so many substances that the physician prefers to indicate a combination of substances, rather than list each specific substance.

e Could be dilated from anoxia from severe overdose.

g Or can occur after administration of Opioid antagonist following briefer period of use.

h Or chills.

j Persecutory delusions.

m Tobacco use for several weeks at least at a level equivalent to more than 10 cigarettes per day with each cigarette containing at least 0.5 mg of nicotine.

n Usually in excess of 250 mg of caffeine.

1 "Chronic schizophrenia means continuous periods of illness of two years or more. When the duration of illness is more than six months but less than two years, it is known as subchronic schizophrenia. Any patient who has been in a residual state for six or more months, who has reoccurrence of active phase, is said to have either subchronic schizophrenia with acute exacerbation or chronic schizophrenia with acute exacerbation depending on how long they have been in the residual state."

MAJOR DISORDERS OF DSM III

Group	Disorder	Cardinal manifestations present for: at least	not more than	Age of onset limits by definition	Exclusion of other disorders that could pre-empt diagnosis	Cardinal manifestations characteristic of long term functioning and are pervasive	Cardinal manifestations cause social or occupational impairment or subjective distress
Organic brain syndromes and organic mental disorders	Psychosis						
	Delirium						
	Dementia				Delirium, delusions, depression can occur & are not excluded		
	Amnestic syndrome						
	Organic delusional syndrome						
	Organic hallucinosis						
	Organic affective syndrome { depressed / manic						
	Organic personality syndrome	No predominant disturbance of mood					
	Primary degenerative dementia				Delirium, delusions or depression can occur also and are not excluded {		
	Multi-infarct dementia						
Affective disorders and affective syndromes	Major affective disorders and syndromes — Manic episode { euphoric mood / irritable mood	1 wk if not in hospital {					
	Major depressive episode { older than 6 / <6	2 weeks {					
	Major depression { single episode / recurrent						
	Bipolar disorder { manic / depressed / mixed						
	Other specific affective disorders — Dysthymic disorder	2 yrs					
	Cyclothymic disorder { hypomanic / depressed	2 yrs {					
	Atypical affective disorders { Atypical bipolar disorder / Atypical depression						
Paranoid disorders	Paranoid disorder	1 week			Schizophrenia, organic mental disorder {		
	Acute paranoid disorder		Less than 6 mo				
	Paranoia	6 months					
	Shared paranoid disorder	1 week					
Psychoses not elsewhere classified	Brief reactive psychosis		2 wks				
	Atypical psychosis		2 wks	$\leqslant 45^W$			
	Schizophreniform disorder	2 wks	6 mo	< 45 yr			
Schizophrenic disorders	Schizophrenia — active phase / prodromal phase / residual phase	6 mos combined {		< 45 yr	Organic mental disorder {		
	paranoid type	6 mo		< 45	Mental retardation {		
	catatonic type	6 mo		< 45			
	disorganized type	6 mo		< 45			
	undifferentiated type	6 mo		< 45			
	residual type[9]	6 mo					
Axis II personality disorders	Schizotypal				Schizophrenia, any	●	●
	Schizoid				Schizophrenia, any	●	●
	Paranoid				Schizophrenia paranoid disorder, any	●	●
	Avoidant					●	●
	Borderline					●	●
	Narcissistic					●	●
	Histrionic					●	●
	Compulsive					●	●
	Dependent					●	●
	Passive-aggressive					●	●
	Antisocial			$\geqslant 18$	Schizophrenia, manic episodes, severe mental retardation {	✪	●

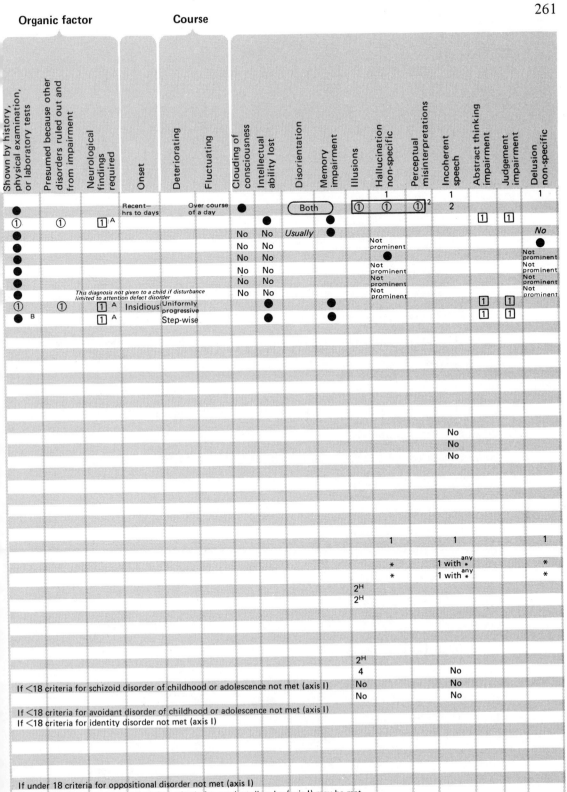

Disorder	Personality change	Impulse control impairment	Paranoid ideas, or suspiciousness	Labile emotions	Sleep-wakefulness cycle disturbance	Psychomotor activity increased or decreased	Mood — Depressed, dysphoric	Mood — Elevated euphoric	Mood — Irritable	Appetite or body weight increased or decreased
Organic brain syndromes and organic mental disorders										
Psychosis										
Delirium					2	2				
Dementia										
Amnestic syndrome										
Organic delusional syndrome										
Organic hallucinosis							No	No	No	
Organic affective syndrome — depressed						2	●			2
Organic affective syndrome — manic								①	①	
Organic personality syndrome	●	1	1	1			No	No	No	
Primary degenerative dementia										
Multi-infarct dementia										
Affective disorders and syndromes										
Major affective disorders — Manic episode / euphoric mood							Can alternate or intermingle with manic ●[D]	●		
Manic episode / irritable mood									●	
Major depressive episode / older than 6						4	●			4
Major depressive episode / <6						3	●[C]			3
Major depression / single episode						4 or 3[F]	●			4 or 3[F]
Major depression / recurrent						4 or 3[F]	●			4 or 3[F]
Bipolar disorder / manic								①	①	
Bipolar disorder / depressed						4 or 3[F]	●			4 or 3[F]
Bipolar disorder / mixed	Depressive symptoms are prominent and last a full day, current or most recent episode									
Other specific affective disorders — Dysthymic disorder							●[E]			
Cyclothymic disorder / hypomanic								①[E]	①[E]	
Cyclothymic disorder / depressed							●[E]			
Atypical affective disorders — Atypical bipolar disorder										
Atypical depression										
Paranoid disorders										
Paranoid disorder										
Acute paranoid disorder										
Paranoia										
Shared paranoid disorder										
Psychoses not elsewhere classified										
Brief reactive psychosis										
Atypical psychosis										
Schizophreniform disorder										
Schizophrenic disorders										
Schizophrenia — active phase										
prodromal phase										
residual phase										
paranoid type										
catatonic type										
disorganized type										
undifferentiated type										
residual type[9]										
Axis II personality disorders										
Schizotypal			4							
Schizoid			No							
Paranoid			●[M]							
Avoidant										
Borderline										
Narcissistic										
Histrionic										
Compulsive										
Dependent										
Passive-aggressive										
Antisocial										

Insomnia or hypersomnia	Loss of energy or fatigue	Complaints of being slowed down	Complaint or evidence of diminished ability to think clearly, concentrate or indecisiveness	Loss of interest or pleasure in usual activities or sex	Feelings of guilt, worthlessness, self-reproach, inadequacy	Recurrent thoughts of wishing to be dead, suicide, death or suicide attempts	Tearfulness	Pessimism about future or brooding over past	Loss of interest in or enjoyment of sex	Decreased activity	Decreased effectiveness at work, school, home	Irritable or excessive anger (or inappropriate anger or tantrums)
2	2		2	2	2	2						*Could*
				1^G								
												Could
Hypomanic episode is same cardinal manifestations but less severe												
4	4		4	4	4	4						
3				3^G								
4 or 3^F	4		4	4 or 3^{FG}	4	4						
4 or 3^F	4		4	4 or 3^{FG}	4	4						*Could*
4 or 3^F	4		4	4 or 3^{FG}	4	4						
involves full manic and major depressive pictures intermixed or alternating												
3	3	3	3		3	3	3	3	3	3^H	3	3
												Could
3	3	3	3		3		3	3	3		3	
												5
												3^H
												—

MAJOR DISORDERS OF DSM III—*cont.*

			Restriction of involvement in pleasurable activities	Less talkative	Social withdrawal (or social isolation)	Increased activity at work, socially sexually	Physical restlessness	Hypersexuality without recognition of possibility of painful consequences	Increased productivity often with unusual and self-imposed hours	Sharpened thinking unusually creative thinking	More talkative or pressured speech
Organic brain syndromes and organic mental disorders		Psychosis									
		Delirium									
		Dementia									
		Amnestic syndrome									
		Organic delusional syndrome									
		Organic hallucinosis									
		Organic affective syndrome { depressed									
		manic				2^H	2^H				2
		Organic personality syndrome									
		Primary degenerative dementia									
		Multi-infarct dementia									
Affective disorders and affective syndromes	Major affective disorders and syndromes	Manic episode { euphoric mood				3^H					3
		irritable mood				4^H	4^H				4
		Major depressive episode { older than 6									
		< 6									
		Major depression { single episode									
		recurrent									
		Bipolar disorder { manic				3 or 4^{HK}	3 or 4^{HK}				3 or 4^K
		depressed									
		mixed									
	Other specific affective disorders	Dysthymic disorder		3^H							
		Cyclothymic disorder { hypomanic						3	3	3	3
		depressed	3	3	3						
	Atypical affective disorders	Atypical bipolar disorder									
		Atypical depression									
Paranoid disorders		Paranoid disorder									
		Acute paranoid disorder									
		Paranoia									
		Shared paranoid disorder									
Psychoses not elsewhere classified		Brief reactive psychosis									
		Atypical psychosis									
		Schizophreniform disorder									
Schizophrenic disorders	Schizophrenia	active phase									
		prodromal phase			2						
		residual phase			2						
		paranoid type									
		catatonic type									
		disorganized type									
		undifferentiated type									
		residual type[9]			2						
Axis II personality disorders		Schizotypal			4						
		Schizoid			● Close friendships with no more than 2 people including family members						
		Paranoid			*Could*						
		Avoidant			●ᵁ						
		Borderline									
		Narcissistic									
		Histrionic									
		Compulsive									
		Dependent									
		Passive-aggressive									
		Antisocial									

Flight of ideas feeling that thoughts are racing	Grandiosity, inflated self-esteem	Distractibility	Unable to respond with pleasure to praise and reward	Decreased need for sleep	Excessive involvement in activities with high risk of self-harm	Increased energy	Extreme gregariousness	Overoptimism or exaggeration of past achievements	Inappropriate laughing, joking [J]	Psychotic features can occur	Previous manic episode if not now manic	Previous major depressive episode	Mood disturbance occurs after psychosis appears —or— mood disturbance brief compared with psychosis
										●			
										●			
										●			
										●			
										Could			
2	2	2			2					Could			
										Could			
										●			
3	3	3			3					●			No
4	4	4			4					●			No
										●			No
										●			No
										●	No		No
										●	No		No
3 or 4 [K]	3 or 4 [K]	3 or 4 [K]			3 or 4 [K]					●	● [I]		No
										●	●	I	No
										●			No
			Every few days							No			
	3			3	3	3	3	3	3	No			
										No			
										Could			
										Could			
										●			●
										●			●
										●			●
										●			●
										●			●
										●			●
										●			●
										Could			
										Could			
										●			●
										●			●
										●			●
										●			●
										Could			
										No			
										No			
										No			
										No			
										No			
	● [H]							Could		No			
										No			
										No			
										No			
										No			

	Preoccupation with mood incongruent delusion or hallucination, or bizarre behavior is present	Mood disturbance can be interrupted by periods of normal mood lasting up to few months	Mood alternates between major depression and hypomania without mania (bipolar II)	Blunted, flat or inappropriate affect	Silly affect	Emotions and behavior appropriate to delusional system
Organic brain syndromes and organic mental disorders						
Psychosis				1		
Delirium						
Dementia						
Amnestic syndrome						
Organic delusional syndrome						
Organic hallucinosis						
Organic affective syndrome — depressed						
Organic affective syndrome — manic						
Organic personality syndrome						
Primary degenerative dementia						
Multi-infarct dementia						
Affective disorders and affective syndromes						
Manic episode — euphoric mood	●					
Manic episode — irritable mood	●					
Major depressive episode — older than 6	●					
Major depressive episode — <6	●					
Major depression — single episode	●					
Major depression — recurrent	●					
Bipolar disorder — manic	●					
Bipolar disorder — depressed	●					
Bipolar disorder — mixed	●					
Dysthymic disorder	✪	●				
Cyclothymic disorder — hypomanic	✪	●				
Cyclothymic disorder — depressed	✪	●				
Atypical bipolar disorder			●			
Atypical depression						
Paranoid disorders						
Paranoid disorder				No	No	●
Acute paranoid disorder				No	No	●
Paranoia				No	No	●
Shared paranoid disorder				No	No	●
Psychoses not elsewhere classified						
Brief reactive psychosis				*Could*		
Atypical psychosis				*Could*		
Schizophreniform disorder				*		
Schizophrenic disorders						
Schizophrenia — active phase	*Could*			*		
Schizophrenia — prodromal phase				2		
Schizophrenia — residual phase				2		
Schizophrenia — paranoid type	*Could*					
Schizophrenia — catatonic type	*Could*					
Schizophrenia — disorganized type	*Could*			●	●	
Schizophrenia — undifferentiated type	*Could*					
Schizophrenia — residual type[9]				2		
Axis II personality disorders						
Schizotypal				No		
Schizoid				No		
Paranoid				No		
Avoidant						
Borderline						
Narcissistic						
Histrionic						
Compulsive						
Dependent						
Passive-aggresive						
Antisocial						

If affective syndrome is absent, neither dominates

Voice gives running commentary on patients thoughts or behavior	Two or more voices talk to each other	Several times of more than 1 or 2 words not related to depression or elation	Hallucinations with persecutory or jealous content	Bizarre delusions	Thought insertion	Thought withdrawal	Thought broadcasting	Delusions of being controlled	Persecutory or jealous delusions	Grandiose delusion	Somatic, grandiose, nihilistic, religious or other delusion without persecutory or jealous content	Formal thought disorder loose associations, markedly illogical thinking, poverty of speech	Grossly disorganized behavior
												No	
												No	
												No	
No^L	No^L	No^L	No^L	No	No	No	No	No	●				
No^L	No^L	No^L	No^L	No	No	No	No	No	●				
No^L	No^L	No^L	No^L	No	No	No	No	No	●				
No^L	No^L	No^L	No^L	No	No	No	No	No	●			1	1
1	1	1		1	1	1	1	1	1 With any hallucination			1	1 with *any
1	1	1		1	1	1	1	1	1 With any hallucination			1	1 with *any
1	1	1	①	1	1	1	1	1	①	①		1	
												1 with *any	
										No			

MAJOR DISORDERS OF DSM III—*cont.*

	Catatonic stupor	Catatonic negativism	Catatonic rigidity	Catatonic excitement	Catatonic posturing	Deterioration from previous level of functioning	Impairment of occupational functioning	Impairment of self-care	Markedly peculiar behavior	Odd speech digressive, vague, over elaborate, metaphorical, circumstantial
Organic brain syndromes and organic mental disorders										
Psychosis										
Delirium										
Dementia										
Amnestic syndrome										
Organic delusional syndrome										
Organic hallucinosis										
Organic affective syndrome — depressed										
Organic affective syndrome — manic										
Organic personality syndrome										
Primary degenerative dementia										
Multi-infarct dementia										
Affective disorders and affective syndromes										
Manic episode — euphoric mood										
Manic episode — irritable mood										
Major depressive episode — older than 6										
Major depressive episode — <6										
Major depression — single episode										
Major depression — recurrent										
Bipolar disorder — manic										
Bipolar disorder — depressed										
Bipolar disorder — mixed										
Dysthymic disorder										
Cyclothymic disorder — hypomanic										
Cyclothymic disorder — depressed										
Atypical bipolar disorder										
Atypical depression										
Paranoid disorders										
Paranoid disorder										
Acute paranoid disorder										
Paranoia										
Shared paranoid disorder										
Psychoses not elsewhere classified										
Brief reactive psychosis	1	1	1	1	1	Could				
Atypical psychosis						Could				
Schizophreniform disorder	*	*	*	*	*	●				
Schizophrenic disorders — Schizophrenia										
active phase	*	*	*	*	*	●				
prodromal phase						●	2	2		2
residual phase						●	2	2	2	2
paranoid type						●				
catatonic type	①	①	①	①	①	●				
disorganized type						●				
undifferentiated type						●				
residual type[9]						●	2	2	2	2
Axis II personality disorders										
Schizotypal										4
Schizoid										No
Paranoid										
Avoidant										
Borderline										
Narcissistic										
Histrionic										
Compulsive										
Dependent										
Passive-aggresive										
Antisocial										

Odd ideas, magical thinking, ESP, superstitiousness, overvalued ideas	Delusional system develops as result of close association with person or persons with disorder with persecutory delusion	Systematized delusions	Meets criteria for schizoprenia	Unusual perceptual experiences	Inadequate rapport in face-to-face interaction due to constricted or inappropriate affect	Hypersensitivity (to real or imagined criticism)	Ideas of reference	Expectation of trickery or harm	Hypervigilance—scanning environment for threat, taking unneeded precautions	Guardedness or secretiveness	Avoidance of accepting blame when warrented	Questioning loyalty of others	Loss of appreciation of total context
	No		No										
	No		No										
	No	●	No										
	●		No										
			Could except for duration^X										
			Could except for duration^X										
			● Except for duration										
2^Z			●	2^H			2^Z						
2^Z			●	2^H			2^Z						
			●										
			●										
		No	●										
			●										
2^Z			●	2^H			2^Z						
4			No		4^H	4	4						
No			No			No	No						
			No			●^{P}		3^N	3^N	3^N	3^N	3^N	3^{YN}

	Due to narrow search for confirmation of ideas	Overconcern with hidden motives and special meanings	Pathological jealousy	Onset related to stress	Tendency to be easily slighted and takes offense quickly	Exaggeration of difficulties	Readiness to counter-attack to perceived threat	Inability to relax	Restricted affectivity
Organic brain syndromes and organic mental disorders									
Psychosis									
Delirium									
Dementia									
Amnestic syndrome									
Organic delusional syndrome									
Organic hallucinosis									
Organic affective syndrome — depressed									
Organic affective syndrome — manic									
Organic personality syndrome									
Primary degenerative dementia									
Multi-infarct dementia									
Affective disorders and affective syndromes									
Manic episode — euphoric mood									
Manic episode — irritable mood									
Major depressive episode — older than 6									
Major depressive episode — < 6									
Major depression — single episode									
Major depression — recurrent									
Bipolar disorder — manic									
Bipolar disorder — depressed									
Bipolar disorder — mixed									
Dysthymic disorder									
Cyclothymic disorder — hypomanic									
Cyclothymic disorder — depressed									
Atypical bipolar disorder									
Atypical depression									
Paranoid disorders									
Paranoid disorder									
Acute paranoid disorder									
Paranoia									
Shared paranoid disorder									
Psychoses not elsewhere classified									
Brief reactive psychosis				●					
Atypical psychosis				No[X]					
Schizophreniform disorder									
Schizophrenic disorders									
Schizophrenia — active phase									
Schizophrenia — prodromal phase									
Schizophrenia — residual phase									
Schizophrenia — paranoid type									
Schizophrenia — catatonic type									
Schizophrenia — disorganized type									
Schizophrenia — undifferentiated type									
Schizophrenia — residual type[9]									
Axis II personality disorders									
Schizotypal									
Schizoid									
Paranoid	3[YN]	3[N]	3[N]		2[R]	2[R]	2[R]	2[R]	●[S]
Avoidant									
Borderline									
Narcissistic									
Histrionic									
Compulsive									
Dependent									
Passive-aggressive									
Antisocial									

Appears cold, unemotional	Pride taken in being objective, rational unemotional	Lack of true sense of humor	Absence of soft, tender and sentimental feelings	Indifference to praise or criticism	Indifference to feelings of others	Hypersensitivity ro rejection	Has peripheral social contacts (occupationally too)	Unwilling to enter relationship unless guaranteed uncritical acceptance	Desire for affection and acceptance	Impulsivity or unpredictability in at least 2 self-damaging areas	Unstable	Intense	Idealization	Devaluation	Manipulation (using others for own ends)	Marked shifts of attitude, between extremes of over-idealization & devaluation
4^H																
●^{V}				●^{U}	●^{U}	No	No	No— doesn't care	No							
2^T	2^T	2^T	2^T													
				No		●	●^{U}	●	●	5	5^H	5^H	5^H	5^H	5^H	5^H
															2	2
															2^H	

MAJOR DISORDERS OF DSM III — *cont.*

Disorder			Identity disturbance (uncertainty about variety of issues of identity)	Affective instability (brief sudden mood shifts)	Physically self damaging acts	Intolerance of being alone	Chronic feelings of emptiness or boredom	Grandiose sense of self-importance or uniqueness	Preoccupation with fantasies of power unlimited success brilliance, beauty, ideal love	Exhibitionism: needs constant attention & admiration
Organic brain syndromes and organic mental disorders		Psychosis								
		Delirium								
		Dementia								
		Amnestic syndrome								
		Organic delusional syndrome								
		Organic hallucinosis								
	Organic affective syndrome	depressed								
		manic								
		Organic personality syndrome								
		Primary degenerative dementia								
		Multi-infarct dementia								
Affective disorders and affective syndromes	Major affective disorders and syndromes	Manic episode { euphoric mood								
		irritable mood								
		Major depressive episode { older than 6								
		<6								
		Major depression { single episode								
		recurrent								
		Bipolar disorder { manic								
		depressed								
		mixed								
	Other specific affective disorders	Dysthymic disorder								
		Cyclothymic disorder { hypomanic								
		depressed								
	Atypical affective disorders	Atypical bipolar disorder								
		Atypical depression								
Paranoid disorders		Paranoid disorder								
		Acute paranoid disorder								
		Paranoia								
		Shared paranoid disorder								
Psychoses not elsewhere classified		Brief reactive psychosis								
		Atypical psychosis								
		Schizophreniform disorder								
Schizophrenic disorders	Schizophrenia	active phase								
		prodromal phase								
		residual phase								
		paranoid type								
		catatonic type								
		disorganized type								
		undifferentiated type								
		residual type[9]								
Axis II personality disorders		Schizotypal								
		Schizoid								
		Paranoid								
		Avoidant								
		Borderline	5	5	5	5	5			
		Narcissistic						●H	●	●
		Histrionic								
		Compulsive								
		Dependent								
		Passive-aggressive								
		Antisocial								

Cool indifference or marked rage, shame, inferiority, emptiness to criticism, defeat, or indifference of others	Entitlement expects special favors without reciprocal responsibility	Lack of empathy	Overly dramatic reactive intensly expressed behavior	Self dramatization exaggerated expression of emotions	Incessant drawing of attention to self	Craving for activity and excitement	Overreaction to minor events	Perceived by others as shallow, insincere (may seem warm, charming superficially)	Vain and demanding	Dependent, helpless seeks reassurance	Egocentric, self indulgent, inconsiderate	Prone to manipulative suicidal threats, attempts	Restricted ability to express warm, tender emotions, formal, serious, stiff
●	2	2	●^{M}	3^N	3^N	3^N	3^N	2	2	2	2^H	2	
		Could 4^H											4

MAJOR DISORDERS OF DSM III— *cont.*

	Perfectionistic with preoccupation with trivial details, misses big picture	Insists that others submit to own way of doing things	Excessive devotion to work, productivity, to exclusion of recreation and relationships	Indecisiveness by postponing, avoiding, can be fear of making mistake	Inability to function independently	Allows others to assume responsibility for major areas of life	Subordinates own needs to person depended on, to avoid relying on self	Resistance to demands for adequate performance
Organic brain syndromes and organic mental disorders								
Psychosis								
Delirium								
Dementia								
Amnestic syndrome								
Organic delusional syndrome								
Organic hallucinosis								
Organic affective syndrome — depressed								
Organic affective syndrome — manic								
Organic personality syndrome								
Primary degenerative dementia								
Multi-infarct dementia								
Affective disorders and affective syndromes								
Manic episode — euphoric mood								
Manic episode — irritable mood								
Major depressive episode — older than 6								
Major depressive episode — <6								
Major depression — single episode								
Major depression — recurrent								
Bipolar disorder — manic								
Bipolar disorder — depressed								
Bipolar disorder — mixed								
Dysthymic disorder								
Cyclothymic disorder — hypomanic								
Cyclothymic disorder — depressed								
Atypical bipolar disorder								
Atypical depression								
Paranoid disorders								
Paranoid disorder								
Acute paranoid disorder								
Paranoia								
Shared paranoid disorder								
Psychoses not elsewhere classified								
Brief reactive psychosis								
Atypical psychosis								
Schizophreniform disorder								
Schizophrenic disorders — Schizophrenia								
active phase								
prodromal phase								
residual phase								
paranoid type								
catatonic type								
disorganized type								
undifferentiated type								
residual type[9]								
Axis II personality disorders								
Schizotypal								
Schizoid								
Paranoid								
Avoidant								
Borderline								
Narcissistic								
Histrionic								
Compulsive	4	4H	4	4				
Dependent					●	●	●	
Passive-aggresive								
Antisocial								

Resistance expressed indirectly by							Before age 15											
Procrastination	Dawdling	Stubbornness	Intentional inefficiency	"Forgetfulness"	Resistance causes long-standing social and occupational ineffectiveness	Persists in behavior even when more effective behavior possible	Truancy 5 days/year for 2 years, not including last year of school	Expulsion or suspension from school for behavior	Delinquency in juvenile court for behavior	Runaway from home overnight at least twice	Lying persistently	Sexual intercourse repeatedly in a casual relationship	Repeated drunkenness or substance abuse	Thefts	Vandalism	School grades below expectations or IQ, may have resulted in repeating year	Chronic violation of rules at home and/or school (other than truancy)	Initiation of fights
2	2	2	2	2	●	●	3	3	3	3	3	3	3	3	3	3	3	3

MAJOR DISORDERS OF DSM III— *cont.*

	Antisocial work manifestation				Failure as responsible parent			
	Too frequent job changes 3 or more jobs in last 5 years with no good explanation	Unemployment ≥ 6 mo in 5 years when expected to work	Absenteeism ≥ 3 days of lateness or absense/month	Walking off several jobs with no other jobs in sight	Child's malnutrition	Child's illness from poor hygiene	Failure to get medical attention for seriously ill child	Child's dependence on neighbors or relatives out of the home for food or shelter
Organic brain syndromes and organic mental disorders								
Psychosis								
Delirium								
Dementia								
Amnestic syndrome								
Organic delusional syndrome								
Organic hallucinosis								
Organic affective syndrome { depressed								
manic								
Organic personality syndrome								
Primary degenerative dementia								
Multi-infarct dementia								
Affective disorders and affective syndromes								
Major affective disorders and syndromes — Manic episode { euphoric mood								
irritable mood								
Major depressive episode { older than 6								
< 6								
Major depression { single episode								
recurrent								
Bipolar disorder { manic								
depressed								
mixed								
Other specific affective disorders — Dysthymic disorder								
Cyclothymic disorder { hypomanic								
depressed								
Atypical affective disorders { Atypical bipolar disorder								
Atypical depression								
Paranoid disorders								
Paranoid disorder								
Acute paranoid disorder								
Paranoia								
Shared paranoid disorder								
Psychoses not elsewhere classified								
Brief reactive psychosis								
Atypical psychosis								
Schizophreniform disorder								
Schizophrenic disorders — Schizophrenia								
active phase								
prodromal phase								
residual phase								
paranoid type								
catatonic type								
disorganized type								
undifferentiated type								
residual type[9]								
Axis II personality disorders								
Schizotypal								
Schizoid								
Paranoid								
Avoidant								
Borderline								
Narcissistic								
Histrionic								
Compulsive								
Dependent								
Passive-aggresive								
Antisocial								

Antisocial work manifestation any one — 4

Failure as responsible parent

No care taker for child < 6 when parent away	Repeated squandering on self of money needed for household necessities	Failure to accept social norms of lawful behavior				Failure to maintain enduring attachment to sexual partner			Irritability or aggressiveness				Failure to honor financial obligations		
		Repeated thefts	Illegal occupation	Multiple arrests	Felony conviction	2 or more divorces and/or separations whether or not legally married	Desertion of spouse	Promiscuity > 10 sexual partners/year	Physical fights	Assault	Spouse beating	Child beating	Defaulting on debts	Failure to provide child support	Failure to support other dependents on regular basis

any one　4　｜　Failure to accept social norms of lawful behavior　any one　4　｜　Failure of attachment to sex partner　any one　4　｜　Aggressivness　any one　4　｜　Failure to honor financial obligations　any one　4

Failure to accept social norms of lawful behavior　any one

MAJOR DISORDERS OF DSM III—*cont.*

Category	Disorder		Impulsivity or failure to plan ahead		Dishonesty			Recklessness		Continuous pattern of antisocial behavior where rights of others are violated with no period of at least 5 years without such behavior from age 15 to present
			Traveling from place to place with no goal or no definite end to travel	Lack of fixed address for month or more	Repeated lying	Use of aliases	Conning others for personal profit	Driving while intoxicated	Recurrent speeding	
Organic brain syndromes and organic mental disorders	Psychosis									
	Delirium									
	Dementia									
	Amnestic syndrome									
	Organic delusional syndrome									
	Organic hallucinosis									
	Organic affective syndrome	depressed								
		manic								
	Organic personality syndrome									
	Primary degenerative dementia									
	Multi-infarct dementia									
Affective disorders and affective syndromes	Major affective disorders and syndromes — Manic episode	euphoric mood								
		irritable mood								
	Major depressive episode	older than 6								
		<6								
	Major depression	single episode								
		recurrent								
	Bipolar disorder	manic								
		depressed								
		mixed								
	Other specific affective disorders — Dysthymic disorder									
	Cyclothymic disorder	hypomanic								
		depressed								
	Atypical affective disorders — Atypical bipolar disorder									
	Atypical depression									
Paranoid disorders	Paranoid disorder									
	Acute paranoid disorder									
	Paranoia									
	Shared paranoid disorder									
Psychoses not elsewhere classified	Brief reactive psychosis									
	Atypical psychosis									
	Schizophreniform disorder									
Schizophrenic disorders	Schizophrenia — active phase									
	prodromal phase									
	residual phase									
	paranoid type									
	catatonic type									
	disorganized type									
	undifferentiated type									
	residual type[9]									
Axis II personality disorders	Schizotypal									
	Schizoid									
	Paranoid									
	Avoidant									
	Borderline									
	Narcissistic									
	Histrionic									
	Compulsive									
	Dependent									
	Passive-aggressive									
	Antisocial									●

Impulsivity any one 4   Dishonesty any one 4   Recklessness any one 4

SO-CALLED "MINOR" DISORDERS DSM-III

		Duration of cardinal manifestations at least:	not more than:	Age of onset limits by definition	Other disorders excluded by definition	Occurs in relation to psychosocial stressor	If related to stressor, how long until onset of disorder
Adjustment disorder	with depressed mood					●	Within 3 mos
	with anxious mood					●	Within 3 mos
	with mixed emotional features				Every other disorder and uncomplicated bereavement	●	Within 3 mos
	with disturbance of conduct					●	Within 3 mos
	with mixed disturbance of emotions and conduct					●	Within 3 mos
	with work (or academic) inhibition					●	Within 3 mos
	with withdrawal					●	Within 3 mos
	with atypical features					●	Within 3 mos
post-traumatic stress disorder	acute		< 6 mo			●	Within 6 mos
	delayed					●	At least 6 mos after
	chronic	6 mos				●	
	delayed and chronic	6 mos				●	At least 6 mos after
Anxiety disorders	panic attack						
	agoraphobia with panic attacks				Major depressive episode, schizophrenia paranoid personality disorder, obsessive compulsive disorder		
	agoraphobia without panic attacks						
	social phobia				Agoraphobia		
	simple phobia				Agoraphobia social phobia		
	panic disorder	3 weeks	At least 3 attacks in 3 weeks not precipitated by circumscribed phobic				
	generalized anxiety disorder	1 month			Panic disorder		
	obsessive compulsive disorder				Any other mental disorder		
	atypical anxiety disorder	This is the residual catagory					
Somatiform disorders	conversion disorder				Schizophrenia somatization disorder	Could	
	psychogenic pain disorder				Any mental (other) disorder	Could	
	somatization disorder			< 30 yr	Can coexist with most other disorders		
	hypochondriasis				Any other mental disorder		
Axis I & axis III	psychological factors affecting physical condition				Somatization disorder		
Dissociative disorders	psychogenic amnesia				Organic mental disorder	Could	
	psychogenic fugue				Organic mental disorder	Could	
	multiple personality						
	depersonalization disorder				any other disorder		
Factitious disorders	factitious disorder with psychological symptoms				Malingering		
	chronic factitious disorder with physical symptoms				Malingering		
	atypical factitious disorder with physical symptoms				Malingering		
V65.20	malingering - not a mental disorder				Every other disorder	Could	
Disorders of impulse control not elsewhere classified	pathological gambling				Antisocial pers. dis.		
	kleptomania				Conduct disorder antisocial pers. dis.		
	pyromania				Organic mental dis. schizophrenia conduct dis., antisocial pers. dis.		
	intermittent explosive disorder					Could	
	isolated explosive disorder					Could	

Ω – Panic attack can occur when in contact with feared object, situation, or when obsessio

○ – But when organic factor does exist it's not enough to account for patient's complaint o

Violation of

Maladaptive reaction to stressor	Impairment in social or occupational functioning	Symptoms that are in excess of normal and expectable reaction	Disturbance is not merely one instance of an overreaction to stress	Disturbance not merely exacerbation of another mental disorder	It is assumed that disturbance will eventually remit when stressor ceases, or if stressor persists, when a new level of adaptation is achieved	Features of depressed mood	Features of anxious mood	Rights of others	Age-appropriate norms & rules	Inhibition in work (or academic) functioning	Social withdrawal
●	1	1	●	●	●	●	No	No	No	No	Could
●	1	1	●	●	●	No	●	No	No	No	No
●	1	1	●	●	●	●	●	No	No	No	Could
●	1	1	●	●	●	No	No	①	①	No	No
●	1	1	●	●	●	①	①	[1]	[1]	No	No
●	1	1	●	●	●	No	No	No	No	●	No
●	1	1	●	●	●	No	No	No	No	No	●
●	1	1	●	●	●	Any mixture of these cardinal manifestations					
							● Discrete periods				
	Could	Could									
	Could	Could									
		Could									
		Could									
stimulus							● Discrete periods / ●				
	[1]										
Could be	Could	Could be	Could	Could							
Could be	Could	Could be	Could	Could							
	●										
Could											
Could											
Could		Could									
								Could	Could	Could	Could
										Could	
										Could	Could
Could		●								Could	Could
Could		●								Could	Could

occurs or when compulsive act resisted or prevented

disability

Y — 14 symptoms in men
12 symptoms in women
this is largely a female disorder

		Psychosis occurs	Meets criteria for schizophrenia	Organic factor shown by history, physical lab exam, or presumed from disorders ruled out	Meets criteria for mood disorder	Panic attacks occur	Stressor would evoke significant distress in almost anyone	Reexperiencing of the trauma	Recurrent, intrusive recollections of the event	Recurrent dreams of the event
Adjustment disorder	with depressed mood	No	No	No	Could					
	with anxious mood	No	No	No	No					
	with mixed emotional features	No	No	No	Could					
	with disturbance of conduct	No	No	No	No					
	with mixed disturbance of emotions and conduct	No	No	No	No					
	with work (or academic) inhibition	No	No	No	No					
	with withdrawal	No	No	No	No					
	with atypical features	No	No	No	No					
Anxiety disorders — post-traumatic stress disorder	acute	No	No	No	No	● [Q]	●	● [M]	1 [N]	1 [N]
	delayed	No	No	No	No	● [Q]	●	● [M]	1 [N]	1 [N]
	chronic	No	No	No	No	● [Q]	●	● [M]	1 [N]	1 [N]
	delayed and chronic	No	No	No	No	● [Q]	●	● [M]	1 [N]	1 [N]
	panic attack	No	No	No	No	●				
agoraphobia	with panic attacks	No	No	No	No	●				
	without panic attacks	No	No	No	No					
	social phobia	No	No	No	No	● [Q]				
	simple phobia	No	No	No	No	● [Q]				
	panic disorder	No	No	No	No	●				
	generalized anxiety disorder	No	No	No	No	No				
	obsessive compulsive disorder	No	No	No	No	● [Q]				
	atypical anxiety disorder									
Somatiform disorders	conversion disorder	No	No	No! [O]	No	No	Could be			
	psychogenic pain disorder	No	No	No! [O]	No	No	Could be			
	somatization disorder	Could	Could	Real disease could exist	Could	Could				
	hypochondriasis	No	No	No [O]	No					
Axis I & axis III	psychological factors affecting physical condition	No	No	●	No					
Dissociative disorders	psychogenic amnesia	No	No	No	No					
	psychogenic fugue	No	No	No	No					
	multiple personality	No	No	No	No					
	depersonalization disorder	No	No	No	No	Could				
Factitious disorders	factitious disorder with psychological symptoms	No	No	No	No					
	chronic factitious disorder with physical symptoms	No	No	No	No					
	atypical factitious disorder with physical symptoms		No	No	No					
V65.20	malingering - not a mental disorder	No	No	No	No					
Disorders of impulse control not elsewhere classified	pathological gambling	No	No		No	No				
	kleptomania	No	No		No	No				
	pyromania	No	No		No	No				
	intermittent explosive disorder	No	No	Could put on axis III	No	No				
	isolated explosive disorder	No	No	Could put on axis III	No	No				

Q — Panic attack can occur when in contact with feared object, situation, or when obse

O — But when organic factor does exist it's not enough to account for patient's compla

Sudden acting or feeling as if traumatic event were reoccuring because of an association	Numbing of responsiveness or reduced involvement with external world, starting some time after trauma	Markedly diminished interest in at least one activity (significant)	Feeling detached or estranged from others	Constricted affect (narrowed range)	Hyperalertness or exaggerated startle response	Sleep disturbance	Guilt about surviving when others did not, or about one's survival behavior	Memory impairment or trouble concentrating	Avoiding activities that arouse memory of trauma	Events that symbolize or resemble trauma intensify symptoms	Dyspivea or shortness of breath	Palpitations	Chest pain or discomfort
1^N	●^{P}	1^R	1^R	1^R	2	2	2	2	2	2			
1^N	●^{P}	1^R	1^R	1^R	2	2	2	2	2	2			
1^N	●^{P}	1^R	1^R	1^R	2	2	2	2	2	2			
1^N	●^{P}	1^R	1^R	1^R	2	2	2	2	2	2			
											4	4	4
											Could^a	Could^a	No
											No	No	Could^a
											12^Y	12^Y	12^Y

occurs or when compulsive act resisted or prevented

disability

	Choking or smothering sensations	Dizziness vertigo or unsteady feelings	Feelings of unreality or depersonalization	Paresthesias	Hot and cold flashes	Sweating	Trembling or shaking	Fear of dying, going crazy or doing something uncontrolled during an attack	Faintness
Adjustment disorder — with depressed mood									
with anxious mood									
with mixed emotional features									
with disturbance of conduct									
with mixed disturbance of emotions and conduct									
with work (or academic) inhibition									
with withdrawal									
with atypical features									
post-traumatic stress disorder — acute									
delayed									
chronic									
delayed and chronic									
panic attack	4	4	4	4	4	4	4	4	4
Anxiety disorders — agoraphobia with panic attacks									
agoraphobia without panic attacks									
social phobia									
simple phobia									
panic disorder									
generalized anxiety disorder									
obsessive compulsive disorder									
atypical anxiety disorder									
Somatiform disorders — conversion disorder		Could[a]							
psychogenic pain disorder		No							
somatization disorder		12[Y]							
hypochondriasis									
Axis I & axis III — psychological factors affecting physical condition									
Dissociative disorders — psychogenic amnesia									
psychogenic fugue									
multiple personality									
depersonalization disorder									
Factitious disorders — factitious disorder with psychological symptoms									
chronic factitious disorder with physical symptoms									
atypical factitious disorder with physical symptoms									
V65.20 — malingering - not a mental disorder									
Disorders of impulse control not elsewhere classified — pathological gambling									
kleptomania									
pyromania									
intermittent explosive disorder									
isolated explosive disorder									

Q – Panic attack can occur when in contact with feared object, situation, or when obses

O – But when organic factor does exist it's not enough to account for patient's complai

Fears and avoids being in, or being alone in public places from which they could not escape or obtain help in the event they became incapacitated	Fears and avoids situation where they may possibly be scrutinized and fear they may act to humiliate or embarrass themselves	Fears and avoids object or situation other than agoraphobia or social phobia (fears dogs)	Significant distress because of fear recognizes fear is unreasonable	Increasing constriction of activities until fears or avoidance dominate life	Shakiness, jitteryness, jumpiness, trembling, tension, muscle aches, fatiguability, can't relax, eyelid twitch, furrowed brow, strained face, fidgeting, restleness, easy startle (any of these)	Sweating, pounding or racing heart, cold clammy hands, dry mouth, dizziness, light-headedness, upset stomach, parasthesias, hot or cold spells, frequent urination, diarrhea, flushing pallor, discomfort in pit of stomach, high resting pulse and respiration rate (any of these)	Anxiety, worry, fear, rumination, anticipation of misfortune to self or others (any of these)
●	No	No	Could	●			
●	No	No	Could	●			
No	●	No	●	No			
No	No	●	●	No			
					3	3	3

The physical condition goes on axis III

occurs or when compulsive act resisted or prevented

disability

SO-CALLED "MINOR" DISORDERS OF DSM-III—*cont.*

Psychological factors judged to be etiologically involved in the system

	Hyperattentiveness resulting in distractability, difficulty in concentrating, insomnia, feeling on "edge", irritability, impatience (any of these)	Obsessions	Compulsions	Significant distress because of symptom	Loss of, or alteration in physical functioning suggesting physical disorder (other than pain or sexual functioning)	Severe, prolonged pain (other than headache) is predominant disturbance	Psychological factor, conflict or need related in time to onset or exacerbation of symptom	Symptom allows person to avoid some activity that is noxious to him or her
Adjustment disorder with depressed mood								
with anxious mood								
with mixed emotional features								
with disturbance of conduct								
with mixed disturbance of emotions and conduct								
with work (or academic) inhibition								
with withdrawal								
with atypical features								
Anxiety disorders — post-traumatic stress disorder: acute				●				
delayed				●				
chronic				●				
delayed and chronic				●				
agoraphobia: panic attack								
with panic attacks				●				
without panic attacks				●				
social phobia								
simple phobia								
panic disorder				●				
generalized anxiety disorder	3			●				
obsessive compulsive disorder		①	①	[1]				
atypical anxiety disorder				●				
Somatiform disorders — conversion disorder				●	●		1	1
psychogenic pain disorder				●		●	1	1
somatization disorder				●				
hypochondriasis				●				
Axis I & axis III — psychological factors affecting physical condition				●	Could	Could	●	
Dissociative disorders — psychogenic amnesia								
psychogenic fugue								
multiple personality				●				
depersonalization disorder				●				
Factitious disorders — factitious disorder with psychological symptoms								
chronic factitious disorder with physical symptoms								
atypical factitious disorder with physical symptoms								
V65.20 malingering - not a mental disorder								
Disorders of impulse control not elsewhere classified — pathological gambling								
kleptomania								
pyromania								
intermittent explosive disorder								
isolated explosive disorder								

Q — Panic attack can occur when in contact with feared object, situation, or when obses

O — But when organic factor does exist it's not enough to account for patient's complai

Symptom enables person to get support or sympathy from the environment that they might otherwise not get	Symptom is not under voluntary control	Symptom cannot be explained by known physical disorder or pathophysiologic mechanism or physical injury	Symptom is inconsistent with anatomic distribution of nervous system or other structures	Symptom, even when there is some related organic pathology (physical disorder) is in excess of what the known disorder could cause	Symptoms are not side effects of medication drugs or alcohol	Physical symptoms, each, or complaints of, caused alteration of life pattern, caused patient to take medicine (other than aspirin), or caused them to see a physician	Symptoms can become a pattern that can dominate patient's life	Sickly: Believes he or she has been sickly a good part of their life	Difficulty swallowing	Loss of voice	Deafness
	●				●						
	●				●						
	●				●						
	●				●						
	●				●						
	●				●						
	●				●						
	●				●		●				
	●				●		●				
	●				●		●				
	●				●		●				
	●				●						
	●				●		●				
	●				●		●				
	●				●						
	●				●		●				
	●				●		●				
1	●	①	①	①	●		●	No	Could[a]	Could[a]	Could[a]
1	●	①	①	①	●		●	No	No	No	No
	●	①	①	①	●	●	●	12^Y	12^Y	12^Y	12^Y
	●	①	①	①	●		●				
	●	No	No	No	●	Could	●				
	●										
	●						●				
	●						●				
No		①	①	①			●	Could	Could	Could	Could
No		①	①	①			●	Could	Could	Could	Could
No		①	①	①			●	Could	Could	Could	Could
No		①	①	①				Could	Could	Could	Could
	●										
	●										
	●										
	●										
	●										

occurs or when compulsive act resisted or prevented

disability

SO-CALLED "MINOR" DISORDERS OF DSM-III—*cont.*

Conversion or pseudoneurological symptoms

	Double vision	Blurred vision	Blindness	Fainting or loss of consciousness	Memory loss	Seizures or convulsions	Trouble walking	Paralysis or muscle weakness	Urinary retention or difficulty urinating	Abdominal pain	Nausea (other than pregnancy)
Adjustment disorder with depressed mood											
with anxious mood											
with mixed emotional features											
with disturbance of conduct											
with mixed disturbance of emotions and conduct											
with work (or academic) inhibition											
with withdrawal											
with atypical features											
post-traumatic stress disorder acute											
delayed											
chronic											
delayed and chronic											
Anxiety disorders panic attack											
agoraphobia with panic attacks											
without panic attacks											
social phobia											
simple phobia											
panic disorder											
generalized anxiety disorder											
obsessive compulsive disorder											
atypical anxiety disorder											
Somatiform disorders conversion disorder	Could[a]	Could[a]	Could[a]	Could[a]	Could[a]	Could[a]	Could[a]	Could[a]	Could[a]	No	Could[a]
psychogenic pain disorder	No	No	No	No	No	No	No	No	No	Could[a]	No
somatization disorder	12^Y	12^Y	12^Y	12^Y	12^Y	12^Y	12^Y	12^Y	12^Y	12^Y	12^Y
hypochondriasis											
Axis I & axis III psychological factors affecting physical condition											
Dissociative disorders psychogenic amnesia					●						
psychogenic fugue					Usually						
multiple personality					Could[b]						
depersonalization disorder											
Factitious disorders factitious disorder with psychological symptoms	Could	Could	Could	Could	Could	Could	Could	Could	Could	Could	Could
chronic factitious disorder with physical symptoms	Could	Could	Could	Could	Could	Could	Could	Could	Could	Could	Could
atypical factitious disorder with physical symptoms	Could	Could	Could	Could	Could	Could	Could	Could	Could	Could	Could
V65.20 malingering - not a mental disorder	Could	Could	Could	Could	Could	Could	Could	Could	Could	Could	Could
Disorders of impulse control not elsewhere classified pathological gambling											
kleptomania											
pyromania											
intermittent explosive disorder											
isolated explosive disorder											

b — one personality may not recall what another personality can remember

Gastrointestinal symptoms				Female reproductive symptoms judged by the patient as more severe or more frequent than occurs in other women				Pain					
Vomiting spells (other than pregnancy)	Bloating (gassy)	Intolerance of a variety of foods (gets sick on them)	Diarrhea	Painful menstruation	Menstrual irregularity	Excessive bleeding	Severe vomiting during pregnancy or causing hospitalization during pregnancy	Back pain	Joint pain	Pain in extremities	Pain in genital area (other than during intercourse)	Pain on urination	Other pain (other than headaches)
Could[a]	Could[a]	Could[a]	Could[a]	No	Could[a]	Could[a]	Could[a]	No	No	No	No	No	No
No	No	No	No	Could[a]	No	No	No	Could[a]	Could[a]	Could[a]	Could[a]	Could[a]	Could[a]
12^Y	12^Y	12^Y	12^Y	12^Y	12^Y	12^Y	12^Y	12^Y	12^Y	12^Y	12^Y	12^Y	12^Y
Could	Could	Could	Could	Could	Could	Could	Could	Could	Could	Could	Could	Could	Could
Could	Could	Could	Could	Could	Could	Could	Could	Could	Could	Could	Could	Could	Could
Could	Could	Could	Could	Could	Could	Could	Could	Could	Could	Could	Could	Could	Could
Could	Could	Could	Could	Could	Could	Could	Could	Could	Could	Could	Could	Could	Could

SO-CALLED "MINOR" DISORDERS OF DSM-III—*cont.*

Psychosexual symptoms for major part of life after opportunities for sexual activity

		Psychosexual symptoms for major part of life after opportunities for sexual activity						
		Sexual indifference	Lack of pleasure during intercourse	Pain during intercourse	Preoccupation with physical signs or physical sensations as abnormal leading to preoccupation with fear or belief of having serious disease	Unrealistic fear persists despite medical reassurance	Physical condition has demonstrable organic pathology or known pathophysiologic mechanism	Sudden inability to recall important information that is too extensive to be explained by ordinary forgetfulness
Adjustment disorder	with depressed mood							
	with anxious mood							
	with mixed emotional features							
	with disturbance of conduct							
	with mixed disturbance of emotions and conduct							
	with work (or academic) inhibition							
	with withdrawal							
	with atypical features							
Anxiety disorders	post-traumatic stress disorder: acute							
	delayed							
	chronic							
	delayed and chronic							
	panic attack							
	agoraphobia: with panic attacks							
	without panic attacks							
	social phobia							
	simple phobia							
	panic disorder							
	generalized anxiety disorder							
	obsessive compulsive disorder							
	atypical anxiety disorder							
Somatiform disorders	conversion disorder						No^O	
	psychogenic pain disorder						No^O	
	somatization disorder	12^Y	12^Y	12^Y			No^O	
	hypochondriasis				●	●	No	
Axis I & axis III	psychological factors affecting physical condition						●	
Dissociative disorders	psychogenic amnesia							●
	psychogenic fugue							
	multiple personality							
	depersonalization disorder							
Factitious disorders	factitious disorder with psychological symptoms							
	chronic factitious disorder with physical symptoms							
	atypical factitious disorder with physical symptoms							
V65.20	malingering - not a mental disorder							
Disorders of impulse control not elsewhere classified	pathological gambling							
	kleptomania							
	pyromania							
	intermittent explosive disorder							
	isolated explosive disorder							

Sudden unexpected travel away from one's home or customary place of work with inability to recall one's past	Assumption of a new identity (partial or complete)	Two or more distinct personalities each of which is dominant at a particular time	The personality that is dominant at a particular time determines behavior	Each personality is complex, integrated, with own behavior and social relationships	At least one episode of depersonalization significantly impairing social or occupational functioning	Goal is to assume role of patient and not otherwise understanding given person's circumstances	Psychological symptoms	Symptoms under voluntary control	Physical symptoms requiring hospitalization	Physical symptoms not requiring hospitalization	Symptoms produced in pursuit of a goal recognizable and understandable given the circumstances
						No		No	Could	Could	No
						No		No	Could	Could	No
						Could		No	Could	Could	No
						Could		No	Could	Could	No
						No		No	Could	Could	No
						No	●	No	Could	Could	No
●	●					No	●	No			No
		●	●	●		No	●	No			No
					●	No	●	No			No
						●	●	●	No	No	No
						●	No	●	●	No	No
						●	No	●	No	●	No
						No	①	●	①	①	●

Stealing without long term planning or assistance from others

Fire setting not from monetary gain or sociopolitical ideology

	Suspicion (not diagnosis) of malingering should occur when:				Failure to resist impulses to:			
	Medicolegal context of presentation (patient refered by lawyer)	Marked discrepency between distress or disability and the medical facts	Lack of cooperation with diagnostic evaluation or prescribed treatment	Presence of antisocial personality disorder	Gamble (chronically and progressively)	Steal objects not for immediate use or monetary value	Set fires	Increasing sense of tension before the act
Adjustment disorder with depressed mood								
with anxious mood								
with mixed emotional features								
with disturbance of conduct								
with mixed disturbance of emotions and conduct								
with work (or academic) inhibition								
with withdrawal								
with atypical features								
post-traumatic stress disorder acute								
delayed								
chronic								
delayed and chronic								
panic attack								
agoraphobia with panic attacks								
without panic attacks								
social phobia								
simple phobia								
panic disorder								
generalized anxiety disorder								
obsessive compulsive disorder								
atypical anxiety disorder								
Somatiform disorders conversion disorder	Could	●	Could					
psychogenic pain disorder	Could	●	Could					
somatization disorder	Could	Could	Could					
hypochondriasis	Could	●	Could					
Axis I & axis III psychological factors affecting physical condition	Could	No	Could					
Dissociative disorders psychogenic amnesia	Could	Could	Could					
psychogenic fugue		Could	Could					
multiple personality			Could					
depersonalization disorder			Could					
Factitious disorders factitious disorder with psychological symptoms		●	Could	Could				
chronic factitious disorder with physical symptoms		●	Could	Very rare				
atypical factitious disorder with physical symptoms		●	Could	Could				
V65.20 malingering - not a mental disorder	1	1	1	1				
Disorders of impulse control not elsewhere classified pathological gambling				No	●			
kleptomania				No		●		●
pyromania				No			●	●
intermittent explosive disorder				No				
isolated explosive disorder				No				

Disruption of family, personal, vocational pursuits due to gambling

Experience of pleasure or release at time of committing act	Arrest for forgery, fraud, embezzlement, income tax evasion, to get money to gamble	Default on debts or other financial responsibilities	Family or spouse relationship disrupted by gambling	Borrowing money from illegal sources (loan sharks)	Can't account for lost money or show evidence of claimed winnings	Loss of work due to absenteeism in order to gamble	Necessary for another person to provide money to help bad financial situation	Several discrete episodes of loss of control of aggressive impulses resulting in serious assault or destruction of property	Single discrete episode where failure to resist an impulse led to a single violent externally directed act that had a catastrophic impact on others
	3	3	3	3	3	3	3		
●									
●									
								●	No
								No	●

	The degree of aggresivity in the episode is grossly out of proportion to any precipitating psychosocial stressor	Signs of generalized impulsivity or aggressivness are absent before or between episodes of violence
Adjustment disorder — with depressed mood		
with anxious mood		
with mixed emotional features		
with disturbance of conduct		
with mixed disturbance of emotions and conduct		
with work (or academic) inhibition		
with withdrawal		
with atypical features		
Anxiety disorders — post-traumatic stress disorder — acute		
delayed		
chronic		
delayed and chronic		
agoraphobia — panic attack		
with panic attacks		
without panic attacks		
social phobia		
simple phobia		
panic disorder		
generalized anxiety disorder		
obsessive compulsive disorder		
atypical anxiety disorder		
Somatiform disorders — conversion disorder		
psychogenic pain disorder		
somatization disorder		
hypochondriasis		
Axis I & axis III — psychological factors affecting physical condition		
Dissociative disorders — psychogenic amnesia		
psychogenic fugue		
multiple personality		
depersonalization disorder		
Factitious disorders — factitious disorder with psychological symptoms		
chronic factitious disorder with physical symptoms		
atypical factitious disorder with physical symptoms		
V65.20 — malingering - not a mental disorder		
Disorders of impulse control not elsewhere classified — pathological gambling		
kleptomania		
pyromania	●	●
intermittent explosive disorder	●	●
isolated explosive disorder		

DISORDERS USUALLY FIRST EVIDENT IN CHILDHOOD OR ADOLESCENCE

	Duration of cardinal manifestations at least:	not more than:	Age of onset limits by definition	Other disorders excluded by definition	Occurs in relation to psychosocial stressor
Axis II specific developmental disorders					
Developmental reading disorder					
Developmental arithmetic disorder				Mental retardation hearing impairment childhood onset pervasive devel. dis. injury or physical dis.	
Developmental language disorder — expressive type					
Developmental language disorder — receptive type					
Developmental articulation disorder					
Mixed specific developmental disorder	More than one specific developmental disorder is present but one is not				
Atypical specific developmental disorder	Specific developmental disorder present not covered by any of the other types				
Mental retardation			Before 18		
Mild mental retardation			Before 18		
Moderate mental retardation			Before 18		
Severe mental retardation			Before 18		
Profound mental retardation			Before 18		
Unspecified mental retardation			Before 18		
V62.89 borderline intellectual functioning not a mental disorder					
Attention deficit disorder with hyperactivity	6 mo		Before 7	Schizoprenia, affective disorder, severe or profound mental retardation	
Attention deficit disorder without hyperactivity	6 mo		Before 7		
Attention deficit disorder residual type	6 mo		Before 7		
Stuttering					
Elective mutism				Not due to any other disorder	
Conduct disorder, undersocialized, aggressive	6 mo			If older than 18, doesn't meet criteria for anti-social personality disorder	
Conduct disorder, undersocialized, nonaggressive	6 mo				
Conduct disorder, socialized, aggressive	6 mo				
Conduct disorder, socialized, nonaggressive	6 mo				
Infantile autism			Before 30 mos	No delusions hallucinations incoherence marked loose associations	
Infantile autism residual state					
Childhood onset pervasive developmental disorder			Before 12 yr. after 30 mos		
Childhood onset pervasive developmental disorder residual state					
Separation anxiety disorder	2 weeks			Pervasive devel. dis. schizophrenia, psychosis	
Avoidant disorder of childhood or adolescence	6 mos		2½–18 yr		
Schizoid disorder of childhood or adolescence	3 mos			Pervasive devel. dis. conduct dis. psychosis	
Overanxious disorder	6 mos			Any other mental disorder	
Oppositional disorder	6 mos		After, before 3–18	Any other mental disorder	
Identity disorder	3 mos			Any other mental disorder	
Anorexia nervosa				Any physical disorder	
Bulimia				Anorexia nervosa or any physical dis.	
Pica	1 mo			Any other disorder	
Rumination disorder of infancy	1 mo				
Reactive attachment disorder of infancy			Before 8 mos	Physical disorder, mental retardation infantile autism	●
Transient tic disorder	1 mo	1 year	Childhood or early adolescence		
Chronic motor tic disorder	1 year				
Tourette's disorder	1 year		2–15 yr		
Atypical tic disorder					
Atypical stereotyped movement disorder					
Functional enuresis			5 yr	Physical disorder	
Functional encopresis			4 yr	Physical disorder	
Sleepwalking disorder					
Sleep terror disorder					

Performance on standardized individually administered tests of reading skill are significantly below expected level, given the individual's schooling, chronological age, mental age (as determined by an individually administered IQ test)	In school, performance on tasks requiring reading skills is significantly below their mental capacity	Disorder can be diagnosed in older adolescent or in an adult	Performance on standardized individually administered tests of arithmetic achievement is significantly below expected level given schooling, chronological age, mental age (as determined by an individually administered IQ test)	In school performance on tasks requiring arithmetic skills is significantly below their mental capacity	Failure to develop vocal expression (encoding) of language	Failure to develop comprehension (decoding) of language
●	●	●	●	●		
		●			●	No
					●	●
						No

predominant, when skills are impared to varying degrees, each should be recorded

					No	No

Any predominant disturbance involving pattern of conduct where basic rights of others or major age appropriate societal norms or rules are violated and that cannot be classified as one of these four should be classified as atypical conduct disorder

					Could	Could

If over 18, doesn't meet criteria for agoraphobia
If over 18, doesn't meet criteria for avoidant personality disorder
If over 18, doesn't meet criteria for schizoid personality disorder
If over 18, doesn't meet criteria for generalized anxiety disorder
If over 18, doesn't meet criteria for passive-aggressive personality disorder
If over 18 doesn't meet criteria for borderline personality disorder

DISORDERS USUALLY FIRST EVIDENT IN CHILDHOOD OR ADOLESCENCE — *cont.*

	Presence of inner language (age appropriate concepts) i.e. understanding purpose and use of a particular household object	Failure to develop consistent articulations of later acquired speech sounds (R, SH, TH, F, Z, L, CH)	Significantly subaverage intellectual functioning, IQ of 70 or below on individually administered IQ test (in infants, clinical judgement is made, test unreliable)	IQ score on individually administered IQ test
Developmental reading disorder				
Developmental arithmetic disorder				
Developmental language disorder — expressive type	●			
Developmental language disorder — receptive type				
Developmental articulation disorder		●		
Mixed specific developmental disorder				
Atypical specific developmental disorder				
Mental retardation			●	<70
Mild mental retardation			●	50-70
Moderate mental retardation			●	39-49
Severe mental retardation			●	20-34
Profound mental retardation			●	<20
Unspecified mental retardation			●	Too impaired, too young to test
V62.89 borderline intellectual functioning not a mental disorder			● or Could	71-84
Attention deficit disorder with hyperactivity				
Attention deficit disorder without hyperactivity				
Attention deficit disorder residual type				
Stuttering				
Elective mutism	●			
Conduct disorder, undersocialized, aggressive				
Conduct disorder, undersocialized, nonaggressive				
Conduct disorder, socialized, aggressive				
Conduct disorder, socialized, nonaggressive				
Infantile autism	Maybe not	Could	Could	
Infantile autism residual state				
Childhood onset pervasive developmental disorder				
Childhood onset pervasive developmental disorder residual state				
Separation anxiety disorder				
Avoidant disorder of childhood or adolescence				
Schizoid disorder of childhood or adolescence				
Overanxious disorder				
Oppositional disorder				
Identity disorder				
Anorexia nervosa				
Bulimia				
Pica				
Rumination disorder of infancy				
Reactive attachment disorder of infancy				
Transient tic disorder				
Chronic motor tic disorder				
Tourette's disorder				
Atypical tic disorder				
Atypical stereotyped movement disorder				
Functional enuresis				
Functional encopresis				
Sleepwalking disorder				
Sleep terror disorder				

Axis II specific developmental disorders

Concurrent deficits in adaptive behavior taking chronological age into consideration	Inattention	Often fails to finish things he or she starts	Often doesn't seem to listen	Easily distracted	Has difficulty concentrating on school work or other tasks requiring sustained attention	Has difficulty sticking to a play activity	Impulsivity	Often acts before thinking	Shifts excessively from one activity to another	Has difficulty organizing work not due to cognitive or intellectual impairment	Needs a lot of supervision	Frequently calls out in class
●												
●												
●												
●												
●												
●												
●												
	●M	3^N	3^N	3^N	3^N	3^N	●P	3^R	3^R	3^R	3^R	3^R
	●M	3^N	3^N	3^N	3^N	3^N	●P	3^R	3^R	3^R	3^R	3^R
	●M	1^N	1^N	1^N	1^N	1^N	●P	1^R	1^R	1^R	1^R	1^R

Could

	Has difficulty awaiting turn in group situations or games	Hyperactivity	Runs about or climbs on things excessively	Has difficulty sitting still or fidgets excessively	Has difficulty staying seated	Moves about excessively during sleep	Is always "on the go" or acts as if "driven by a motor"
Developmental reading disorder							
Developmental arithmetic disorder							
Developmental language disorder — expressive type							
Developmental language disorder — receptive type							
Developmental articulation disorder							
Mixed specific developmental disorder							
Atypical specific developmental disorder							
Mental retardation							
Mild mental retardation							
Moderate mental retardation							
Severe mental retardation							
Profound mental retardation							
Unspecified mental retardation							
V62.89 borderline intellectual functioning not a mental disorder							
Attention deficit disorder with hyperactivity	3^R	●^{S}	2^T	2^T	2^T	2^T	2^T
Attention deficit disorder without hyperactivity	3^R	No	No	No	No	No	No
Attention deficit disorder residual type	1^R	No	No	No	No	No	No
Stuttering							
Elective mutism							
Conduct disorder, undersocialized, aggressive							
Conduct disorder, undersocialized, nonaggressive							
Conduct disorder, socialized, aggressive							
Conduct disorder, socialized, nonaggressive							
Infantile autism							
Infantile autism residual state							
Childhood onset pervasive developmental disorder							
Childhood onset pervasive developmental disorder residual state							
Separation anxiety disorder							
Avoidant disorder of childhood or adolescence							
Schizoid disorder of childhood or adolescence							
Overanxious disorder							
Oppositional disorder							
Identity disorder							
Anorexia nervosa							
Bulimia							
Pica							
Rumination disorder of infancy							
Reactive attachment disorder of infancy							
Transient tic disorder							
Chronic motor tic disorder							
Tourette's disorder							
Atypical tic disorder							
Atypical stereotyped movement disorder							
Functional enuresis							
Functional encopresis							
Sleepwalking disorder							
Sleep terror disorder							

Axis II specific developmental disorders

Symptoms result in some degree of social or occupational (or academic) functioning	Once met the criteria of attention deficit disorder with hyperactivity	Frequent repetitions or prolongation of sounds syllables or words or frequent or unusual hesitations and pauses that disrupt the rhythmic flow of speech	Continuous refusal to talk in almost all social situations including at school	Ability to comprehend spoken language	Ability to speak	Repetitive, persistent pattern of aggressive conduct where basic rights of others violated	Physical violence against persons or property	Thefts outside the home involving confrontation with the victim	Repetitive persistent pattern of nonaggressive conduct where basic rights of others or major age appropriate norms or rules violated
●									
●									
●					No				
●				●	No				
●				No	No				
●				●	●				
●									
●									
●									
●									
Could									
Could									
Could									
●	●								
		●							
				●	●				
			●						
Could									
Could						●	1	1	
Could									●
Could						●	1	1	
									●
●									
●									
●									
Could									
●									
●									
Could									
Could						No	No	No	No
●									

DISORDERS USUALLY FIRST EVIDENT IN CHILDHOOD OR ADOLESCENCE — cont.

	Chronic violations of important rules at home and at school where rules are reasonable and age appropriate for child	Repeated running away from home overnight	Persistent serious lying in and out of the home	Stealing not involving confrontation with a victim	Has at least one peer-group friendship that has lasted over 6 months
Developmental reading disorder					
Developmental arithmetic disorder					
Developmental language disorder — expressive type					
Developmental language disorder — receptive type					
Developmental articulation disorder					
Mixed specific developmental disorder					
Atypical specific developmental disorder					
Mental retardation					
Mild mental retardation					
Moderate mental retardation					
Severe mental retardation					
Profound mental retardation					
Unspecified mental retardation					
V62.89 borderline intellectual functioning not a mental disorder					
Attention deficit disorder with hyperactivity					
Attention deficit disorder without hyperactivity					
Attention deficit disorder residual type					
Stuttering					
Elective mutism					
Conduct disorder, undersocialized, aggressive				No	No more than 1
Conduct disorder, undersocialized, nonaggressive	1	1	1	1	No more than 1
Conduct disorder, socialized, aggressive				No	2
Conduct disorder, socialized, nonaggressive	1	1	1	1	2
Infantile autism					
Infantile autism residual state					
Childhood onset pervasive developmental disorder					
Childhood onset pervasive developmental disorder residual state					
Separation anxiety disorder					
Avoidant disorder of childhood or adolescence					
Schizoid disorder of childhood or adolescence					
Overanxious disorder					
Oppositional disorder	No	No	No	No	
Identity disorder					
Anorexia nervosa					
Bulimia					
Pica					
Rumination disorder of infancy					
Reactive attachment disorder of infancy					
Transient tic disorder					
Chronic motor tic disorder					
Tourette's disorder					
Atypical tic disorder					
Atypical stereotyped movement disorder					
Functional enuresis					
Functional encopresis					
Sleepwalking disorder					
Sleep terror disorder					

Axis II specific developmental disorders

Attachment criterion of conduct disorder

Extends self for others even when no immediate advantage likely	Feels guilt or remorse when the reaction is appropriate and not just when caught or in trouble	Avoids blaming or informing on companions	Shows concern for welfare of friends or companions	Pervasive lack of responsiveness to others (autism)	Gross deficits in language development	When speech present peculiar speech patterns such as immediate and delayed echolalia metaphorical language pronominal reversal	Bizarre responses such as resistance to change, peculiar interest in, or attachments to animate or inanimate objects	Gross and sustained impairments in social relationships, lack of response, empathy inappropriate clinging
				Could				
				Could				
				Could				
				Could				
No more than 1	No more than 1	No more than 1	No more than 1					
No more than 1	No more than 1	No more than 1	No more than 1					
2	2	2	2					
2	2	2	2					
				●	●	●	●	Could
								●

Disorder	Sudden excessive anxiety such as free-floating anxiety catastrophic reactions to everyday occurrences inability to be consoled when upset, unexplained panic attacks	Constricted or inappropriate affect	Resistance to change in the environment	Oddities of motor movement, posturing	Speech abnormalities such as questionlike melody, monotonous voice
Developmental reading disorder					
Developmental arithmetic disorder					
Developmental language disorder — expressive type					
Developmental language disorder — receptive type					
Developmental articulation disorder					
Mixed specific developmental disorder					
Atypical specific developmental disorder					
Mental retardation					
Mild mental retardation					
Moderate mental retardation					
Severe mental retardation					
Profound mental retardation					
Unspecified mental retardation					
V62.89 borderline intellectual functioning not a mental disorder					
Attention deficit disorder with hyperactivity					
Attention deficit disorder without hyperactivity					
Attention deficit disorder residual type					
Stuttering					
Elective mutism					
Conduct disorder, undersocialized, aggressive					
Conduct disorder, undersocialized, nonaggressive					
Conduct disorder, socialized, aggressive					
Conduct disorder, socialized, nonaggressive					
Infantile autism	Could	Could	Could	Could	Could
Infantile autism residual state					
Childhood onset pervasive developmental disorder	3	3	3	3	3
Childhood onset pervasive developmental disorder residual state					
Separation anxiety disorder					
Avoidant disorder of childhood or adolescence					
Schizoid disorder of childhood or adolescence					
Overanxious disorder					
Oppositional disorder					
Identity disorder					
Anorexia nervosa					
Bulimia					
Pica					
Rumination disorder of infancy					
Reactive attachment disorder of infancy					
Transient tic disorder					
Chronic motor tic disorder					
Tourette's disorder					
Atypical tic disorder					
Atypical stereotyped movement disorder					
Functional enuresis					
Functional encopresis					
Sleepwalking disorder					
Sleep terror disorder					

Axis II specific developmental disorders

Once had an illness that met criteria for infantile autism	Some signs of illness persist to present although doesn't meet full criteria	Once had an illness that met the criteria for childhood onset pervasive devel. dis.	Persistent and excessive shrinking from contact with strangers	Desire for affection and acceptance and generally warm relations with family and familiars	Symptoms interfere with social functioning in peer relationships	No close friend of similar age other than relative or similarly socially isolated child	No apparent interest in making friends	No pleasure from usual peer interactions	General avoidance of nonfamilial social contacts especially with peers	No interest in activity that involves other children (team sport clubs)
					Could					
					Could					
					Could					
					Could					
					Could					
			Could		Could	Could	Could	Could	Could	Could
●	●		Could		Could	Could	Could	Could	Could	Could
			Could		Could	Could	Could	Could	Could	Could
	●	●	Could		Could	Could	Could	Could	Could	Could
			●	●	●	Could	Could	Could	Could	Could
			Could	No!	●	●	●	●	●	●

DISORDERS USUALLY FIRST EVIDENT IN CHILDHOOD OR ADOLESCENCE — *cont.*

	Unrealistic worry about possible harm befalling major attachment figures or fear that they will not return	Unrealistic worry that an untoward calamity will separate child from attachment figure	Persistent reluctance or refusal to go to school in order to stay home or with attachment figures	Persistent reluctance or refusal to go to sleep without being next to attachment figure, or to go to sleep away from home
Developmental reading disorder				
Developmental arithmetic disorder				
Developmental language disorder — expressive type				
Developmental language disorder — receptive type				
Developmental articulation disorder				
Mixed specific developmental disorder				
Atypical specific developmental disorder				
Mental retardation				
Mild mental retardation				
Moderate mental retardation				
Severe mental retardation				
Profound mental retardation				
Unspecified mental retardation				
V62.89 borderline intellectual functioning not a mental disorder				
Attention deficit disorder with hyperactivity				
Attention deficit disorder without hyperactivity				
Attention deficit disorder residual type				
Stuttering				
Elective mutism				
Conduct disorder, undersocialized, aggressive				
Conduct disorder, undersocialized, nonaggressive				
Conduct disorder, socialized, aggressive				
Conduct disorder, socialized, nonaggressive				
Infantile autism				
Infantile autism residual state				
Childhood onset pervasive developmental disorder				
Childhood onset pervasive developmental disorder residual state				
Separation anxiety disorder	3	3	3	3
Avoidant disorder of childhood or adolescence				
Schizoid disorder of childhood or adolescence				
Overanxious disorder				
Oppositional disorder				
Identity disorder				
Anorexia nervosa				
Bulimia				
Pica				
Rumination disorder of infancy				
Reactive attachment disorder of infancy				
Transient tic disorder				
Chronic motor tic disorder				
Tourette's disorder				
Atypical tic disorder				
Atypical stereotyped movement disorder				
Functional enuresis				
Functional encopresis				
Sleepwalking disorder				
Sleep terror disorder				

Axis II specific developmental disorders

| | | | | | Generalized or persistent worry not related to concerns over separation | | | | | | |
Persistent avoidance of being alone at home and upset if cannot follow attachment figure around the home	Repeated nightmares involving themes of separation	Complaints of physical symptoms on school days	Signs of excessive distress at separation or when anticipating separation (when age < 6 distress = panic)	Social withdrawal apathy, sadness or difficulty concentrating at work or play when not with attachment figure	Unrealistic worry about future events	Preoccupation with appropriateness of behavior in the past	Overconcern about competence in a variety of areas	Excessive need for reassurance about a variety of worries	Somatic complaints with no physical basis	Marked self-consciousness susceptibility to embarrassment, humiliation	Marked feelings of tension or inability to relax
3	3	3	3	3							
					4	4	4	4	4	4	4

DISORDERS USUALLY FIRST EVIDENT IN CHILDHOOD OR ADOLESCENCE — *cont.*

	Disobedient negativistic provocative opposition to authority figures	Violation of minor rules	Temper Tantrums	Argumentativeness	Provocative behavior	Stubbornness	Long term goals	Career choice
Developmental reading disorder								
Developmental arithmetic disorder								
Developmental language disorder — expressive type								
Developmental language disorder — receptive type								
Developmental articulation disorder								
Mixed specific developmental disorder								
Atypical specific developmental disorder								
Mental retardation								
Mild mental retardation								
Moderate mental retardation								
Severe mental retardation								
Profound mental retardation								
Unspecified mental retardation								
V62.89 borderline intellectual functioning not a mental disorder								
Attention deficit disorder with hyperactivity		Could						
Attention deficit disorder without hyperactivity		Could						
Attention deficit disorder residual type								
Stuttering								
Elective mutism								
Conduct disorder, undersocialized, aggressive	Could	Could	Could	Could	Could	Could		
Conduct disorder, undersocialized, nonaggressive	Could	Could	Could	Could	Could	Could		
Conduct disorder, socialized, aggressive	Could	Could	Could	Could	Could	Could		
Conduct disorder, socialized, nonaggressive	Could	Could	Could	Could	Could	Could		
Infantile autism								
Infantile autism residual state								
Childhood onset pervasive developmental disorder								
Childhood onset pervasive developmental disorder residual state								
Separation anxiety disorder								
Avoidant disorder of childhood or adolescence								
Schizoid disorder of childhood or adolescence								
Overanxious disorder								
Oppositional disorder	● M	2^N	2^N	2^N	2^N	2^N		
Identity disorder							3	3
Anorexia nervosa								
Bulimia								
Pica								
Rumination disorder of infancy								
Reactive attachment disorder of infancy								
Transient tic disorder								
Chronic motor tic disorder								
Tourette's disorder								
Atypical tic disorder								
Atypical stereotyped movement disorder								
Functional enuresis								
Functional encopresis								
Sleepwalking disorder								
Sleep terror disorder								

Axis II specific developmental disorders

Severe subjective distress about a variety of issues related to identity including:

Friendship patterns	Sexual orientation and behavior	Religious identification	Moral value systems	Group loyalties	Intense fear of becoming obese which doesn't diminish with progressive weight loss	Disturbance of body image (feels fat even when emaciated)	Weight loss of at least 25% of body weight (including adjustments for growth)	Refusal to maintain body weight over minimum normal wt. for age and height	Recurrent episodes of binge eating (rapid consumption in usually less than 2 hours)	Eating high caloric easily ingested food during binge	Inconspicuous eating during a binge
3	3	3	3	3	●	●	●	●	●	3	3

DISORDERS USUALLY FIRST EVIDENT IN CHILDHOOD OR ADOLESCENCE — cont.

Disorder	Termination of binge by abdominal pain, sleep, self-induced vomiting social interruption	Repeated attempts to lose weight by severely restrictive diets, self-induced vomiting diuretics or cathartics	Frequent weight changes larger than 10 lb. due to alternate binges and fasts	Awareness that eating pattern abnormal and fear of not being able to stop voluntarily	Depressed mood and self-deprecating thought after binges
Axis II specific developmental disorders					
Developmental reading disorder					
Developmental arithmetic disorder					
Developmental language disorder — expressive type					
Developmental language disorder — receptive type					
Developmental articulation disorder					
Mixed specific developmental disorder					
Atypical specific developmental disorder					
Mental retardation					
Mild mental retardation					
Moderate mental retardation					
Severe mental retardation					
Profound mental retardation					
Unspecified mental retardation					
V62.89 borderline intellectual functioning not a mental disorder					
Attention deficit disorder with hyperactivity					
Attention deficit disorder without hyperactivity					
Attention deficit disorder residual type					
Stuttering					
Elective mutism					
Conduct disorder, undersocialized, aggressive					
Conduct disorder, undersocialized, nonaggressive					
Conduct disorder, socialized, aggressive					
Conduct disorder, socialized, nonaggressive					
Infantile autism					
Infantile autism residual state					
Childhood onset pervasive developmental disorder					
Childhood onset pervasive developmental disorder residual state					
Separation anxiety disorder					
Avoidant disorder of childhood or adolescence					
Schizoid disorder of childhood or adolescence					
Overanxious disorder					
Oppositional disorder					
Identity disorder					
Anorexia nervosa					
Bulimia	3	3	3	●	●
Pica					
Rumination disorder of infancy					
Reactive attachment disorder of infancy					
Transient tic disorder					
Chronic motor tic disorder					
Tourette's disorder					
Atypical tic disorder					
Atypical stereotyped movement disorder					
Functional enuresis					
Functional encopresis					
Sleepwalking disorder					
Sleep terror disorder					

Repeated eating of non-nutritive substances	Repeated regurgitation without nausea or associated gastro-intestinal disturbance	Weight loss or failure to make expected weight gains	Lack of the type of care that ordinarily results in affectional bonds	Lack of developmentally appropriate signs of social responsivity	Lack of visual tracking of eyes and faces at > 2 mo	Lack of smiling response to faces at > 2 mo	Lack of visual reciprocity at > 2 mo or lack of vocal reciprocity with caretaker at > 5 mo	Lack of alerting and turning toward caretaker's voice > 4 mo	Lack of spontaneous reaching for mother > 4 mo
		Could							
●	●	● ●	●	●ᴹ	1ᴺ	1ᴺ	1ᴺ	1ᴺ	1ᴺ

	Lack of anticipatory reaching when approched to be picked up at $>$ 5 mo	Lack of participation in playful games with caretaker at $>$ mo	Weak cry	Excessive sleep	Lack of interest in the environment	Hypomotility
Axis II specific developmental disorders						
Developmental reading disorder						
Developmental arithmetic disorder						
Developmental language disorder — expressive type						
Developmental language disorder — receptive type						
Developmental articulation disorder						
Mixed specific developmental disorder						
Atypical specific developmental disorder						
Mental retardation						
Mild mental retardation						
Moderate mental retardation						
Severe mental retardation						
Profound mental retardation						
Unspecified mental retardation						
V62.89 borderline intellectual functioning not a mental disorder						
Attention deficit disorder with hyperactivity						
Attention deficit disorder without hyperactivity						
Attention deficit disorder residual type						
Stuttering						
Elective mutism						
Conduct disorder, undersocialized, aggressive						
Conduct disorder, undersocialized, nonaggressive						
Conduct disorder, socialized, aggressive						
Conduct disorder, socialized, nonaggressive						
Infantile autism						
Infantile autism residual state						
Childhood onset pervasive developmental disorder						
Childhood onset pervasive developmental disorder residual state						
Separation anxiety disorder						
Avoidant disorder of childhood or adolescence						
Schizoid disorder of childhood or adolescence						
Overanxious disorder						
Oppositional disorder						
Identity disorder						
Anorexia nervosa						
Bulimia						
Pica						
Rumination disorder of infancy						
Reactive attachment disorder of infancy	1N	1N	3	3	3	3
Transient tic disorder						
Chronic motor tic disorder						
Tourette's disorder						
Atypical tic disorder						
Atypical stereotyped movement disorder						
Functional enuresis						
Functional encopresis						
Sleepwalking disorder						
Sleep terror disorder						

Recurrent, involuntary, repetitive, rapid, purposeless:

Weak rooting and grasping in response to feeding attempts	Poor muscle tone	Motor movements (tics)	Tics, involving no more than 3 muscle groups at any one time	Tics, multiple muscle groups	Multiple vocal tics	Ability to suppress tics for minutes to hours	Variation in intensity over weeks or months	Unvarying intensity over weeks or months	Repeated involuntary voiding of urine by day or by night	Events per month (how many times)	Repeated voluntary or involuntary passage of feces of normal or near normal consistency into places not appropriate
3	3										
		●				●	●	No			
			●			●	No	●			
				●	●	●	●	No			

Any tic disorder not fitting one of above

Not for tics: for headbanging, rocking, repetitive voluntary movements

									●	2 at age 5-6 1/mo after	
										1/mo	●

DISORDERS USUALLY FIRST EVIDENT IN CHILDHOOD OR ADOLESCENCE — *cont.*

	Repeated episodes of arising from bed during sleep and walking about for several minutes to ½ hour	Has blank staring face unresponsive to efforts to influence or communicate can be woken only with difficulty	Has amnesia for the episode	Within several minutes after awakening from episode no impairment of mental activity or behavior (may be brief confusion)	Episode did not occur in REM sleep or occur with abnormal EEG
Axis II specific developmental disorders					
Developmental reading disorder					
Developmental arithmetic disorder					
Developmental language disorder — expressive type					
Developmental language disorder — receptive type					
Developmental articulation disorder					
Mixed specific developmental disorder					
Atypical specific developmental disorder					
Mental retardation					
Mild mental retardation					
Moderate mental retardation					
Severe mental retardation					
Profound mental retardation					
Unspecified mental retardation					
V62.89 borderline intellectual functioning not a mental disorder					
Attention deficit disorder with hyperactivity					
Attention deficit disorder without hyperactivity					
Attention deficit disorder residual type					
Stuttering					
Elective mutism					
Conduct disorder, undersocialized, aggressive					
Conduct disorder, undersocialized, nonaggressive					
Conduct disorder, socialized, aggressive					
Conduct disorder, socialized, nonaggressive					
Infantile autism					
Infantile autism residual state					
Childhood onset pervasive developmental disorder					
Childhood onset pervasive developmental disorder residual state					
Separation anxiety disorder					
Avoidant disorder of childhood or adolescence					
Schizoid disorder of childhood or adolescence					
Overanxious disorder					
Oppositional disorder					
Identity disorder					
Anorexia nervosa					
Bulimia					
Pica					
Rumination disorder of infancy					
Reactive attachment disorder of infancy					
Transient tic disorder					
Chronic motor tic disorder					
Tourette's disorder					
Atypical tic disorder					
Atypical stereotyped movement disorder					
Functional enuresis					
Functional encopresis					
Sleepwalking disorder	●	●	●	●	●
Sleep terror disorder					●

Recurrent episodes of abrupt awakening (1–10 min) usually 30 to 200 min. after onset of sleep	Usually beginning with a panicky scream	Intense anxiety during episode	Tachycardia	Rapid Breathing	Dilated pupils	Sweating	Piloerection	Relative unresponsiveness to efforts to console and comfort usually with confusion disorientation and perseverative motor movements
●	●	●	3	3	3	3	3	●

SUBSTANCE USE DISORDERS

Pathological pattern of use

	Need for daily use for adequate functioning	Inability to cut down or stop use	Repeated efforts to control or reduce excess use by periods of abstinence or by restricting use to certain times of the day	Amnestic periods for events while intoxicated (blackouts)	Intoxication throughout the day	Continuation of use despite a serious physical disorder aggravated by use	Occasional consumption of a fifth of spirits or equivalent in
Alcohol abuse	◇①	◇①	◇①	◇①	◇①	◇①	◇①
Alcohol Dependence (alcoholism)	◇①	◇①	◇①	◇①	◇①	◇①	◇①
Barbiturate or similarly acting sedative or hypnotic — abuse		◇①		◇①	◇①		
Barbiturate or similarly acting sedative or hypnotic — dependence		◇①		◇①	◇①		
Opioid abuse		◇①					
Opioid dependence		◇①					
Cocaine abuse		◇①			◇①		
Amphetamine or similarly acting sympathomimetic — abuse		◇①			◇①		
Amphetamine or similarly acting sympathomimetic — dependence		◇①			◇①		
Phencyclidine or similarly acting arylcyclohexylamine (PCP) abuse					◇①		
Hallucinogen abuse		◇①			◇①		
Cannabis abuse					◇①		
Cannabis dependence					◇①		
Tobacco dependence			①			①	
Other, mixed or unspecified substance abuse	"Other" used when abused substance is none of above, "mixed"						
Other specified substance dependence	"Other specified" is known drug but none of above						
Unspecified substance dependence	Used as initial diagnosis when specific substance not yet known						
Dependence on combination of opioid and other non alcoholic substance	Used when there is dependence both on opioid and unknown						
Dependence on combination of substances, excluding opioids and alcohol	{ Used when there is dependence on more than one non-identifiable non-opioid, non-alcoholic substances[d]						

[d]-or where there are so many substances that the physician

Impairment in social or occupational functioning

Drinking of non-beverage alcohol	Frequent use of equivalent of 600 mg of Secobarbital or 60 mg of diazepam	Use of drug nearly every day for at least a month	Episode of opioid overdose-intoxication so severe that respiration and consciousness are impaired	Episodes of opioid overdose-intoxication so severe that hallucinations and delusions occur in a clear sensorium (state of consciousness)	Episodes of delirium due to drug	Episodes of delusional disorder due to drug	Episodes of hallucinosis due to drug	Episodes of affective disorder due to drug	Violence while intoxicated	Absence from work	Loss of job
◇①		◇①							①	①	①
◇①		◇①							①	①	①
	◇①								①	①	①
	◇①								①	①	①
		◇①	◇①						①	①	①
		◇①	◇①						①	①	①
				◇①					①	①	①
		◇①			◇①	◇①			①	①	①
		◇①			◇①	◇①			①	①	①
					◇①	◇①	◇①		①	①	①
						◇①		◇①	①	①	①
		◇①				◇①			①	①	①
		◇①				◇①			①	①	①
		●									

used when they are two or more of above and, nonalcoholic, and cannot be identified[d]

non-opioid, non alcoholic substance[d]

prefers to indicate a combination of substances rather than list each specific substance

SUBSTANCE USE DISORDERS—*cont.*

	Impairment in social or occupational functioning						
	Arguments or difficulties with family or friends over excessive substance use	Fights, loss of friends	Marked loss of interest in activities previously engaged in	Legal difficulties arrest for intoxicated behavior, traffic accidents while intoxicated, more than one arrest for sale, purchase or possession of substance	Duration of problem of at least one month	Tolerance—need for markedly increased amount to get same effect or regular use of same amount leads to markedly diminished effect	Withdrawal—cessation or reduction in use causes drug-specific withdrawal
Alcohol abuse	①	①		①	●		
Alcohol Dependence (alcoholism)	①	①		①	●	[1]	[1]
Barbiturate or similarly acting sedative or hypnotic { abuse		①		①	●		
Barbiturate or similarly acting sedative or hypnotic { dependence		①		①	●	[1]	[1]
Opioid abuse		①		①	●		
Opioid dependence		①		①	●	[1]	[1]
Cocaine abuse		①		①	●		
Amphetamine or similarly acting sympathomimetic { abuse		①		①	●		
Amphetamine or similarly acting sympathomimetic { dependence		①		①	●	[1]	[1]
Phencyclidine or similarly acting arylcyclohexylamine (PCP) abuse		①		①	●		
Hallucinogen abuse		①		①	●		
Cannabis abuse		①	①	①	●		
Cannabis dependence		①	①	①	●	●	
Tobacco dependence					●		①
Other, mixed or unspecified substance abuse							
Other specified substance dependence							
Unspecified substance dependence							
Dependence on combination of opioid and other non-alcoholic substance							
Dependence on combination of substances, excluding opioids and alcohol							

SUBSTANCE-INDUCED ORGANIC MENTAL DISORDERS

	Time after use when symptoms start	End	Problem not due to any other mental or physical disorder	Problem occurs from cessation or reduction of drug use	Problem occurs in context of prolonged, heavy drug use
Alcohol intoxication			●		
Alcohol idiosyncratic intoxication			●		
Alcohol withdrawal	Several hours		●	●	
Alcohol withdrawal delirium	Within 1 week		●	●	
Alcohol hallucinosis	Within 48 hours		●	●	
Alcohol amnestic disorder			●		●
Dementia associated with alcoholism		At least 3 weeks	●		●
Barbiturate or similarly acting sedative or hypnotic Intoxication			●		
Barbiturate or similarly acting sedative or hypnotic Withdrawal			●	●	●
Barbiturate or similarly acting sedative or hypnotic Withdrawal delirium	Within 1 week		●	●	
Barbiturate or similarly acting sedative or hypnotic Amnestic disorder			●		●
Opioid intoxication			●		
Opioid withdrawal			●	●	● g
Cocaine intoxication	Within 1 hour		●		
Amphetamine or similarly acting sympathomimetic — Intoxication	Within 1 hour		●		
Amphetamine or similarly acting sympathomimetic — Delirium	Within 24 hours		●		
Amphetamine or similarly acting sympathomimetic — Delusional disorder			●		●
Amphetamine or similarly acting sympathomimetic — Withdrawal			●	●	●
Phencyclidine (PCP) or similarly acting arylcyclohexylamine — Intoxication	Within 1 hour		●		
Phencyclidine (PCP) or similarly acting arylcyclohexylamine — Delirium			●		
Phencyclidine (PCP) or similarly acting arylcyclohexylamine — Mixed organic mental disorder			●		
Hallucinogen hallucinosis			●		
Hallucinogen affective disorder		More than 24 hours	●		
Hallucinogen delusional disorder		More than 24 hours	●		
Cannabis intoxication	Within 2 hours		●		
Cannabis delusional disorder	Within 2 hours	6 hours	●		
Tobacco withdrawal	Within 24 hours		●	●	
Caffeine intoxication			●		
Other, or unspecified substance — Intoxication					
Other, or unspecified substance — Withdrawal				●	
Other, or unspecified substance — Delirium					
Other, or unspecified substance — Dementia					
Other, or unspecified substance — Amnestic disorder					
Other, or unspecified substance — Delusional disorder					
Other, or unspecified substance — Hallucinosis					
Other, or unspecified substance — Affective disorder					
Other, or unspecified substance — Personality disorder					
Other, or unspecified substance — Atypical or mixed organic mental disorder					

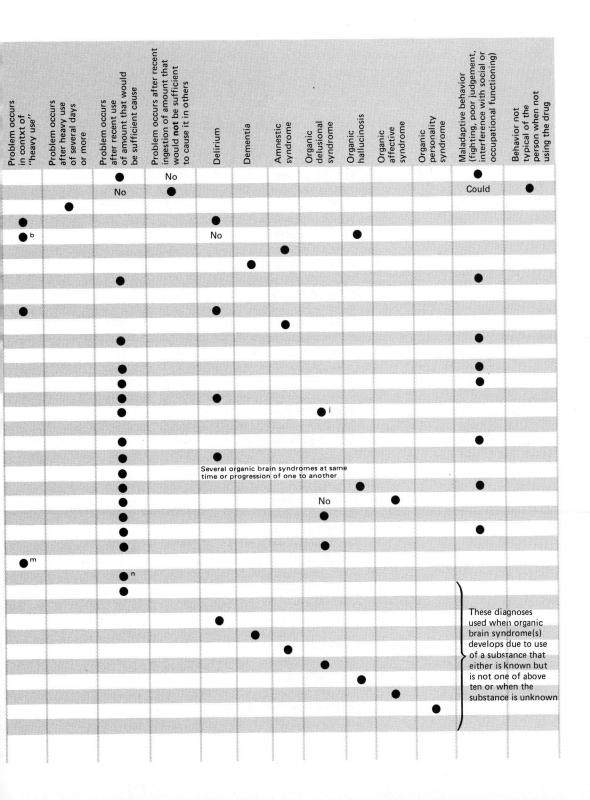

SUBSTANCE-INDUCED ORGANIC MENTAL DISORDERS — *cont.*

	Marked behavioral change	Drowsiness	Insomnia	Irritability	Restlessness	Nervousness	Excitement	Hypervigilance
Alcohol intoxication				[1]				
Alcohol idiosyncratic intoxication	●							
Alcohol withdrawal				1				
Alcohol withdrawal delirium								
Alcohol hallucinosis								
Alcohol amnestic disorder								
Dementia associated with alcoholism								
Barbiturate or similarly acting sedative or hypnotic Intoxication				①				
Barbiturate or similarly acting sedative or hypnotic Withdrawal								
Barbiturate or similarly acting sedative or hypnotic Withdrawal delirium								
Barbiturate or similarly acting sedative or hypnotic Amnestic disorder								
Opioid intoxication	[1]							
Opioid withdrawal			4					
Cocaine intoxication								①
Amphetamine or similarly acting sympathomimetic — Intoxication								①
Amphetamine or similarly acting sympathomimetic — Delirium								
Amphetamine or similarly acting sympathomimetic — Delusional disorder								
Amphetamine or similarly acting sympathomimetic — Withdrawal								
Phencyclidine (PCP) or similarly acting arylcyclohexylamine — Intoxication								
Phencyclidine (PCP) or similarly acting arylcyclohexylamine — Delirium								
Phencyclidine (PCP) or similarly acting arylcyclohexylamine — Mixed organic mental disorder								
Hallucinogen hallucinosis								
Hallucinogen affective disorder								
Hallucinogen delusional disorder								
Cannabis intoxication								
Cannabis delusional disorder								
Tobacco withdrawal		4			4	4		
Caffeine intoxication			5		5	5	5	
Other, or unspecified substance — Intoxication								
Other, or unspecified substance — Withdrawal								
Other, or unspecified substance — Delirium								
Other, or unspecified substance — Dementia								
Other, or unspecified substance — Amnestic disorder								
Other, or unspecified substance — Delusional disorder								
Other, or unspecified substance — Hallucinosis								
Other, or unspecified substance — Affective disorder								
Other, or unspecified substance — Personality disorder								
Other, or unspecified substance — Atypical or mixed organic mental disorder								

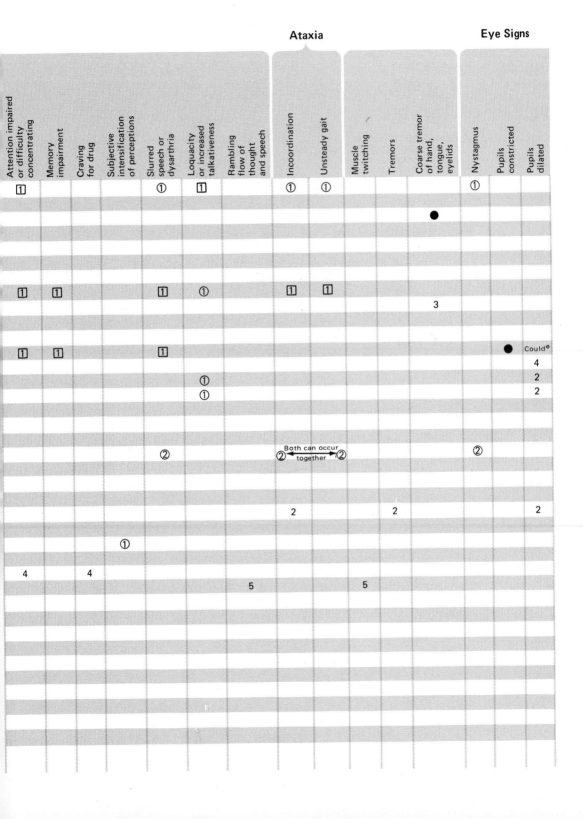

SUBSTANCE-INDUCED ORGANIC MENTAL DISORDERS — *cont.*

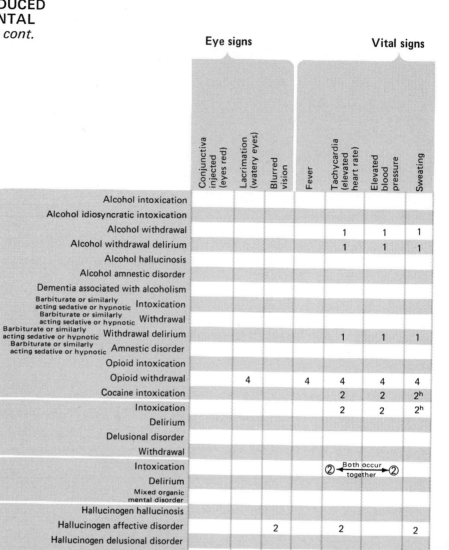

	Eye signs			Vital signs			
	Conjunctiva injected (eyes red)	Lacrimation (watery eyes)	Blurred vision	Fever	Tachycardia (elevated heart rate)	Elevated blood pressure	Sweating
Alcohol intoxication							
Alcohol idiosyncratic intoxication							
Alcohol withdrawal					1	1	1
Alcohol withdrawal delirium					1	1	1
Alcohol hallucinosis							
Alcohol amnestic disorder							
Dementia associated with alcoholism							
Barbiturate or similarly acting sedative or hypnotic Intoxication							
Barbiturate or similarly acting sedative or hypnotic Withdrawal							
Barbiturate or similarly acting sedative or hypnotic Withdrawal delirium					1	1	1
Barbiturate or similarly acting sedative or hypnotic Amnestic disorder							
Opioid intoxication							
Opioid withdrawal		4		4	4	4	4
Cocaine intoxication					2	2	2h
Amphetamine or similarly acting sympathomimetic Intoxication					2	2	2h
Amphetamine or similarly acting sympathomimetic Delirium							
Amphetamine or similarly acting sympathomimetic Delusional disorder							
Amphetamine or similarly acting sympathomimetic Withdrawal							
Phencyclidine (PCP) or similarly acting arylcyclohexylamine Intoxication					② ←Both occur together→	②	
Phencyclidine (PCP) or similarly acting arylcyclohexylamine Delirium							
Phencyclidine (PCP) or similarly acting arylcyclohexylamine Mixed organic mental disorder							
Hallucinogen hallucinosis							
Hallucinogen affective disorder			2		2		2
Hallucinogen delusional disorder							
Cannabis intoxication	1				●		
Cannabis delusional disorder							
Tobacco withdrawal							
Caffeine intoxication							
Other, or unspecified substance Intoxication							
Other, or unspecified substance Withdrawal							
Other, or unspecified substance Delirium							
Other, or unspecified substance Dementia							
Other, or unspecified substance Amnestic disorder							
Other, or unspecified substance Delusional disorder							
Other, or unspecified substance Hallucinosis							
Other, or unspecified substance Affective disorder							
Other, or unspecified substance Personality disorder							
Other, or unspecified substance Atypical or mixed organic mental disorder							

Orthostatic hypotension	Palpitations	Cardiac arrhythmia	Flushed face	Autonomic Hyperactivity	Rhindrrhea	Piloerection	Dry mouth	Nausea and vomiting	Diarrhea	Gastrointestinal disturbances or complaints	Diuresis	Numbed or diminished responsiveness to pain	Sensation of slowed time	Synesthesias	Illusions	Vivid auditory hallucinations
			①													
1				1				1								
				1												
																●
3				3				3								
				●												
					4	4			4							
								2								
								2								
												②	②̣	②̣		
														1	1	
	2															
							1̣						①			
										4						
		5	5							5	5					

SUBSTANCE-INDUCED ORGANIC MENTAL DISORDERS — *cont.*

	Response to hallucination appropriate to content	Depersonalization or derealization	Ideas of reference	Mood change	Mood lability	Disinhibition of sexual and aggressive impulses	Aggressiveness and hostility
Alcohol intoxication				[1]			
Alcohol idiosyncratic intoxication							
Alcohol withdrawal							
Alcohol withdrawal delirium							
Alcohol hallucinosis							
Alcohol amnestic disorder	●						
Dementia associated with alcoholism							
Barbiturate or similarly acting sedative or hypnotic Intoxication					①	①	
Barbiturate or similarly acting sedative or hypnotic Withdrawal							
Barbiturate or similarly acting sedative or hypnotic Withdrawal delirium							
Barbiturate or similarly acting sedative or hypnotic Amnestic disorder							
Opioid intoxication							
Opioid withdrawal							
Cocaine intoxication							
Amphetamine or similarly acting sympathomimetic — Intoxication							
Amphetamine or similarly acting sympathomimetic — Delirium							
Amphetamine or similarly acting sympathomimetic — Delusional disorder			3				3
Amphetamine or similarly acting sympathomimetic — Withdrawal							
Phencyclidine (PCP) or similarly acting arylcyclohexylamine — Intoxication					[2]		
Phencyclidine (PCP) or similarly acting arylcyclohexylamine — Delirium							
Phencyclidine (PCP) or similarly acting arylcyclohexylamine — Mixed organic mental disorder							
Hallucinogen hallucinosis		1					
Hallucinogen affective disorder							
Hallucinogen delusional disorder							
Cannabis intoxication							
Cannabis delusional disorder							
Tobacco withdrawal							
Caffeine intoxication							
Other, or unspecified substance — Intoxication							
Other, or unspecified substance — Withdrawal							
Other, or unspecified substance — Delirium							
Other, or unspecified substance — Dementia							
Other, or unspecified substance — Amnestic disorder							
Other, or unspecified substance — Delusional disorder							
Other, or unspecified substance — Hallucinosis							
Other, or unspecified substance — Affective disorder							
Other, or unspecified substance — Personality disorder							
Other, or unspecified substance — Atypical or mixed organic mental disorder							

Depressed or dysphoric mood	Psychomotor retardation	Apathy	Euphoria	Grandiosity	Elation	Psychomotor agitation	Periods of inexhaustibility	Anxiety	Headache	Malaise or weakness	Fatigue	Disturbed sleep	Increased dreaming	Yawning	Increased appetite
1								1		1					
3								3		3					
①	①	①	①											4	
				①	①	①									
				①	①	①									
						3		3							
●											2	2	2		
			②	②		②		②							
		①	①												1
								4	4						
						5	5								

PSYCHOSEXUAL DISORDERS

	Duration of cardinal manifestations		Age of onset limits, by definition	Exclusion of other disorders
	At least	Not more than		
Gender identity disorders				
Transsexualism	2 yrs			Any other mental disorder
Gender identity disorder of childhood in females			Before puberty	
Gender identity disorder of childhood in males			Before puberty	
Atypical gender identity disorder			Any gender identity disorder that	
Paraphilias				
Fetishism				
Transvestism			Transsexualism	
Zoophilia				
Pedophilia			If the patient is an adult—the about age difference and sexual	
Exhibitionism				
Voyeurism				
Sexual masochism				
Sexual sadism				
Atypical paraphilia			This is the residual catagory	
Psychosexual dysfunctions				
Inhibited sexual desire				Not due exclusively to physical factors or another axis I disorder
Inhibited sexual excitement				
Inhibited female orgasm				
Inhibited male orgasm				
Premature ejaculation				Any axis I disorder
Functional dyspareunia				Not due to lack of lubrication, functional vaginismus
Functional vaginismus				Not exclusively a physical disorder not due to any other axis I disorder
Atypical psychosexual dysfunction			This is the residual catagory	
Other Psychosexual Disorders				
Ego-dystonic homosexuality				
Psychosexual disorder not elsewhere classified			This is the residual category	

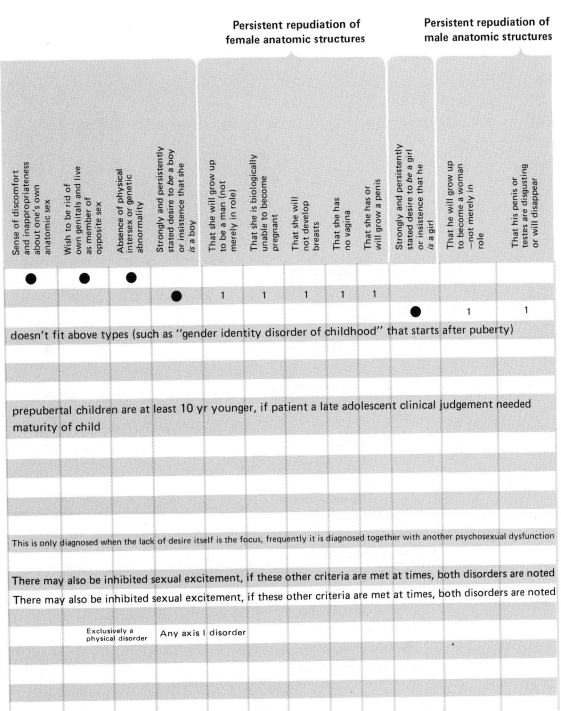

| | That it would be better not to have a penis or testes | Preoccupation with Female Stereotypical Activity | | Use of non-living objects (fetishes) is repeatedly preferred or exclusive method of achieving sexual excitement | Fetishes not limited to female clothing used in cross-dressing (transvestism) or objects designed to be used for sexual stimulation (vibrator) |
		Preference for cross-dressing or simulating female attire	Compelling desire to participate in games or pastimes of girls		
Gender identity disorders					
Transexualism					
Gender identity disorder of childhood in females					
Gender identity disorder of childhood in males	1	1	1		
Atypical gender identity disorder					
Paraphilias					
Fetishism				●	●
Transvestism					
Zoophilia					
Pedophilia					
Exhibitionism					
Voyeurism					
Sexual masochism					
Sexual sadism					
Atypical paraphilia					
Psychosexual dysfunctions					
Inhibited sexual desire					
Inhibited sexual excitement					
Inhibited female orgasm					
Inhibited male orgasm					
Premature ejaculation					
Functional dyspareunia					
Functional vaginismus					
Atypical psychosexual dysfunction					
Other psychosexual disorders					
Ego-dystonic homosexuality					
Psychosexual disorder not elsewhere classified					

Recurrent and persistent cross-dressing by a heterosexual male	Use of cross-dressing for the purpose of sexual excitement (at least early in the disorder)	Intense frustration when cross-dressing is interfered with	Act or fantasy of engaging in sexual activity with animals is a repeatedly preferred or exclusive method of achieving sexual excitement	Act or fantasy of engaging in sexual activity with pre-pubertal children as preferred or exclusive method of achieving sexual excitement	Repetitive acts of exposing genitals to unsuspecting stranger for purpose of achieving sexual excitement and no attempt at sexual activity with stranger	Repeatedly observes unsuspecting people who are naked, in the act of disrobing, or engaging in sexual activity with the observed strangers is sought	The observing is the preferred or exclusive method of achieving sexual excitement	Preferred or exclusive mode of producing sexual excitement is to be humiliated bound, beaten, or otherwise made to suffer
●	●	●						
			●					
				●				
					●			
						●	●	

1

And both are noted

PSYCHOSEXUAL DISORDERS—*cont.*

Category	Disorder	Has intentionally participated in activity where own life was threatened, or was physically harmed, for purpose of producing sexual excitement	On non-consenting partner, has repeatedly intentionally inflicted psychological or physical suffering in order to produce sexual excitement	With consenting partner repeatedly preferred or exclusive mode of sexual excitement combines humiliation with simulated or mildly injurious bodily suffering
Gender identity disorders	Transexualism			
	Gender identity disorder of childhood in females			
	Gender identity disorder of childhood in males			
	Atypical gender identity disorder			
Paraphilias	Fetishism			
	Transvestism			
	Zoophilia			
	Pedophilia			
	Exhibitionism			
	Voyeurism			
	Sexual masochism	1		
	Sexual sadism		1	1
	Atypical paraphilia			
Psychosexual dysfunctions	Inhibited sexual desire			
	Inhibited sexual excitement			
	Inhibited female orgasm			
	Inhibited male orgasm			
	Premature ejaculation			
	Functional dyspareunia			
	Functional vaginismus			
	Atypical psychosexual dysfunction			
Other psychosexual disorders	Ego-dystonic homosexuality			
	Psychosexual disorder not elsewhere classified			

On a consenting partner bodily injury that is extensive, permanent or possibly mortal is inflicted in order to achieve sexual excitement	Sexual activity that is judged adequate in intensity, focus and duration	Persistent and pervasive inhibition of sexual desire, taking into account factors that affect sexual desire like age, health, intensity and frequency of sexual desire and context of life	Recurrent and persistent inhibition of sexual excitement during sexual activity—in males: partial or complete failure to attain or maintain erection until completion of the sexual act—in females: partial or complete failure to attain or maintain the lubrication-swelling response of sexual excitement until completion of the sexual act	Recurrent and persistent inhibition of the female orgasm, as manifested by delay or absence of orgasm following a normal sexual excitement phase	Recurrent and persistent inhibition of the male orgasm as manifested by a delay or absense of ejaculation following an adequate phase of sexual excitement
1					
		•			
	•		•		
	•			•	
	•				•
	•				

	Ejaculation occurs before the patient wishes it, because of recurrent and persistent absence of reasonable voluntary control of ejaculation and orgasm the judgement of reasonable control takes account of age, novelty of sexual partner, frequency and duration of coitus and other factors that affect duration of the excitement phase of sexual activity	Coitus is associated with recurrent and persistent genital pain in either the male or the female	History of recurrent and persistent involuntary spasm of the musculature of the outer third of the vagina that interferes with coitus
Gender identity disorders Transexualism			
Gender identity disorder of childhood in females			
Gender identity disorder of childhood in males			ı
Atypical gender identity disorder			
Paraphilias Fetishism			
Transvestism			
Zoophilia			
Pedophilia			
Exhibitionism			
Voyeurism			
Sexual masochism			
Sexual sadism			
Atypical paraphilia			
Psychosexual dysfunctions Inhibited sexual desire			
Inhibited sexual excitement			
Inhibited female orgasm			
Inhibited male orgasm			
Premature ejaculation	●		
Functional dyspareunia		●	
Functional vaginismus			●
Atypical psychosexual dysfunction			
Other psychosexual disorders Ego-dystonic homosexuality			
Psychosexual disorder not elsewhere classified			

Complaint that heterosexual arousal is persistently absent or weak and significantly interferes with initiating or maintaining wanted heterosexual relationships

There is a sustained pattern of homosexual arousal that has been unwanted and a persistent source of distress

Index

Intensity of affective (or emotional) expression, 101
Interest, 101
International Congress on Infant Psychiatry, 212
Interpersonal relations, 32
Intoxication, 176
IQ, 212
Isolated explosive disorder, 16

Jealousy, delusions of, 84
Judgment, 61

Labile affect, 102
Laceration, 7
Language development and disturbances in children, 71, 72
Learning disabilities, 212
Leisure time, use of, 22, 36
Lithium, 177, *204*
  history of, 191, 192, 193
Localized or circumscribed amnesia, 55
Loneliness, 45
Loosening of association, 77, 79, 171, 176, 185
Loquacity, 71
Low IQ, 60
Low mood, elevated mood, relationship, 189
Low self-esteem, 27

Magical thinking, 89, *208*
Major depression, 193, *199*
  recurrent, 194
  recurrent, in remission, 11
  single episode, 194
Major disorders in DSM-III, *199*
Major versus minor mental illness, 173
Major tranquilizers, 189, 190-193, 198, 204
Malingering, 139, *141*
Mandatory axes, 6
Mania, 193
  and depression, comparison, 105
    treatment, 190, 191
  severe, 177, 178, 187, 188, 194
Manic depressive psychosis, 171, 172, 184, *215*
Manic episode, 194, 195
Manic mood, 104, *105,* 150, 177, 187
Manipulation of others, 33, 44, *209*
Marital problems, (V61.10), 4
Masochism, sexual, 154
Melancholia, 188, 191
Memory, 182
  disturbance, 52
  long term (or remote), 54
  and orientation, alertness, attention, 51-52
  recent, 53
  short term, 53
Mental disorder, 3, 27, *162,* 167, 178, 179, 184, *187*
  cardinal manifestation of, 28
  in children, 213
  divided by psychosis, 162
  versus reaction to stress, 6
Mental retardation in children, 212

Metaphorical language, 72
Middle insomnia, *121*
Middle zone, 170, 172, 173, 179, 180, 183, 186, *187,* 188, 189, 194, 198, *199,* 200-203, *204,* 207, *215*
Mind versus body, 169
Mistrust, 33
  and suspiciousness of people, 42
Money management, 38
Mood, 100, 101, *105,* 195
  depressive with manic and hypomanic, 104
  elevated, expansive, or irritable, 103
Mood-congruent and mood-incongruent delusions, 87, 106, 195
Mood disorders, 177, 187, 192, *199, 204, 215*
  disturbances, 176
  psychotic distinguished from psychotic with schizophrenia, 192
Mood disturbances, 184, 194
Mood fluctuations, 195
Moral insanity, 170-171
  reconsidered, 173, 180
Multiaxial diagnosis, 5
Multiaxial system, 5
  case illustration, 7
Multiple personality, 93, 182, 203

Narcissistic personality, *204,* 206, 207, *209, 215*
Neurosis, 201, 202, 203
  anxiety, 181, 198
  conversion, 198
  depressive, 181
  dissociative, 198
  history, 180
  hypochondriacal, 203
  hysteria, 181-182
  obsessive-compulsive, 203
  phobic, 181
  types, 181
  why dropped, 198
Neurotic disorders, 180, 183, *187,* 200, *204, 215*
Neurotic symptom, 180, 181, 186
Neurotransmitter theory, defined, 192, 193
Nightmares, sleep terror, sleepwalking, 122, *123*
Nihilistic delusions, 86, 88
No diagnosis or condition on Axis I (V 71.09), 9, 10
No diagnosis or condition on Axis II (V 71.09), 10
No mental disorder on Axis I (V 71.09), 13
No mental disorder on Axis II (V 71.09), 13
Non-aggressive violation of rights of others, 40, 205
Noncompliance with medical treatment (V 15.81), 16
No physical disorder, 13
NREM sleep, 119, *123*
Nystagmus, 133

Obsessions, 78
Obsessive-compulsive neurosis, 203